Essentials of Clinical Genetics in Nursing Practice

Felissa R. Lashley (formerly Felissa L. Cohen), RN, PhD, ACRN, FAAN, FACMG, is Dean and Professor, College of Nursing at Rutgers, The State University of New Jersey. Prior to that, she was Dean and Professor at Southern Illinois University Edwardsville and Clinical Professor of Pediatrics at the School of Medicine at Southern Illinois University, Springfield. Dr. Lashley received her BS from Adelphi College, her MA from New York University, and her PhD in human genetics, with a minor in biochemistry, from Illinois State University. She is certified as a PhD Medical Geneticist by the American Board of Medical Genetics, the first nurse to be so certified, and is a founding fellow of the American College of Medical Genetics. She began her practice of genetic evaluation and counseling in 1973.

Dr. Lashley has authored more than 300 publications, including three editions of *Clinical Genetics in Nursing Practice*, the first two editions of which received Book of the Year awards from the *American Journal of Nursing*. Other books have also received *AJN* Book of the Year Awards, including *The Person with AIDS: Nursing Perspectives* (Durham and Cohen, editors), *Women Children and HIV/AIDS* (Cohen and Durham, editors), and *Emerging Infectious Diseases: Trends and Issues* (Lashley and Durham, editors). *Tuberculosis: A Sourcebook for Nursing Practice* (Cohen and Durham, editors) received a Book of the Year award from *Nurse Practitioner*. Dr. Lashley has received several million dollars in external research funding and has served as a member of the charter AIDS Research Review Committee, National Institute of Allergy and Infectious Diseases, National Institutes of Health.

Dr. Lashley has been a distinguished lecturer for Sigma Theta Tau International and served as Associate Editor of *Image: The Journal of Nursing Scholarship*. She is a fellow of the American Academy of Nursing. She received an Exxon Education Foundation Innovation Award for her article on integrating genetics into community college nursing curricula. She is a member of the International Society of Nurses in Genetics and the American Society of Human Genetics. She was a member of the steering committee of the National Coalition for Health Professional Education in Genetics sponsored by the National Human Genome Research Institute, National Institutes of Health. She served as President of the HIV/AIDS Nursing Certification Board. Dr. Lashley received the 2000 Nurse Researcher Award from the Association of Nurses in AIDS Care, the 2001 SAGE Award by the Illinois Nurse Leadership Institute for outstanding mentorship, and the 2003 Distinguished Alumni Award from Illinois State University. In 2005, she was inducted into the Illinois State University's College of Arts and Sciences Hall of Fame. She served as a member of the PKU Consensus Development Panel, National Institutes of Health. She was selected as a Woman of Excellence by the New Jersey Women in AIDS Network in March 2005. Dr. Lashley serves as a board member at Robert Wood Johnson University Hospital in New Brunswick, New Jersey.

Essentials of Clinical Genetics in Nursing Practice

Felissa R. Lashley, RN, PhD, ACRN, FAAN, FACMG

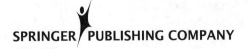

SPRINGER PUBLISHING COMPANY

New York

To my wonderful family who make it all possible and worthwhile: my F_1 generation: Peter, Heather, and Neal and their spouses, Julie, Chris, and Anne; and especially my loving F_2 generation: Benjamin, Hannah, Jacob, Grace, and Lydia Cohen. You brighten my every day.

Springer Publishing Company, LLC
11 West 42nd Street
New York, NY 10036
www.springerpub.com

Acquisitions Editor: James Costello
Production Editor: Gail Farrar
Cover Design: Mimi Flow
Composition: Publishers' Design and Production Services, Inc.

07 08 09 10 / 5 4 3 2 1

Library of Congress Cataloging-in-Publication Data

Lashley, Felissa R., 1941–
    Essentials of clinical genetics in nursing practice / Felissa R. Lashley.
       p. cm.
    Includes bibliographical references and index.
    ISBN 0-8261-0222-0
    1. Medical genetics. 2. Nursing. I. Title.
    [DNLM: 1. Genetics, Medical—methods. 2. Genetic Diseases, Inborn—nursing.
   3. Nursing Care—methods. QZ 50 L343e 2006]
   RB155.L372 2006
   616'.042—dc22

                       2006049780

Printed in the United States of America by Bang Printing.

Contents

Preface

Being able to look at clients and families with a "genetic eye" has become critical for all nurses. Advances from genetic and genomic research have influenced all areas of health care and cross all periods of the life cycle. Genetic factors are responsible in some way for both indirect and direct disease causation; for variation that determines predisposition, susceptibility, and resistance to disease; and for response to treatment. When we look into the future of health care, we can see that genetic knowledge will have direct influences, including genetic screening and testing and personalized drug therapy.

Nurses must be able to "think genetically" to help individuals and families in all practice areas who are affected in some way by genetic disease or are contemplating genetic testing. Each person has his or her own state of health and is at varying risks for developing diseases because of variation in his or her genetic makeup. This includes not only diseases thought of as genetic but the common disorders such as cancer and heart disease.

The call for the inclusion of genetics in the curricula of the health professions, especially nursing and medicine, has been long standing. More recently, activities of the National Coalition for Health Professional Education in Genetics have helped to focus on the need for health professional competency in genetics. The lay public has become better informed about genetic advances applied to genetic testing and health care, and nurses must be able to understand genetic material and use their knowledge appropriately in practice.

Becoming competent in the use of genetic content begins in nursing education programs. It was with this in mind that this book, *The Essentials of Clinical Genetics in Nursing Practice*, was written. Part I of the book discusses the place of genetics in health care and the health care trends that are related to genetics. This is followed by a review of basic and molecular biology, a discussion of human variation and diversity, and gene action and types of inheritance. The topics of prevention of genetic disease, genetic testing, and treatment are presented, including aspects of genetic counseling. Part II applies these principles to nursing courses. Specific application of genetics and genomics in regard to pharmacology, history taking and physical assessment, maternal-child nursing, adult health and illness and medical-surgical nursing, psychiatric mental health nursing, community and public health nursing, and trends, policies, and social and ethical issues are all discussed. The broad concepts are presented in a nursing context with selected disease examples and case examples. Many illustrations, figures, key concepts and questions, and examples from my own practice appear liberally throughout the book.

In this book, the term *normal* is used as it is by most geneticists—to mean free from the disorder or condition in question. Genetic terminology does not generally use apostrophes (for example, Down syndrome instead of Down's syndrome), and this pattern has been followed.

The writing of this book in a manner to allow students to apply genetics throughout their nursing program is an important step in preparing nurses early to think inclusively about genetics in all types of disease conditions and in preserving optimum health. This book grew out of the one I began over 25 years ago and has also been a labor of love. All nurses, as health care providers and as citizens, need to understand the advances in genetics and the implications for health care and social decisions. No health care professional can practice without such knowledge.

Felissa R. Lashley, RN, PhD, ACRN, FAAN, FACMG

I

The Basics

1

Genomics in Health Care

Genetic knowledge has had a major impact on both society and health care. It affects our daily lives, from routinely discussing deoxyribonucleic acid (DNA) evidence in the forensic sense to eating genetically modified foods. The health care impact spans prevention, detection, diagnosis, and treatment. The influence of genetics is seen in every part of the human lifespan, from prenatal through old age. As we look at where we are now and what the future holds, we can already realize what some of the genetically related basic knowledge, underpinnings, and applications that will influence health care will be. These include the following:

- Most, if not all, disorders are now known to have a genetic basis to some extent. This includes conditions that, on the surface, appear to be wholly brought about by environmental factors. An example is fractures of the bone, which are at least partly dependent on bone density, which is largely genetically determined. Therefore, a mutant gene to some extent can be thought of as an etiologic agent. Thus, all health care providers must understand genes and gene interactions to manage patients with common disorders.
- Many genetic disorders that appear to follow Mendelian patterns of inheritance and were ascribed to a single mutant gene are now known to be more complex than formerly thought.
- Different mutational changes within a gene may produce different phenotypic outcomes with varying responses to treatment and prognosis linked to genotype. Persons with specific genotypic mutations already are known to

have preferential responses to certain medications or therapeutic approaches.
- The so-called traditional genetic disorders are seen across the lifespan from conception through old age, and the signs and symptoms may vary depending on the stage of the lifespan at which they manifest. Many inherited single gene disorders have infant, childhood, and adult forms; other disorders typically appear or are noticed in adulthood, such as Huntington disease and hemochromatosis.
- Nontraditional modes of inheritance such as mitochondrial (mt) inheritance will assume additional importance as they become increasingly understood and associated with disease conditions. A recent example is one type of infertility that results from possessing a high percentage of immotile sperm due to a mutation of mtDNA in some men.
- The so-called common or complex diseases such as cancer, chronic obstructive pulmonary disease, diabetes mellitus, and heart disease have varying genetic components that are evident in etiology, diagnosis, treatment, management, or preventive approaches.
- Humans have various polymorphisms and variations in their make-up that do not manifest themselves as diseases per se but influence how we all respond to agents, including infectious agents, and chemicals in the environment, foods, and medications. This profoundly affects how people will respond to health care interventions because all people have different degrees of possible health.
- Technological advances have been such that persons with genetic disorders appearing in infancy or childhood who formerly died early

are living beyond early adulthood. For example, there are adults with sickle cell anemia who have lived into their eighties. A person's previously identified existing genetic condition such as cystic fibrosis and, eventually, total genetic make-up will influence the choice of care and treatment for the new health problems associated with normal aging as well as the long-term outlook for the genetic disorder. Therefore, health care providers must deal with how the genetic disorder bears on the appearance of common health problems and the aging process, as well as vice versa. For example, how will co-illness with type 2 diabetes mellitus influence the course of disease and response in an adult with cystic fibrosis? How will common conditions such as hypertension be managed against the background of a previously existing genetic disease?

- The nature and manifestations of previously existing genetic conditions will influence the choice of care and treatment for health problems associated with midlife and aging.
- As those with genetic disorders who formerly died in childhood live longer lives, the manifestations and effects of those genetic disorders will be described across the lifespan.
- Ways of thinking about health promotion and disease prevention will change because of new genetic knowledge.
- Communicable disease outbreaks are and will continue to be traced using molecular methods.
- Gene mutations in microbes will be studied for information on microbial resistance and to figure out why certain organisms are more virulent and take a larger toll than others.
- Genetic testing for detection, diagnosis, and choice of drug therapy will expand in utilization.
- Many disorders will be treated using knowledge from genetics both directly and indirectly, and the use of gene therapy will become more widespread.
- Drug therapy will be tailored to a person's genetic make-up for a particular disorder or for one or more underlying variations or mutations, and the field of pharmacogenomics (see Glossary) will continue to grow.

- Genetic information that predicts the development of disease and influences health care will be available prenatally for all individuals.
- Assessment for genetic risk for specific conditions preceding options of testing followed by counseling will become more prevalent and include persons at risk for common disorders such as heart disease, various types of cancers, Alzheimer disease, and others in addition to ones in common use such as tests used as part of prenatal diagnosis.
- All of the above will spawn complex legal, ethical, social, and policy issues.

Many of the challenges and applications of new genetic information are still not known, but we can be sure that nurses, and indeed all other health professionals in all areas of practice, will encounter clients with the traditional genetic disorders as well as common disorders with a genetic component. This increased recognition of the role of genetics in many types of conditions and the application of gene-based diagnostic tests and therapies mean that practitioners must be prepared not only to offer and provide genetic testing but also the appropriate accompanying risk assessment, education, interpretation, and counseling.

EXTENT AND IMPACT

Results of surveys on the extent of genetic disorders vary based on the definitions used, the time of life at which the survey is done, and the composition of the population examined. Estimates of the incidence are shown in Table 1.1. This does not include the impact of genes on the common disorders or on

TABLE 1.1 Incidence of Genetic Disorders

Type of Disorder	Incidence
Chromosome aberrations	0.5–0.6% in newborns, 5–7% in stillbirths and perinatal deaths, 50% in spontaneous abortions
Single gene disorders	2–3% by 1 year of age
Major malformations	4–7%
Minor malformations	10–12%

TABLE 1.2 Burden of Genetic Disease to Family and Community

- Financial cost to the family
- Decreases in planned family size
- Loss of geographic mobility
- Decreased opportunities for siblings
- Loss of family integrity
- Loss of career opportunities and job flexibility
- Social isolation
- Lifestyle alterations
- Reduction in contributions to their communities by families
- Disruption of husband-wife or partner relationship
- Threatened family self-concept
- Coping with intolerant public attitudes
- Psychological effects
- Stresses and uncertainty of treatment
- Physical health problems
- Loss of dreams and aspirations
- Cost to society of institutionalization or home or community care
- Cost to society because of additional problems and needs of other family members
- Cost of long-term care
- Housing and living arrangement changes

susceptibility. In addition to the impact by prevalence, genetic disorders exact emotional, financial, and physical tolls on the affected individual his/her family, and to some extent the community and society (Table 1.2). Perhaps nowhere else is it as important to focus on the family as the primary unit of care, because identification of a genetic disorder in one member affects others in the family.

GENETIC DISEASE THROUGH THE LIFESPAN

Genetic alterations leading to disease are present at birth but may not be manifested clinically until a later age, or even not at all if the alteration is a harmless biochemical variation. The time of manifestation depends on the following factors:

- Type and extent of the alteration
- Exposure to external environmental agents
- Influence of other specific genes possessed by the individual and by his/her total genetic make-up
- Internal environment of the individual

Characteristic times for the clinical manifestation and recognition of selected genetic disorders are shown in Table 1.3. These times do not mean that manifestations cannot appear at other times, but rather that the time span shown is typical. For example, Huntington disease, usually manifesting after 35 years of age, may be manifested in the older child, but this is very rare. Other disorders may be diagnosed in the newborn period or in infancy instead of at their usual later time because of participation in screening programs (e.g., medium-chain acyl-CoA dehydrogenase (MCAD) deficiency), or because of the systematic search for affected relatives due to the occurrence of the disorder in another family member, rather than because of the occurrence of signs or symptoms (e.g., Duchenne muscular dystrophy). Milder forms of inherited single gene disorders are being increasingly recognized in adults.

HUMAN GENOME PROJECT

The Human Genome Project was begun in 1990. In the United States, it was centered in the National Center for Human Genome Research at the National Institutes of Health (NIH) and the Department of Energy. David Smith directed the program at the Department of Energy, and James Watson and Francis Collins were the first and second directors at NIH, respectively. There were major endeavors associated with this. Among the most important were

- Genetic mapping;
- Physical mapping;
- Sequencing the 3 billion DNA base pairs of the human genome;

TABLE 1.3   Usual Stage of Manifestation of Selected Genetic Disorders

Disorder	Newborn	Infancy	Childhood	Adolescence	Adult
			Life Cycle Stage		
Achondroplasia	X				
Down syndrome	X				
Spina bifida	X				
Urea cycle disorders	X				
Tay-Sachs disease		X			
Lesch-Nyhan syndrome		X	X		
Cystic fibrosis		X	X		
Ataxia-telangiectasia			X		
Hurler disease			X		
Duchenne muscular dystrophy			X		
Homocystinuria			X		
Gorlin syndrome			X	X	
Acute intermittent porphyria				X	
Klinefelter syndrome				X	
Refsum disease				X	X
Wilson disease			X	X	X
Acoustic neuroma (bilateral)				X	X
Polycystic renal disease (adult)					X
Huntington disease					X

- Development of improved technology for genomic analysis;
- The identification of all genes and functional elements in genomic DNA, especially those associated with human diseases;
- Informatics development, including sophisticated databases and automating the management and analysis of data
- Establishment of the Ethical, Legal, and Social Implications (ELSI) programs as an integral part of the project.

ELSI issues included research on "identifying and addressing ethical issues arising from genetic research, responsible clinical integration of new genetic technologies, privacy and the fair use of genetic information, and professional and public education about ELSI issues."

The Human Genome Project finished sequencing 99% of the gene-containing part of the human genome sequence in April 2003. A variety of themes and challenges for the future build on the foundation of the Human Genome Project. (Detailed information about these can be found at http://www.genome.gov.) Future research will include gene expression and the study of proteomics, which studies the interaction of all proteins in the genome. In summary, future directions of the Human Genome Project most relevant to nursing include

- Understanding and cataloguing common heritable variants in human populations;
- Identifying genetic contributions to disease and drug response;
- Developing strategies to identify gene variants that contribute to good health and resistance to disease;
- Developing genome-based approaches to prediction of disease susceptibility, drug response, and early detection of illness;
- Developing molecular taxonomy of disease states including the possibility of reclassifying

illness on the basis of molecular characterization;

- Using these understandings to develop new therapeutic approaches to disease;
- Investigating how genetic risk information is conveyed in clinical practice, including how it influences health behaviors and affects outcomes and costs;
- Developing genome-based tools to improve health for all;
- Developing policy options for the uses of genomics that include genetic testing and genetic research with human subject protection and appropriate use of genomic information;
- Understanding the relationships between genomics, race, and ethnicity as well as of uncovering the genomic contributions to human traits and behaviors and the consequences of uncovering these types of information;
- Assessing how to define the appropriate and inappropriate uses of genomics.

NURSING ROLES IN A GENOMIC ERA

What should nurses know relevant to genetics and genomics? Various groups have identified core competencies for the health professions, including the National Coalition for Health Professional Education in Genetics. (Detailed ones may be found at http://www.nchpeg.org.) All nurses need to be able to understand the language of genetics and be able to communicate with others using it appropriately, interview clients and take an accurate history over three generations, recognize the possibility of a genetic disorder in an individual or family, and appropriately refer that person or family for genetic evaluation or counseling. They should also be prepared to explain and interpret correctly the purpose, implications, and results of genetic tests in such disorders as cancer and Alzheimer disease. Nurses will be seeing adults with childhood genetic diseases and will have to deal with how those disorders will influence and be influenced by the common health problems that occur in adults as they age, as well as seeing the usual health problems of adults superimposed on the genetic background of a childhood genetic disorder such as cystic fibrosis. Nurses will also see more persons with identified

adult-onset genetic disorders, such as hemochromatosis and some types of Gaucher disease. The precise role played by the nurse in relation to genetics and genomics varies depending on the disorder, the needs of the client and family, and the nurse's expertise, role, education, and job description. Advanced-practice nurses will have additional skills to offer. Depending on these, nurses may be providing any of the following in relation to genetic disorders and variations, many of which are extensions of usual nursing practice:

- Providing direct genetic counseling (requires advanced education and certification)
- Planning, implementing, administering, or evaluating genetic screening or testing programs
- Monitoring and evaluating clients with genetic disorders
- Working with families under stress engendered by problems related to a genetic disorder
- Coordinating care and services for clients affected by genetic disorders
- Managing home care and therapy of persons affected by genetic disorders
- Following up on positive newborn screening tests
- Interviewing clients with a genetic disorder
- Assessing needs and interactions in clients and families affected by genetic disorders
- Taking comprehensive and relevant family histories
- Drawing and interpreting pedigrees
- Assessing genetic risk, especially in conjunction with genetic testing options
- Assessing the client and family's cultural/ethnic health beliefs and practices as they relate to the genetic problem
- Assessing the client and family's strengths and weaknesses and family functioning
- Providing health teaching and education related to genetics and genetic testing
- Serving as an advocate for a client and family affected by a genetic disorder
- Participating in public education about genetics
- Developing an individualized plan of care
- Reinforcing and interpreting genetic counseling and testing information
- Supporting families when they are receiving counseling and making decisions

- Recognizing the possibility of a genetic component in a disorder and taking appropriate referral action
- Appreciating and ameliorating the social impact of a genetic problem on the client and family
- Advocating for patients and families

Additionally, there is an organization for nurses interested in genetics, the International Society of Nurses in Genetics (ISONG; http://www.isong.org). Various certifications are available for nurses related to genetics depending on their education and experience, including those through ISONG and the American Board of Medical Genetics.

Recognizing the importance of genetics in health care and policy allows new ways to think about health and disease. In those affected by a genetic disorder, it is particularly important to focus on the family as the primary unit of care, because identification of a genetic disorder in one member can allow others in the family to receive appropriate preventive measures, detection, and diagnosis or treatment and to choose reproductive and life options concordant with their personal beliefs. The demand for genetic services continues to grow. Only a small percentage of those who should receive them are actually receiving them. Health disparities, especially among the poor and disadvantaged of various ethnic backgrounds, may also occur in regard to genetic services and need to be addressed.

Nurses as a professional group are in an ideal position to apply principles of health promotion, maintenance, and disease prevention coupled with an understanding of cultural differences, technical skills, family dynamics, growth and development, and other professional skills to the person and family unit threatened by a genetic disorder in ways that can ensure an appropriate outcome.

END NOTES

Genomics will be to the 21st century what infectious disease was to the 20th century for public health (Gerard, Hayes, & Rothstein, 2002). In addition to the affected individual, genetic disorders exact a toll on all members of the family, as well as on the community and society. Although mortality

from infectious disease and malnutrition has declined in the United States, the proportion due to disorders with a genetic component has increased, assuming a greater relative importance. Genetic disorders can occur as the result of a chromosome abnormality, mutations in a single gene, mutations in more than one gene, disturbance in the interaction of multiple genes with the environment, and the alteration of genetic material by environmental agents. Depending on the type of alteration, the type of tissue affected (somatic or germline), the internal environment, the genetic background of the individual, the external environment, and other factors, the outcome can result in no discernible change, structural or functional damage, aberration, deficit, or death. Effects may be apparent immediately or may be delayed. Outcomes can be manifested in many ways, including abnormalities in biochemistry, reproduction, growth, development, immune function, or behavior or combinations of these.

A mutant gene, an abnormal chromosome, or a teratologic agent that causes harmful changes in genetic material is as much an etiologic agent of disease as is a microorganism. Genes set the limits for the responses and adaptations that individuals can make as they interact with their environments. Genes never act in isolation; they interact with other genes against the individual's genetic background and internal milieu and with agents and factors in the external environment.

KEY POINTS

- Health care and society are increasingly influenced by genetics and genomics.
- Nurses will encounter clients/patients with genetically influenced disorders in every area of clinical nursing practice.
- Genetic disorders may appear in any phase of the lifespan.
- The Human Genome Project resulted in gene sequencing of the human genome.
- Nurses play many roles in caring for persons and families affected by genetically influenced disorders.
- Nurses should have basic knowledge and competencies relating to genetics and genomics.

2

Basic and Molecular Concepts in Biology

Basic terms and genetic processes are introduced in this chapter. This includes basic information about genes and chromosomes and the process of transmitting genetic information. Cell division, including mitosis and meiosis, is reviewed briefly. The following chapters in this section build on the material here to discuss the classifications of genetic disease and the types of inheritance.

GENES, CHROMOSOMES, AND TERMINOLOGY

Genes are the basic units of heredity. A *gene* can be defined as a segment of deoxyribonucleic acid (DNA) that encodes or determines the structure of an amino acid chain or polypeptide. A *polypeptide* is a chain of amino acids connected to one another. It may be a complete protein or enzyme molecule, or one of several subunits that are modified before completion. There are about 20,000 to 25,000 genes in a person's genome (total genetic complement or makeup). The vast majority of genes are located in the cell nucleus, but genes are also present in the mitochondria (power plants) of the cells. Genes direct the process of protein synthesis; thus, they are responsible for the determination of such products as structural proteins shown in Box 2.1.

Genes are also concerned with the regulation of proteins and enzymes and guide the development of the embryo. One consequence of altered enzyme or protein structure can be altered function. The capacity of genes to function in these ways means

that they are significant determinants of structural integrity, cell function, and the regulation of biochemical, developmental, and immunological processes.

CHROMOSOMES AND GENES

Chromosomes are structures present in the cell nucleus that are composed of DNA, histones (a basic protein), nonhistone (acidic) proteins, and a small amount of ribonucleic acid (RNA). This chromosomal material is known as *chromatin*. Genes are located on chromosomes. Chromosomes can be seen under the light microscope and appear threadlike during certain stages of cell division, but they shorten and condense into rodlike structures during other stages, such as metaphase. Each chromosome can be individually identified by means of its size, staining qualities, and morphological characteristics. Chromosomes have a centromere, which is a region in the chromosome that can be seen as a constriction. *Telomeres* are specialized structures at the ends of chromosomes; they have been likened to the caps on shoelaces. They consist of multiple tandem repeats (many adjacent repetitions) of the same base sequences. Telomeres are currently believed to have important functions in cell aging and cancer.

The normal human chromosome number in most somatic (body) cells and in the zygote is 46. This is known as the diploid (2N) number. Chromosomes occur in pairs; normally one of each pair is derived from the individual's mother and one of each pair is derived from the father. There are 22 pairs of autosomes (non-sex chromosomes common to both sexes) and a pair of sex chromosomes. The sex chromosomes present in the normal female are two X chromosomes (XX). The sex chromosomes present in the normal male are one X chromosome and one Y chromosome (XY). Gametes (ova and sperm) each contain one member of a chromosome pair, for a total of 23 chromosomes (22 autosomes and one sex chromosome). This is known as the haploid (N) number or one chromosome set. The fusion of male and female gametes during fertilization restores the diploid number of chromosomes (46) to the zygote, normally contributing one maternally derived chromosome and one paternally derived chromosome to each pair, along with its genes.

Genes are arranged in a linear fashion on a chromosome, each with its specific locus (place). However, less than 5% of the DNA in the genome consists of gene-coding sequences. There are also stretches of DNA that are not known to contain genes. These are said to be noncoding DNA. Autosomal genes are those whose loci are on one of the autosomes (non-sex chromosomes). Each chromosome of a pair (homologous chromosomes) normally has the identical number of arrangement of genes, except, of course, for the X and Y chromosomes in the male. Nonhomologous chromosomes are members of different chromosome pairs. Only one copy of a gene normally occupies its given locus on the chromosome at one time. The reason is that in somatic cells, the chromosomes are paired, and two copies of a gene are normally present—one copy of each one of a chromosome pair. The exceptions are the X and Y chromosomes of the male, or certain structural abnormalities of the chromosome. Genes at corresponding loci on homologous chromosomes that govern the same trait may exist in slightly different forms or alleles. Alleles are

therefore alternative forms of a gene at the same locus. A way to think about this is that if a gene were an apple, alleles could be Cortland, Macintosh, Jonathan, Winesap, and so on.

For any given gene under consideration, if the two gene copies or alleles are identical, they are said to be *homozygous*. For a given gene, if one gene copy or allele differs from the other, they are said to be *heterozygous*. The term *genotype* is most often used to refer to the genetic makeup of a person when discussing a specific gene pair, but sometimes it is used to refer to a person's total genetic makeup or constitution. *Phenotype* refers to the observable expression of a specific trait or characteristic that can either be visible or biochemically detectable. Thus, blond hair and blood group A are considered phenotypic features. A trait or characteristic is considered *dominant* if it is expressed or phenotypically apparent when one copy or dose of the gene is present. A trait is considered *recessive* when it is expressed only when two copies or doses of the gene are present or if one copy is missing, as occurs in X-linked recessive traits in males. *Codominance* occurs when each one of the two alleles present is expressed when both are present, as in the case of the AB blood group. Those genes located on the X chromosome (X-linked) are present in two copies in the female but only one copy in males, since males have only one X chromosome. Therefore, in the male, the genes of his X chromosome are expressed for whatever trait they determine. Genes on the X chromosome of the male are often referred to as *hemizygous*, because no partner is present. In the female, a process known as X-inactivation occurs so that there is only one functioning X chromosome in each somatic cell. Very few genes are known to be located on the Y chromosome, but they are only present in males. These terms are summarized in Box 2.2.

Standards for both gene and chromosome nomenclature are set by international committees. To describe known genes at a specific locus, genes are designated by uppercase Latin letters, sometimes in combinations with arabic numbers, and they are italicized or underlined. Alleles of genes are preceded by an asterisk. Some genes have many or multiple alleles that are possible at its locus. This can lead to slightly different variants of the same basic gene product. For any given gene, any individual would still normally have only two alleles present in

BOX 2.2

Selected Definitions

Term	Definition
Alleles	Alternative forms of a gene at a given locus.
Codominant	When each of two alleles present is expressed when both are present.
Dominant	A trait that is apparent or expressed when one copy or dose of the gene is present.
Genotype	Refers to person's genetic make-up for a specific gene pair or total genetic make-up.
Hemizygous	Having one copy of a particular gene.
Heterozygous alleles	One allele of the same gene pair differs from the other.
Homologous chromosomes	Members of the chromosome pairs with same gene number and arrangement.
Homozygous alleles	Ones that are identical.
Phenotype	Observable expression of a specific trait or characteristic.
Recessive	A trait that is apparent or expressed only when two types or doses of the gene are present or if one copy is missing.

somatic cells—one on each chromosome. Thus, in referring to the genes for the ABO blood groups, *ABO*A1*, *ABO*O*, and *ABO*B* are examples of the formal ways for identifying alleles at the ABO locus. As an example, genotypes may be written as *ADA*1/ADA*2* or *ADA*1/*2* to illustrate a sample genotype for the enzyme adenosine deaminase. Further shorthand is used to more precisely describe mutations and allelic variants. These describe the position of the mutation, sometimes by codon or by the site. For example, one of the cystic fibrosis mutations, deletion of amino acid 508, phenylalanine, is written as PHE508DEL or ΔF508.

However, to explain patterns of inheritance more simply, geneticists often use capital letters to represent genes for dominant traits and small letters to represent recessive ones. Thus, a person who is heterozygous for a given gene pair can be represented as Aa, one who is homozygous for two dominant alleles AA, and one who is homozygous for two recessive alleles aa. For autosomal recessive traits, the homozygote (AA) and the heterozygote (Aa) may not be distinguishable on the basis of phenotypic appearance, but they may be distinguishable biochemically because they may make different amounts or types of gene products. This information can often be used in carrier screening for recessive disorders to determine genetic risk and for

genetic counseling. Using this system, when discussing two different gene pairs at different loci, a heterozygote may be represented as AaBb. When geneticists discuss a particular gene pair or disorder, normality is usually assumed for the rest of the person's genome, and the term *normal* is often used unless stated otherwise. Chromosome nomenclature is discussed in Chapters 4 and 5.

DNA AND RNA

DNA and RNA are both nucleic acids with similar components: a nitrogenous purine or pyrimidine base, a five-carbon sugar, and a phosphate group that together comprise a nucleotide. In DNA and RNA, the purine bases are adenine (A) and guanine (G). In DNA, the pyrimidine bases are cytosine (C) and thymine (T), and in RNA they are C and uracil (U) instead of T. The human genome is believed to contain about 3 billion nucleotide bases. The sugar in DNA is deoxyribose, and in RNA it is ribose. These nucleotides are formed into chains or strands. DNA is double stranded, and RNA is single stranded. Each DNA strand has polarity or direction (5' to 3' and 3' to 5'), and two chains of opposite polarity are antiparallel and complementary. The well-known three-dimensional conformation of DNA is the double helix. This may be visualized as a flexible ladder in which the sides are the phosphate and sugar groups, and the rungs of the ladder are the bases from each strand that form hydrogen bonds with the complementary bases on the opposite strand. This flexible ladder is then twisted into the double helix of the DNA molecule. In DNA, A always pairs with T, forming two bonds (A:T), and G always pairs with C, forming three bonds (G:C), although it does not matter which DNA strand a given base is on. However, a given base on one strand determines the base at the same position in the other DNA strand because they are complementary. If G occurs in one chain, its partner is always C in the other strand. If one thinks of these bases as being similar to teeth in a zipper, then the two sides with the teeth can fit together to zip in only one way—A matched with T and G matched with C. Thus, the sequence of bases in one strand determines the position of the bases in the complementary strand. In RNA, U pairs with A because T is not present.

There are three major classes of RNA involved in protein synthesis: messenger RNA (mRNA), ribosomal RNA (rRNA), and transfer RNA (tRNA). The RNA that receives information from DNA and serves as a template for protein synthesis is mRNA. Ribosomal RNA is one of the structural components of ribosomes—the RNA-protein molecule that is the site of protein synthesis. Transfer RNA is the clover-leaf shaped RNA that brings amino acids to the mRNA and guides them into position during protein synthesis. The middle of the clover leaf contains the anticodon, and one end attaches the amino acid.

DNA template		3′... AAA	TGA	CTG... 5′
mRNA		5′... UUU	ACU	GAC... 3′
tRNA anticodon		3′... AAA	UGA	CUG... 5′
Polypeptide chain	NH$_2$... phe	thr		asp... COOH

Key: A = adenine, C = cytosine, T = thymine,
      U = uracil, phe = phenylalanine,
      thr = threonine, asp = aspartic acid.

FIGURE 2.1   Relationship among the nucleotide base sequence of DNA, mRNA, tRNA, and amino acids in the polypeptide chain produced.

sage. One codon that specifies an amino acid usually begins the message. More than one code word may specify a given amino acid, but only one amino acid is specified by any one codon; thus, the code is said to be degenerate. For example, the codons that code for the amino acid leucine are UAG, UUG, CUU, CUC, CUA, and CUG, but none of these code for any other amino acid. The relationship between the base sequence in DNA, mRNA, the anticodon in tRNA, and the translation into an amino acid is shown in Figure 2.1.

The code is nonoverlapping. Therefore, CACUUUAGA is read as CAC UUU AGA and specifies histidine, phenylalanine, and arginine, respectively. A shorthand way of referring to a specific amino acid is to use either a specified group of three letters or a single letter to denote a specific amino acid. In this system, for example, arginine may be referred to as arg or as simply R, while the symbols for phenylalanine are either phe or F. General genetics referred to in the References provide more information about the code.

THE GENETIC CODE

The position or sequence of the bases in DNA ultimately determines the position of the amino acids in the polypeptide chain whose synthesis is directed by the DNA. Therefore, the structure and properties of body proteins are determined by the DNA base sequence of a person's genes. It does this by means of a code. Each amino acid is specified by a sequence of three bases called a *codon*. There are 20 major amino acids and 64 codons or code words. Sixty-one of the codons specify amino acids, and 3 are "stop" signals that terminate the genetic mes-

DNA REPLICATION

When a cell divides, the daughter cell must receive an exact copy of the genetic information that it contains. Thus, DNA must replicate itself. In order to do this, double-stranded DNA must unwind or relax first, and the strands must separate. Then each parental strand serves as a template or model for the new strand that is formed. After replication of an original DNA helix, two daughter ones will result. Each daughter will have one original parental strand and one newly synthesized one. DNA replication is highly accurate, and needs to be; otherwise, mutations would frequently occur. After replication is complete, a type of "proofreading" for mutations occurs, and repair takes place if needed. Many enzymes, including DNA polymerases, ligases, and helicases, mediate the process. Replication of DNA is an important precursor of cell division. Despite several repair mechanisms, sometimes errors remain and are replicated, passing them to daughter cells.

PROTEIN SYNTHESIS

Information coded within the DNA is eventually translated into a polypeptide chain. The usual pattern of information flow in humans in abbreviated form is as follows:

DNA $\xrightarrow{\text{transcription}}$ primary mRNA
$\circlearrowleft$ transcript
replication

primary mRNA $\xrightarrow{\text{processing}}$ mRNA $\xrightarrow{\text{translation}}$ polypeptide
   transcript

It is known that information can flow in reverse in certain circumstances from RNA to DNA by means of the enzyme reverse transcriptase, a finding of special importance in cancer and human immunodeficiency virus (HIV) research. Basically, protein synthesis is the process by which the sequence of bases in DNA ends up as corresponding sequences of amino acids in the polypeptide chain produced. It is not possible to give a full discussion of protein synthesis here. The process is a complex one that involves many factors (e.g., initiation, elongation, and termination), RNA molecules, and enzymes that will not all be mentioned in the brief discussion below. The process is illustrated in Figure 2.2.

First, the DNA strands that are in the double helix formation must separate. One, the master or antisense strand, acts as template for the formation of mRNA. The nontemplate strand is referred to as the *sense strand*. An initiation site indicates where transcription begins. Transcription is the process by which complementary mRNA is synthesized from a DNA template. This mRNA carries the same genetic information as the DNA template, but it is coded in complementary base sequence. Translation is the process whereby the amino acids in a given poly-

peptide are synthesized from the mRNA template, with the amino acids placed in an ordered sequence as determined by the base sequence in the mRNA.

Not long ago, it was believed that all regions of DNA within a gene were both transcribed and translated. It is now known that in many genes, there are regions of DNA both within and between genes that are not transcribed into mRNA and are therefore not translated into amino acids. In other words, many genes are not continuous but are split. Therefore, transcription first results in an mRNA that must then undergo processing in order to remove intervening regions or sequences that are known as *introns*. Structural gene sequences that are retained in the mRNA and are eventually translated into amino acids are called *exons*. Therefore, transcription first results in a primary mRNA transcript or precursor that then must undergo processing in order to remove the introns. During processing, a "cap" structure is added at one end that appears to protect the mRNA transcript, facilitate RNA splicing, and enhance translation efficiency. A sequence of adenylate residues called the *poly-A tail* is added to the other end that may increase stability and facilitate translation. Splicing then occurs. This all occurs in the nucleus.

The mature mRNA then enters the cell cytoplasm, where it binds to a ribosome. There is a point of initiation of translation, and the coding region of the mRNA is indicated by the codon AUG (methionine). Methionine is usually cleaved from the finished polypeptide chain. Sections at the ends of the mRNA transcript are not translated. Amino acids that are inserted into the polypeptide chain are brought to the mRNA-ribosome complex by activated tRNA molecules, each of which is specific for a particular amino acid. The tRNA contains a triplet of bases that is complementary to the codon in the mRNA that designates the specific amino acid. This triplet of bases in the tRNA is called an *anticodon*. The anticodon of tRNA and the mRNA codon pair at the ribosome complex. The amino acid is placed in the growing chain, and as each is placed, an enzyme causes peptide bonds to form between the contiguous amino acids in the chain. Passage of mRNA through the ribosome during translation has been likened to that of a punched tape running through a computer to direct the operation of machinery. When the termination codon

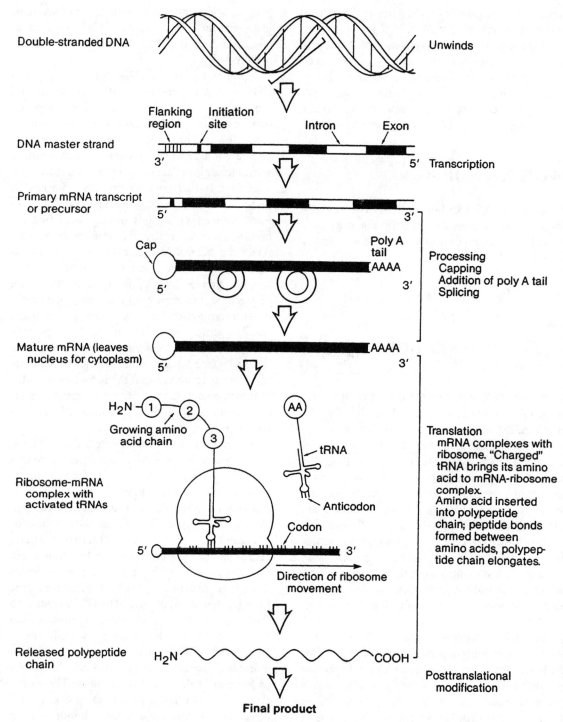

FIGURE 2.2   Abbreviated outline of steps in protein synthesis shown without enzymes and factors.

is reached, the polypeptide chain is released from the ribosome. After release, polypeptides may undergo posttranslational modification (i.e., carbohydrate groups may be added to form a glycoprotein, assembly occurs, as well as folding and new conformations). Proteins that are composed of subunits are assembled, and the quaternary structure (final folding arrangement) is finalized. In addition, epigenetic modifications such as methylation may occur. Alterations in epigenetic processes are increasingly recognized as being important in disease causation.

The study of proteomics, which is defined as the large-scale characterization of the entire protein complement, gives a broader picture of protein modifications and mechanisms involved in protein function and interactions and allows the study of entire complex systems. This is important because it is increasingly realized that neither genes nor proteins function in isolation; they are interconnected in many ways, and so it is important to understand the complex functioning of cells, tissues, and organs.

GENE ACTION AND EXPRESSION

Although the same genes are normally present in every somatic cell of a given individual, they are not all active in all cells at the same time. They are selectively expressed, or "switched" on and off. For example, the genes that determine the various chains that make up the hemoglobin molecule are present in brain cells, but in brain cells hemoglobin is not produced because the genes are not activated. Some genes, known as *housekeeping genes*, are expressed in virtually all cells. As development of the organism proceeds and specialization and differentiation of cells occur, genes that are not essential for the specialized functions are switched off, and others may be switched on. *Epigenetics* refers to alterations of genes that do not involve the DNA sequence. Epigenetic mechanisms may be involved in gene expression control. One type is called *methylation*. The process known as methylation occurs in most genes that are deactivated, and demethylation occurs as genes are activated during differentiation of specific tissues. Methylation plays a role in imprinting, an important concept discussed later.

MUTATION

A mutation may be simply defined as a change (usually permanent) in the genetic material. A mutation that occurs in a somatic cell affects only the descendants of that mutant cell. If it occurs early in division of the zygote, it is present in a larger number of cells than if it appeared late. If it occurred before zygotic division into twins, the twins could differ for that mutant gene or chromosome. If mutation occurs in the germline, the mutation will be transmitted to all the cells of the offspring, both germ and somatic cells. Mutations can arise de novo (spontaneously), or they may be inherited. Mutations can involve large amounts of genetic material, as in the case of chromosomal abnormalities, or they may involve very tiny amounts, such as only the alteration of one or a few bases in DNA. About 40% of small deletions are of 1 base pair (bp), and an additional 30% are two to three bp. Different alleles of a gene can result in the formation of different gene products. These products can differ in qualitative or quantitative parameters, depending on the nature of the change. For example, some mutations of one base in the DNA still result in the same amino acid being present in its proper place, whereas others could cause substitution, deletion, duplication, or termination involving one or more bases. The gene product can be altered in a variety of ways shown in Box 2.3.

Enzymes that differ in electrophoretic mobility (separation of protein by its charge across an electrical field, usually on a gel) because of different alleles at a gene locus are called *allozymes*. Other types of mutations can result in other aberrations. Sometimes

BOX 2.3

Ways Gene Product Can Change After Mutation

- Impairment of its function in some way, such as activity, net charge, or binding capability
- Availability of a decreased or increased amount to varying degrees
- Complete absence of gene product
- No apparent change in gene product

the effects of mutations are mild, and these can have more of an effect on the population at large because they tend to be transmitted, whereas a mutation with a very large effect may be eliminated because the affected person dies or does not reproduce.

Alteration of the gene product may have different consequences, including the following:

- It may be clinically apparent in either the heterozygous or homozygous state (as in the inborn metabolic errors).
- It might not be apparent unless the individual is exposed to a particular extrinsic agent or a different environment (as in exposure to general anesthetics in persons with malignant hyperthermia, as discussed in Chapter 6).
- It may be noticed only when individuals are being screened for variation in a population survey.
- It may be noticed only when a specific variation is being looked for (as in specific screening detection programs among Black populations for sickle cell trait or when specific genetic diagnostic testing among individual family members is done).

Because the codons are read as triplets, an addition or deletion of only one nucleotide shifts the entire reading frame and can cause (1) changes in the amino acids inserted in the polypeptide chain after the shift, (2) premature chain termination, or (3) chain elongation, resulting in a defective or deficient product. A base substitution in one codon may or may not change the amino acid specified because it may change it to another codon that still codes for the specified amino acid. A point mutation is one in which there is a change in only one nucleotide base; it is also called a single nucleotide substitution or polymorphism (SNP). There can be different SNP variations in the two alleles of a different gene. *SNPs* is usually the term used for polymorphisms in noncoding regions. The consequences of these types of mutations are illustrated in Figure 2.3. Other types of mutations can occur. These include expansion of trinucleotide repeats and creating instability (see Chapter 4) such as deletions, insertions, duplications, and inversions that may be visible at the chromosomal level. Complex mutational events may occur as well, such as a combination of a deletion and inversion. Sometimes mutations are described in terms of function. Thus,

a null mutation is one in which no phenotypic effect is seen. A loss of function mutation is said to occur when it results in defective, absent, or deficient function of its products. Mutations that result in new protein products with altered function are often called *gain-of-function mutations.* This term is also used to describe increased gene dosage from gene duplication mutations. Gene duplication has become of greater interest since new genes may be created by this mechanism. New mosaic genes may also be created by duplication from parts of other genes. Mutant alleles may also code for a protein that interferes with the product from the normal one, sometimes by binding to it, resulting in what is known as a *dominant negative* mutation.

CELL DIVISION

It is essential that genetic information be relayed accurately to all cell descendants. This occurs in two ways: through somatic cell division, or *mitosis,* and through germ cell division, or *meiosis,* leading to gamete formation. Meiosis and mitosis are compared in Table 2.1

Mitosis and the Cell Cycle

Mitosis is the process of somatic cell division, whereby growth of the organism occurs, the embryo develops from the fertilized egg, and cells normally repair and replace themselves. Such division maintains the diploid chromosome number of 46. It normally results in the formation of two daughter cells that are exact replicas of the parent cell. Therefore, daughter cells have the identical genetic makeup and chromosome constitution of the parent cell unless a mutation has occurred. Somatic cells have a cell cycle composed of phases whose length varies according to cell type, age, and other factors. These phases are known as G_0, G_1, S, G_2, and M. During the G_1 phase, materials needed by the cell for replication and division, such as nucleotide bases, amino acids, and RNA, are accumulated. During the S phase, DNA synthesis occurs, and the cell content of DNA doubles in preparation for the M phase. Mitosis occurs during the M phase. The term *interphase* is used to describe the phases of the cell cycle except for the M phase. The cell cycle and mitosis are illustrated and further discussed in Figure 2.4.

1. Original or normal pattern

DNA	TTT	AGC	CTG	ATT	
mRNA	AAA	UCG	GAC	UAA	
Amino acid chain	lys	ser	asp	stop	(Chain terminates here)

2. Deletion of T in first triplet of DNA

DNA	TTA	GCC	TGA	TT	
mRNA	AAU	CGG	ACU	AA	
Amino acid chain	ileu	leu	thr	no stop command	(Chain elongates until stop reached)

3. Addition of T in first triplet of DNA

DNA	TTT	TAG	CCT	GAT	T	
mRNA	AAA	AUC	GGA	CUA	A	
Amino acid chain	lys	ileu	gly	his	no stop command	

(Chain elongates until stop reached)

4. Substitution of T for G in second triplet of DNA. This substitution of a pyrimidine for a purine base is called a *transversion*.

DNA	TTT	ATC	CGT	ATT	
mRNA	AAA	UAG	GAC	UAA	
Amino acid chain	lys	stop			(Chain is prematurely terminated)

5. Substitution of G for C in second triplet of DNA. This substitution of one purine base for another is called a *transition*.

DNA	TTT	AGG	CTG	ATT	
mRNA	AAA	UCC	GAC	UAA	
Amino acid chain	lys	ser	asp	stop	(Note that there is no change in the amino acid inserted because both UCC and UCG code for serine.)

Key: Lys = lysine, ser = serine, asp = aspartic acid, ilu = isoleucine, leu = leucine, thr = threonine, gly = glycine, his = histidine. Numbers 2 and 3 are examples of frame-shift mutations. Numbers 4 and 5 are examples of the mechanism for single nucleotide polymorphism (SNP).

FIGURE 2.3 Examples of the consequences of different point mutations.

TABLE 2.1 Comparing Mitosis and Meiosis

Mitosis	Meiosis
Function is for growth and repair	Function is for gamete formation
Happens in most somatic cells	Happens in testes and ovary to form gametes
Preceded by replication of chromosomes	Preceded by replication of chromosomes
Has one cell division	Has two cell divisions
Results in two diploid daughter cells	Results in four haploid daughter cells
Daughter cell chromosome number same as parent (2N, diploid)	Daughter cell chromosome number is half of parent cell (N, haploid)
Daughter cells normally genetically identical	Daughter cells are genetically not the same

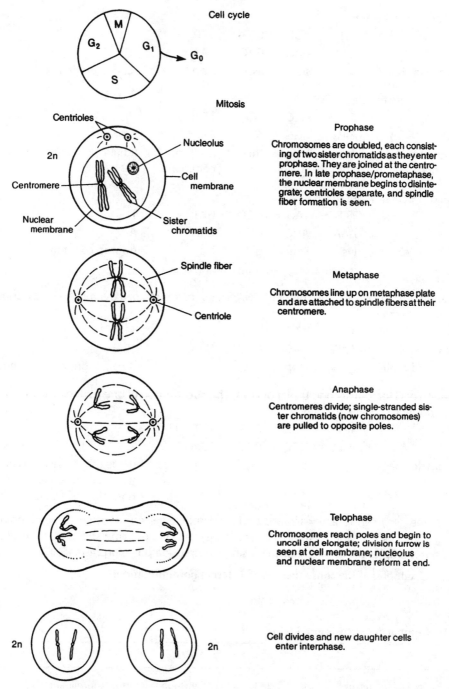

Cell cycle

Mitosis

Prophase

Chromosomes are doubled, each consisting of two sister chromatids as they enter prophase. They are joined at the centromere. In late prophase/prometaphase, the nuclear membrane begins to disintegrate; centrioles separate, and spindle fiber formation is seen.

Metaphase

Chromosomes line up on metaphase plate and are attached to spindle fibers at their centromere.

Anaphase

Centromeres divide; single-stranded sister chromatids (now chromosomes) are pulled to opposite poles.

Telophase

Chromosomes reach poles and begin to uncoil and elongate; division furrow is seen at cell membrane; nucleolus and nuclear membrane reform at end.

Cell divides and new daughter cells enter interphase.

FIGURE 2.4   Mitosis and the cell cycle. (*Top*) Cell cycle. G = gap; S = synthesis; M = mitotic division; G_1 = synthesis of mRNA, rRNA, and ribosomes; S = DNA and histone synthesis, chromosome replication, sister chromatids form; G_2 = spindle formation, G_0, G_1, S, G_2 are all interphase periods. M is the period of mitotic division shown in the bottom figure. The time a cell spends in each phase depends on its age, type, and function. When a cell enters G_0 it is usually in differentiation, not growth, and needs a stimulus such as hormones to enter G_1. (*Bottom*) Mitosis (shown with one autosomal chromosome pair).

Meiosis, Gamete Formation, and Fertilization

Meiosis is the process of germ cell division in which the end result is the production of haploid gametes from one diploid germ cell. Meiosis consists of two sequential divisions: the first is a reduction division, and the second is an equational one. In males, four sperm result from each original germ cell, and in females, the end result after the second meiotic division is three polar bodies and one ovum. As a result of meiosis, the daughter cells that are formed have 23 chromosomes, one of each pair of autosomes, and one sex chromosome, which in normal female ova will always be an X chromosome. Meiosis is shown in Figure 2.5. Fusion of the male and female gametes at fertilization restores the diploid number of chromosomes to 46. The zygote then begins a series of mitotic divisions as embryonic development proceeds.

In the males, meiosis takes place in the seminiferous tubules of the testes and begins at puberty. In females, oogenesis takes place in the ovaries. It is initiated in fetal development and develops through late prophase. It is then dormant until maturation, usually at about 12 years of age, when the first meiotic division is completed at the time of the release of the secondary oocyte from the Graffian follicle at ovulation. The second meiotic division normally is not completed until the oocyte is penetrated by a sperm. During the process of fertilization, the female contributes most of the cytoplasm containing mRNA, the mitochondria, and so forth to the zygote.

In the process of meiosis, each homologous chromosome, with its genes, normally separates from each other (Mendel's Law of Segregation) so that only one of a pair normally ends up in a given gamete. Then each member of the chromosome pair assorts independently. It is normally a matter of chance as to whether, for example, a chromosome number 1, which was originally from the person's mother, and a chromosome number 2, which was originally from the person's father, end up in the same gamete or not, or whether, by chance, all maternally derived chromosomes end up in the same gamete (Mendel's Law of Independent Assortment). During meiosis, the phenomenon of crossing over occurs. This process involves the breaking and rejoining of DNA and allows the exchange of genetic material and recombination to occur. This allows for new combinations of alleles and maintains variation. Assuming heterozygosity at only one locus per chromosome, 2^{23}, more than 8 million possible different gametes could be produced by one individual.

MITOCHONDRIAL GENES

The cell nucleus is not the only site where DNA and genes are present. In humans, they are also present in mitochondria. The mitochondria are bodies located in the cell cytoplasm that are concerned with energy production and metabolism and are thus known as the "power plants" of the cell. One of the functions of the mitochondrial oxidative phosphorylation system (OXPHOS) is to generate adenosine triphosphate (ATP) for cell energy. Cells contain hundreds of mitochondria (mt), and each mitochondrium can contain up to 10 copies of mtDNA, meaning that thousands of copies of mtDNA are present in some cells. The amount of DNA present in mitrochondria is far less than in the nucleus. The mitochondrial genes are virtually only maternally transmitted. It is now known that some genetic disorders are a result of mtDNA mutations. These are discussed further in Chapter 4.

GENE MAPPING AND LINKAGE

The assignment of genes to specific chromosomes, specific sites on those chromosomes, and the determination of the distance between them is known as *gene mapping*. One geneticist has likened the importance of mapping genes to their chromosomal location to the discovery that the heart pumps blood or that the kidney secretes urine. Both genetic and physical approaches have been used to map genes to specific locations on chromosomes. The complete DNA sequence for each chromosome has been determined. Within segments of DNA, the exact identity and order of nucleotides can be determined to sequence a gene.

In the genetic approach to mapping, the distance between genes on the same chromosome is commonly expressed in terms of map units or centimorgans (after the geneticist Thomas Morgan). Physical mapping uses measures such as bases and

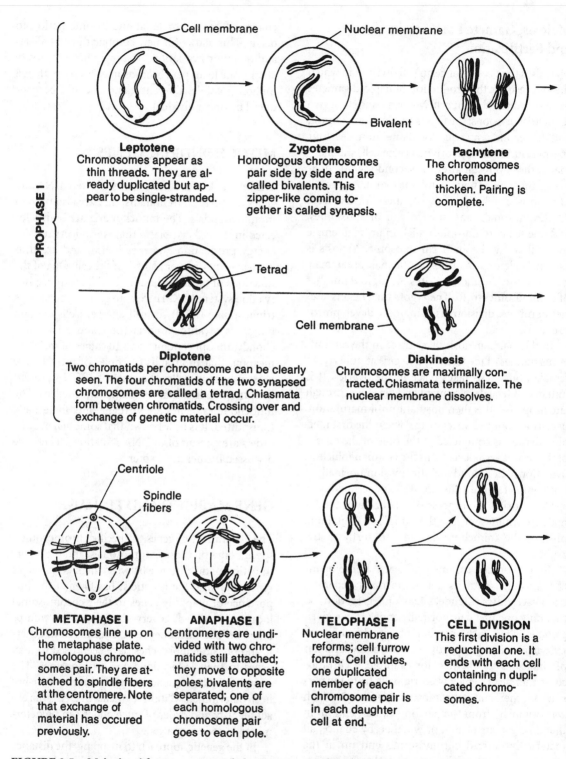

FIGURE 2.5   Meiosis with two autosomal chromosome pairs. (*Top*) Prophase I. (*Bottom*) Prometaphase—nuclear membrane disintegrates, nucleolus disappears, and spindle apparatus forms. This is followed by the rest of meiois I: metaphase I, anaphase I, telophase I, and cell division.

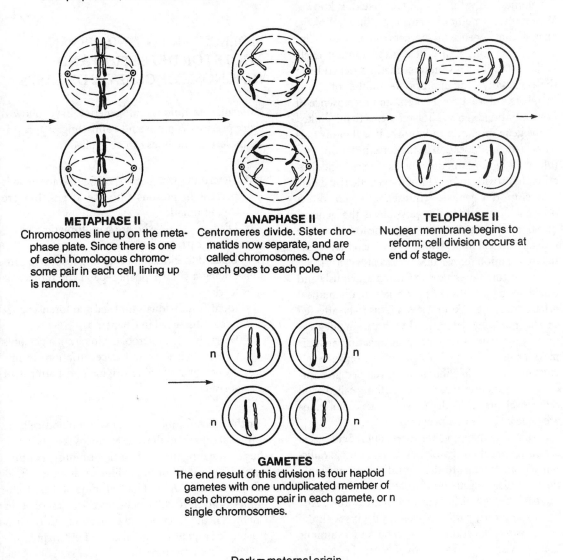

As cells enter the second part of meiosis, chromosomes elongate, the nuclear membrane disintegrates after prophase II; no DNA replication occurs. Each cell contains 1 set (n) of duplicated chromosomes.

METAPHASE II
Chromosomes line up on the metaphase plate. Since there is one of each homologous chromosome pair in each cell, lining up is random.

ANAPHASE II
Centromeres divide. Sister chromatids now separate, and are called chromosomes. One of each goes to each pole.

TELOPHASE II
Nuclear membrane begins to reform; cell division occurs at end of stage.

n   n

n   n

GAMETES
The end result of this division is four haploid gametes with one unduplicated member of each chromosome pair in each gamete, or n single chromosomes.

Dark = maternal origin
Light = paternal origin

FIGURE 2.5 (cont.)   Meiosis with two autosomal chromosome pairs—meiosis II.

kilobases (kb). Many techniques are used to map genes. Genes located on the same chromosome are called *syntenic*. Those located 50 or fewer map units apart are said to be *linked*. Genes that are linked (located on the same chromosome—50 map units or closer) are not likely to assort independently, as discussed in the previous section. The closer together or the more tightly linked they are, the greater the chance is that they will "travel" together during meiosis and end up in the same gametic cell. Although direct detection of mutations, such as through DNA analysis, is the preferred method of diagnosis of genetic disease, this is not always possible. Direct methods can be used to detect many known mutations, such as the one for sickle cell anemia, in which one mutation, the substitution of the amino acid valine for glutamic acid, is known. When direct methods cannot be used, linkage analysis that depends on markers can be used to figure out the inheritance of a given mutant allele within a family. This indirect method depends on the availability of an appropriate number of family members, informative markers, and the absence of nonparenthood. Thus, if the marker is tightly linked to the gene mutation of interest, it will almost always predict the location of the gene mutation. This information can sometimes be used in specific situations to provide information for genetic risk determination and genetic counseling when direct prenatal diagnosis is not possible if the gene in question is known to be linked to one for detectable trait and the parental genotypes are such that essential information for calculating risks is available.

By meeting the criteria discussed previously and others and by making appropriate mathematical calculations, the risk for a given fetus to be affected can be indirectly determined with varying degrees of the probability of accuracy. Segregation analysis plays a role in genetic linkage studies. Linkage calculations use the likelihood of a given pedigree under certain assumptions, and something called a lod score is calculated. Today most linkage calculations are done by computer programs.

In physical mapping, the major approaches used are positional cloning and functional cloning. *Functional cloning* refers to the identification and location of a disease gene on the basis of knowledge of the basic biochemical defect in that disorder. Another technique, *positional cloning*, begins with the chromosome location of the gene and examines that DNA stretch for functional genes. DNA samples from multiple affected families and normals are needed. The located area is treated with restriction enzymes, and patients affected by the disease are compared with those who are not. DNA probes are then used to locate the potential gene, which can then be sequenced. A strategy that somewhat combines these methods is positional-candidate cloning in which a disease is mapped to a small region of a chromosome and that area is searched for a candidate gene for that disease. Newer methods for positional cloning using linkage and linkage dis-

equilibrium are being used for both Mendelian and complex diseases.

MOLECULAR TECHNIQUES AND TOOLS FOR DETECTION AND DIAGNOSIS OF GENETIC DISEASES

Molecular techniques in genetics have allowed more precise diagnosis and counseling. Appropriate molecular methods can be applied to:

- Determine whether a specific mutant gene is present in persons who are at risk but are asymptomatic;
- Diagnose those who are symptomatic;
- Detect carriers;
- Be used to differentiate among disorders producing a similar phenotype at the molecular level;
- Identify individuals for legal and forensic purposes (discussed in Chapter 3);
- Determine the microbial etiology of a person's infectious disease and trace variations in microbes to determine origins and patterns of spread.

For the DNA sample, usually white blood cells or epithelial cells from the buccal mucosa can be used, thus eliminating the need for tissue biopsy. For prenatal diagnosis, chorionic villus or amniotic fluid cells can be used. A brief look at some of these techniques is given next. Genetic tests are described in Chapter 5, and forensic and legal applications such as genetic parenthood are discussed in Chapter 3.

One of the basic tools in molecular genetics is the use of restriction enzymes or restriction endonucleases for recombinant DNA or other technology. These enzymes recognize a specific nucleotide sequence (recognition site) and cut the DNA where that sequence occurs. Different restriction enzymes have different known recognition sites, and thus the number of fragments produced by the process depends on which enzyme is used. In brief, the procedure is as follows: The DNA is extracted from the sample and is incubated with a specific restriction enzyme that digests or cuts the DNA into thousands of fragments of varying lengths (restriction fragment length polymorphisms [RFLPs], as described earlier). The fragment length varies not only in regard to the specific restriction enzyme used but also in regard to individual variation, resulting in differences in the size of segments of DNA when a particular restriction enzyme cut site is present or absent. These are then subjected to another technique such as the Southern Blot or polymerase chain reaction (PCR), depending on the purpose of the analysis.

Among the uses of DNA profiling or fingerprints are criminal and paternity applications. After using a particular restriction enzyme to obtain DNA fragments from a sample, fragments are placed on a gel and into an electrical field to separate the fragments by size. This process, called *electrophoresis*, depends on the more rapid migration of smaller fragments and the slower migrations of larger fragments. Fragments are rendered single stranded. They are then transferred to a membrane or filter, and a specific labeled probe is added; then washing occurs. Hybridization of the labeled probe will occur to the DNA with a complementary sequence. If radioactively labeled, then autoradiography is used to create an X-ray film showing a band pattern. Fluorescent dyes may also be used as labels, with appropriate detectors for fluorescence instead of autoradiography. The process can be repeated for multiple probes. Specific fragments of samples from two or more different sources can be compared to see if they are from the same individual (with certain probabilities). Northern and Western blots are similar but are for mRNA and proteins, respectively. A variation is the use of in situ hybridization. With in situ hybridization, a prepared, labeled DNA probe is incubated with a cell or tissue sample and later examined.

Another major advance has been the ability to clone DNA. When a segment of DNA or a gene is isolated and cloned (copies made), a particular gene or DNA segment can be used as a DNA probe or used in genetic engineering or gene or pharmacological therapy. During the cloning procedure, DNA fragments can be inserted into plasmids or other vectors to produce many copies of the specific fragment or gene, as well as the production of large quantities of products for treatment, such as human growth hormone, insulin, or alpha interferon.

Another technique is PCR, which amplifies a chosen DNA segment rapidly and exponentially with each cell cycle, making up to millions of copies. Its inventor, Kary Mullis, was awarded the 1993 Nobel Prize in chemistry. It can do this rapidly from as little a source of DNA as one nucleated cell. Thus DNA can be obtained from such sources as one hair, dried blood spots, saliva traces, or decayed DNA sources. PCR is so sensitive that it is important that no contamination occur, which can happen if proper precautions are not taken. It uses two oligonucleotide primers complementary to the flanking sequence of the DNA stretch that is of interest in amplification and is usually used for smaller DNA regions. After enough DNA copies are generated, analysis can take place, which can include digesting the amplified DNA with a restriction enzyme, hybridizing the product by using allele-specific oligonucleotides (ASO) (ASOs are short—usually 7 to 30 nucleotide long—probes) or other probes, direct nucleotide sequencing of the PCR product, and others. PCR is also being used in archaeological DNA studies because only very tiny amounts of DNA obtained from sources such as mummies can be used for analysis. *Multiplex PCR* refers to the analysis of more than one sample at the same time. Another application of PCR use is in chronic myeloid leukemia (CML). PCR can be used to detect the presence of *BCR-ABL* transcripts after bone marrow transplant to detect whether minimal residual disease remains. Various advances and variations occur in the types of molecular diagnoses used as new techniques become available.

Microarray (or chip) technology has allowed the detection and analysis of thousands of genes simultaneously as to patterns of expression and interaction of pathways. A microarray consists of a solid surface such as a glass slide or silicon wafer on which each spot on the array corresponds to an immobilized DNA target sample that can represent a gene. A fluorescent labeled sample (usually mRNA or DNA) is then applied and incubated with the microarray, allowing binding or hybridization to the immobilized target DNA. The fluorescent signal is measured so that information about gene expression can be obtained. Gene expression profiles can be developed. This technique is useful in many studies in cancers and infectious diseases. For example, in leukemia, different expression profiles are seen with different genetic mutations and may be used in diagnosis, prognosis, and, we hope, someday, prevention.

KEY POINTS

- There are new understandings of the complexity of the processes of DNA replication, transcription, and translation.
- There is increasing research interest in post-translational modification and epigenetic processes such as methylation and their significance in human variation and disease.
- There is a new emphasis on how proteins and metabolites in the body function not only alone but in combination.
- Elucidating gene expression is important in normal function and in disease states.
- Molecular techniques are increasingly used for detection and diagnosis of genetic variations and disorders, personal identification, and epidemiological and anthropological studies.

3

Human Diversity and Variation
We Are Not All Genetically Identical

CASE EXAMPLE 1

Ellen and Mary are next-door neighbors in Kansas City, Missouri. Both of them have had appointments with the same woman's health nurse practitioner for preconception counseling. Ellen, who is of Ashkenazi Jewish descent, has been asked to consider genetic testing to determine whether she might be a carrier for Tay-Sachs disease as well as certain other conditions but not beta-thalassemia. Tay-Sachs disease is an autosomal recessive disorder resulting in a neurodegenerative disorder. Mary, who is of Greek descent, has been asked to consider genetic testing to determine whether she might be a carrier for beta-thalassemia but not Tay-Sachs disease. Beta-thalassemia is a disorder resulting in deficient or absent synthesis of the beta hemoglobin chains. After reading this chapter, you should be able to answer why the recommended testing was considered appropriate for each woman.

CASE EXAMPLE 2

Joan has a baby boy, Richard, who is now four months old. Two possible men may be the father, Jonas and Dwayne. The geneticist takes samples of blood from Joan, Richard, Jonas, and Dwayne for DNA analysis and possibly other markers to determine genetic parenthood. Why is it ideal to take samples from all of these individuals?

GENETIC INDIVIDUALITY

Each individual has a unique genetic constitution that makes him/her genetically and biochemically distinct from all other individuals (except for monozygous twins, triplets, and other multiples). No individuals, with the exceptions mentioned, have the exact same genotype or phenotype. Even identical twins can show some differences in epigenetic regions. Because a person's genetic constitution determines the limits of the range of responses and potentials within which he/she can interact with the environment, each person has his/her own relative state of health. Thus, individuals are not at equivalent risk for developing a given disease. A person's genetic make-up plays a pivotal role in the maintenance of homeostasis and in susceptibility and resistance to disease.

Most genes in humans are shared by all members of the human species. Differences have more to do with variation in frequency of certain alleles than in whether the gene is present or absent. A genetic variation is called a *polymorphism* when two or more alleles are maintained in a population so that the frequency of one of the uncommon alleles is maintained at a frequency of at least 1%. The ABO, MN, and Rh blood groups and the human leukocyte antigen (HLA) system are some of the best-known examples of classic genetic polymorphisms and are discussed later. The clinical use of the knowledge of these polymorphisms has been amply demonstrated by the ability to perform compatible transfusions and tissue transplants.

The newer polymorphisms being identified may involve only one nucleotide change in a gene and are known as single nucleotide polymorphisms (SNPs, (pronounced *snips*). Information from the Human Genome Project has revealed that there are about 3 million places in the genome where SNPs occur. The reasons for such a high degree of variation are not fully known. Most polymorphisms appear neutral or cause benign variations. It may be that the preservation of individual and population genetic diversity allows humans to adapt to environmental changes and challenges and thus to survive.

SNPs and their constellations can be used to create pattern "maps" across populations in the United States, Asia, and Africa. This can give information about population history; patterns of migration; the evolution of the human genome; the geographic distribution of human variation; the age of populations; disease susceptibility in and among populations; and relationships among genetic, cultural, linguistic, and ecological variables. But there are also ethical concerns regarding these maps, such as informed consent, confidentiality, the possible exploitation of indigenous peoples, and the potential for abuse of the information obtained.

VARIATIONS AND POLYMORPHISMS IN DNA AND CHROMOSOMES

Deoxyribonucleic acid (DNA) varies among individuals and populations. Variation may be seen at the gene and the chromosome levels. At the chromosomal level, variations are especially evident in certain chromosomes, such as 1, 9, and the Y. In most cases, the significance is not known, and some of these may serve as *private* (within a family) markers. Others may be *public*. DNA sequence polymorphisms may occur within the coding (exon) regions or noncoding (such as introns) regions. Polymorphisms may occur in every 1:200 to 1:300 base pairs overall. Polymorphisms occur more often outside coding genes. These polymorphisms may be single or multiple. The more alternate forms that are present, the more useful a polymorphism is for genetic and medical applications. Each person (with the possible exception of identical multiples) has a distinct "fingerprint" of DNA. Overall, humans resemble each other in 99.9% of their DNA. The following variations are among those identified (and are explained in Table 3.1):

TABLE 3.1   Selected DNA Variations

Variation	Description
RFLPs	Single-base pair changes in noncoding DNA areas that result in removal or addition of a recognition site for a restriction enzyme. This causes an increase or decrease in the length of the restriction fragment due to differences in the number of cleavage sites cut by certain restriction endonucleases.
SNPs	Single-nucleotide changes in DNA. Patterns of SNPs are also being used to look at particular phenotypic variations as haplotypes and across populations and ethnic groups. May or may not be associated with disease.
STRs	Usually comprise pairs such as CG of two bases (although three to five pairs have been noted) that are repeated a few to many times.
VNTRs	Short DNA sequences that are repeated in tandem order a varying number of times, usually ranging in size from 5 to 50 or more base pairs. The size can change during cell division, and in some cases, expansion can lead to disease expression such as in fragile X syndrome (see Chapter 9).

- Restriction fragment length polymorphisms (RFLPs)
- Minisatellites or variable number tandem repeats; (VNTRs)
- Microsatellites or short tandem repeats (STRs)
- Single nucleotide polymorphisms (SNPs)
- Variants in mitochondrial DNA

These variants are the basis of various DNA tests used for:

- Determining genetic parentage and other family relationships;
- Individual identification in legal and forensic cases, including disasters and matching DNA in material at crime scenes or on victims with that of suspects on file in data banks;
- Genetic testing for diagnosis of certain disease conditions;

- Distinguishing between similar-appearing genetic diseases at the molecular level;
- Determining carrier status for certain genetic disorders;
- Determining the microbial etiology of a person's infectious disease and tracing variations in microbes to determine origins and patterns of spread.

Genetic testing is discussed in Chapter 5.

MAINTENANCE OF VARIATION AND POLYMORPHISM

The rare, inherited, single gene biochemical disorders are extreme examples of the spectrum of genetic diversity or variation. Variations too rare to meet the criteria for a polymorphism in the general human population may assume higher frequencies within particular population groups. Population groups that have shared a common ancestry may be isolated from the general population for cultural, social, religious, economic, political, linguistic, or geographic reasons. Members of a particular population group often pick mates or intermarry within that same group. They therefore have more specific rare alleles in their gene pool (the collection of genes in a particular population) than that of the general population. Examples of such groups are the Finns, Icelanders, Pacific Islanders, and Ashkenazi (Eastern European) Jews. This has clinical significance—for example:

- Targeting groups for establishing screening or prenatal detection programs
- Identifying individuals who are at the highest risk for adverse outcomes from exposure to certain drugs, foods, or external agents so that preventative measures can be taken

Some of the genetic diseases known to be present in higher frequencies in certain population groups are shown in Table 3.2. The presence of these rare alleles and disorders in higher frequency in some population groups is not "good" or "bad." They probably evolved, in some cases, because in the heterozygous or carrier state, they offered some type of protection (selective advantage) or because

TABLE 3.2 Distribution of Selected Genetic Traits and Disorders by Population or Ethnic Group

Ethnic or Population Group	Genetic or Multifactorial Disorder Present in Relatively High Frequency
Åland Islanders	Ocular albinism (Forsius-Eriksson type)
Amish	Limb-girdle muscular dystrophy (Adams, Allen counties, Ohio)
	Ellis-van Creveld (Lancaster County, Pennsylvania)
	Pyruvate kinase deficiency (Mifflin, Ohio)
Armenians	Familial Mediterranean fever
Asians	Dubin-Johnson syndrome (Iran)
	Ichthyosis vulgaris (Iraq, India)
	Werdnig-Hoffmann disease (Karaite Jews)
	G6PD deficiency, Mediterranean type
	Phenylketonuria (Yemen)
	Metachromatic leukodystrophy (Habbanite Jews, Saudi Arabia)
Blacks (African)	Sickle cell disease
	Hemoglobin C disease
	Hereditary persistence of hemoglobin F
	G6PD deficiency, African type
	Lactase deficiency, adult
	Beta-thalassemia
Burmese	Hemoglobin E disease
Chinese	G6PD deficiency, Chinese type
	Lactase deficiency, adult
Costa Ricans	Malignant osteopetrosis
Druze	Alkaptonuria
English	Cystic fibrosis
	Hereditary amyloidosis, Type III
Finns	Congenital nephrosis
	Generalized amyloidosis syndrome, V
	Polycystic liver disease
	Retinoschisis
	Aspartylglycosaminuria
	Diastrophic dwarfism
French Canadians (Quebec)	Morquio syndrome
Gypsies (Czech)	Congenital glaucoma
Hopi Indians	Tyrosinase positive albinism
Icelanders	Phenylketonuria (PKU)

(continues)

TABLE 3.2   Distribution of Selected Genetic Traits and Disorders by Population or Ethnic Group (*continued*)

Ethnic or Population Group	Genetic or Multifactorial Disorder Present in Relatively High Frequency
Inuit	Congenital adrenal hyperplasis
	Pseudocholinesterase deficiency
	Methemoglobinemia
Irish	Phenylketonuria
	Neural tube defects
Japanese	Acatalasemia
	Cleft lip or palate
	Oguchi disease
Jews	
Ashkenazi	Tay-Sachs disease (infantile)
	Niemann-Pick disease (infantile)
	Gaucher disease (adult type)
	Familial dysautonomia
	Bloom syndrome
	Torsion dystonia
	Factor XI (PTA) deficiency
Sephardic	Familial Mediterranean fever
	Ataxia-telangiectasia (Morocco)
	Cystinuria (Libya)
	Glycogen storage disease III (Morocco)
Lapps	Developmental dysplasia of hip
Lebanese	Dyggve-Melchior-Clausen syndrome
Mediterranean people (Italians, Greeks)	G6PD deficiency, Mediterranean type
	Beta-thalassemia
	Familial Mediterranean fever
Navajo Indians	Ear anomalies
Nova Scotia Acadians	Niemann-Pick disease, type D
Polynesians	Clubfoot
Polish	Phenylketonuria
Portuguese	Joseph disease
Scandinavians (Norwegians, Swedes, Danes)	Cholestasis-lymphedema (Norwegians)
	Sjögren-Larsson syndrome (Swedes)
	Krabbe disease
	Phenylketonuria
Scots	Phenylketonuria
	Cystic fibrosis
	Hereditary amyloidosis, type III
Thailanders	Lactase deficiency, adult
	Hemoglobin E disease
Zuni people	Tyrosinase positive albinism

of founder effects or population "bottlenecks," as described later in this chapter. As members of specific racial and ethnic groups intermarry, intermate, and become less isolated, there will be fewer definable genetic disorders occurring with greater frequency within given groups.

Population geneticists are interested in reasons for the maintenance of certain variations and polymorphisms in populations. Many complicated mathematical formulas are used to determine such things as mutation rates and to measure the effects of migration, for example. One of the fundamental principles in population genetics is that of the Hardy-Weinberg law, which is useful for different types of population problems and has had practical application in genetic counseling. (This topic is beyond the scope of this book.)

Frequencies of alleles in populations change because of such effects as mutation, selection, migration, fitness, random genetic drift, nonrandom mating, and other factors such as meiotic drive, differential gamete survival, and linkage to a favorable or an unfavorable gene (the so-called hitchhiker effect). Some of the factors that alter the frequency of alleles in certain population groups are shown in Table 3.3. Because selection has appeared to be very important in maintaining certain alleles in the population, additional discussion follows.

Selection and Selective Advantage

The fact that some alleles are rapidly eliminated from the gene pool in the homozygous recessive state, but may enjoy a higher frequency in the heterozygous state than could be maintained by mutation alone, suggests that their presence confers some type of selective advantage to the heterozygote over the normal homozygote. In the case of sickle cell disease, various lines of evidence indicate that the sickle cell heterozygotes (SA) in endemic malarial areas in Africa are less severely affected by *Plasmodium falciparum* (one type of malarial parasite) than are either the normal homozygote (AA) or the homozygote with sickle cell disease (SS). A positive correlation between the endemic malarial areas in Africa and the distribution of the hemoglobin (Hb) S gene was demonstrated years ago. The same appears to be true for the Hb C allele in West Africa, the Hb E allele in Southeast Asia, for beta-thalassemia in the formerly endemic malarial areas in parts of Italy and Greece, and for one type of

ABLE 3.3 Factors That Alter Allele requencies in Populations

actor	Definition
ifferential amete survival	Occurs when gametes with a certain composition are favored over the others with a different composition in survival.
itness	The ability of a person to reach reproductive age and pass on his/her genes to the next generation. Individuals who do not are genetically dead. An example is individuals who are homozygous for the gene for infantile Niemann Pick disease (an autosomal recessive disorder characterized by intellectual and physical delay, neurological effects, and hepatosplenomegaly) and who die in childhood. They are said to have genotypes with a low degree of fitness.
ounder effect	A type of genetic drift that occurs when a small group from a large population migrates to another locale and one or more members of the founding group possess a variant allele that is rare in the original population. That variant allele now assumes a greater proportion. Porphyria variegata is an example (see Chapter 6).
inkage	Refers to genes that are located on the same chromosome within 50 map units of each other.
Meiotic drive	Forces that change Mendelian segregation ratios in meiosis.
Migration	Movement of a population into the territory of another with different allelic frequencies from the migrant one, causing altered ratios of alleles in future generations.
Mutation	A change in genetic material that can occur in germ or somatic cells. Usually used to connote harmful effects, but this is not necessarily so.
Random genetic drift	The process that leads to a change in gene frequencies by chance alone.
Selection	The process by which certain alleles become more or less frequent in a population because of the occurrence of events making their possession more or less advantageous. It is a powerful force in evolution.

glucose-6-phosphate dehydrogenase (G6PD) deficiency in Mediterranean populations. Those heterozygotes are not an advantage once they have changed their environment and have settled in a malaria-free area such as the United States. It can be demonstrated that the frequency of the sickle cell gene in Blacks of African descent is decreasing in this country, as would be expected once the heterozygous advantage is removed.

Another polymorphism appears to have developed in response to malaria in Papua New Guinea. There, a defect known as *ovalocytosis*, an erythrocyte membrane defect involving a mutation in erythrocyte band 3, results in rigidity of the membrane. The malarial parasite thus cannot pull the membrane around itself when it enters the blood. Because of this, in heterozygotes, there is resistance to invasion by malarial parasites. This situation has the potential for drug development to protect against malaria by mimicking this defect to some degree.

BLOOD GROUP SYSTEMS

Immunogenetics began in 1900 when Landsteiner discovered the ABO blood group system. At this time, 26 such systems, plus 5 collections and 2 series, are known in humans, but all are not necessarily clinically significant. A six-digit number is given to every blood group antigen, in which the first three digits represent the system, collection, or series and the second three digits represent the antigen. The systems that are best characterized and most important are ABO, Rhesus, Kell, Lewis, Duffy, MNSs, Lutheran, P, Kidd, Diego, Yt, Xg, Dombrock, Chido/Rogers, and Scianna. The functions of the products coded for by some of these genes are not yet completely elucidated, and therefore the full understanding of importance is not known. For example, it is relatively recently that the Kidd gene locus was recognized as coding for the urea transporter of the erythrocyte. The frequency of the ABO blood group varies in different population groups and has been used in human genetics to study diversity, migration, and selection.

ABO System

The ABO system is the most clinically important. The major alleles present at the ABO locus on chromosome 9 are A, B, and O. Both the A and B alleles are dominant to the O but codominant to each other. The A and B alleles code for certain enzymes and glycosyltransferases, and add sugar groups to the H substance precursor to form the A and B glycoprotein antigens. The O allele does not produce an enzyme. These A and B antigens are not confined to the red cell but are widely distributed throughout the body. There are various subtypes of the A, B, and O alleles, with more polymorphisms being revealed by newer DNA techniques, but only A1 and A2 appear to have any antigenic importance. The relationship between genotype and blood group is shown in Table 3.4, and examples of the inheritance of the ABO blood groups are illustrated in Figure 3.1 (top). Persons with blood group O are sometimes said to have a "null" phenotype. Independent of the ABO system are the H and secretor systems.

Persons with the genotype HH or Hh produce the H substance, which is the precursor for the A and B antigens and is modified by the enzymes produced by the A and B alleles. Thus, individuals with A, B, or AB blood groups use up some or all of the H substance. Because the O allele does not produce a transferase, it exerts no effect on this pathway, the H substance is unmodified, and more H antigen remains present. The allele h is a rare silent allele recessive to H. Persons with hh who have the A or B allele do not express them due to the absence of the H substrate. The secretor (Se, se) locus determines whether the ABH antigens will be secreted in body fluids such as saliva. Individuals who are nonsecretors (sese) do not secrete ABH antigens. Approximately 80% of the White population are secretors. The secretor gene appears to have a regulatory function on the H gene.

The clinical significance of these relationships is illustrated by the case of a woman who contacted the genetic counseling center. She was believed to have blood group O, her husband was A, and her child was AB. She had been told by local health professionals that this was not possible unless her husband was not the child's father. The situation was causing considerable stress in their marital relationship. Investigation demonstrated that she in fact had the B allele, but was homozygous for the rare Bombay phenotype known as hh. B antigen production was blocked by the two h alleles, even though she had at least one B gene. This client had contacted the genetic counseling center on her own. The health professionals involved in this case had simply accepted what they considered to be the most likely explanation, without further investigation or consultation. Rare cases of other variance are known. This is an example of why it is necessary to recognize the limits of one's own knowledge. Another approach would have been to do DNA testing to establish parentage, as discussed below.

The Rhesus (Rh) System

It was not until 1940 that Landsteiner and Wiener discovered the rhesus (Rh) system. This system has become increasingly more complex. Many variants and about 45 antigens are known, and various symbols have been used to describe the major components. The most common, the one proposed by Fisher, Race, and Sanger, reflects the existence of three very closely linked loci: C or c, D or d (no antiserum for the d antigen has been found and those who are RhD negative actually lack the gene; however "d" is used here for convenience), and E or e, which are written together as cDe. The C and E alleles are much less antigenic than the D. The D allele is considered responsible for determining Rh positivity (+) in a dominant relationship to d. This inheritance pattern is illustrated in Figure 3.1 (bottom). The percentage of Rh negative individuals in the White population is approximately 15%. Few Native Americans or Asians are Rh negative. In the Black population, approximately 7% are Rh negative.

TABLE 3.4   **Relationships in the ABO Blood Group System**

Blood Group (Phenotype)	Genotype(s)	Red Cell Antigen(s)	Antibodies in Serum
A	AO, AA	A (+H)	Anti-B
B	BO, BB	B (+H)	Anti-A
AB	AB	A, B (+H)	None
O	OO	H	Anti-A Anti-B

ABO system*

Parents	AO × BO	AB × OO	AA × BB	AA × BO	AB × BB	BB × OO
	↓	↓	↓	↓	↓	↓
Offspring genotype	AB,AO,BO,OO	AO,BO	AB	AB,AO	AB,BB	BO
Theoretical proportion for each pregnancy	¼ ¼ ¼ ¼	½ ½	all	½ ½	½ ½	all
Blood group phenotype	AB, A, B, O	A, B	AB	AB, A	AB, B	B

Rh system

Parents	Dd × dd	Dd × dd	Dd × Dd
Offspring	DD	Dd,dd	DD,Dd,dd
Theoretical proportion for each pregnancy	all	½, ½	¼, ½, ¼
Rh type	Rh (+)	Rh (+), Rh (−)	Rh (+), Rh (+), Rh (−)

*Not all possible combinations are shown.

FIGURE 3.1   Examples of transmission of blood group genes.

MATERNAL-FETAL INCOMPATIBILITY

The major importance of the Rh system lies in its application to maternal-fetal incompatibility. When the father is Rh (+) and the mother is Rh (−), a fetus that is Rh (+) induces antibodies in the mother that can readily cross the placenta and cause hemolytic disease of the newborn (erythroblastosis fetalis). Such sensitization can occur through feto-maternal blood exchange in utero or at the time of delivery. Hemolytic disease of the newborn is not usually seen until the second or later pregnancies. An Rh (−) (dd) woman and an Rh (+) man are more likely to have an Rh (+) child if the father is homozygous (DD) than if he is heterozygous (Dd). In the latter case, the chance that the child would be Rh (+) at each pregnancy is 50% as opposed to 100%.

Since the availability of Rh (D) immunoglobulin in 1968, the incidence of hemolytic disease of the newborn has markedly decreased. However, not all women who should be receiving Rh immunoglobulin are. Therefore, nurses need to be aware of events that can cause sensitization and require Rh immunoglobulin administration. These include feto-maternal hemorrhage, spontaneous or induced abortion even in early pregnancy, any previous blood transfusion that was or might have been Rh incompatible, amniocentesis, chorionic villus sampling, fetal blood sampling, fetoscopy, abdominal trauma, and cesarean section. Other factors influence Rh immunization such as ABO compatibility between the fetus and mother.

The current recommendation is to administer 300 μg of Rh immunoglobulin to nonsensitized Rh negative women at 28 weeks gestation, thus reducing the incidence of antenatal alloimmunization to about 0.1%. This same dose should be given after birth if the infant is RhD-positive and as soon as possible, but within 72 hours after delivery. However, it can be given up to the 14th day. The Rh status of every pregnant woman should be determined, and if she is Rh (−), then antibody status must be done. If the Rh of the father of the child is unknown and other conditions indicate the possibility of incompatibility (e.g., mother Rh [−], second pregnancy), Rh immunoglobulin should be administered. Rh incompatibility can be diagnosed through genotyping of amniocytes using PCR.

Although incompatibility in the Rh system is the most important, ABO incompatibility can also cause injury. This occurs when the mother is blood group O; the father is A, B, or AB; and the child is A or B. Although this reaction is not usually too severe in the newborn, the incompatibility is now believed to lead to early embryonic deaths and is often not recognized as a cause. ABO incompatibility may cause severe fetal anemia as well as fetal ascites and polyhydramnios. Erythroblastosis caused by ABO incompatibility may be observed in the first pregnancy, in contrast to the usual situation existing for Rh. It is interesting to note that ABO incompatibility is somewhat protective against Rh immunization. Incompatibilities in the Kell system have also been shown to be responsible for hemolytic disease.

BLOOD GROUPS AND DISEASE

The first association between the ABO blood groups and disease was made in the case of stomach cancer. Persons having blood group A were 1.26 times more likely to develop stomach cancer than persons with other blood types. Other associations were subsequently determined that linked pernicious anemia with type A; rheumatic fever with type A, B, or AB; smallpox with type A or AB; and duodenal or gastric ulcer with type O. The risk of duodenal ulcer in nonsecretors with type O blood is two and a half times that of types A, B, and AB secretors. Nonsecretors appear to have increased oral carriage of *Candida albicans* and increased susceptibility to increased urinary tract infection with *Escherichia coli*. The Duffy (Fy) blood group has three alleles. The null allele *Fy (a-b-)* is found in almost 100% of African Blacks and about 85% of American Blacks. The Duffy antigenic sites on red cells are the receptors for *Plasmodium vivax*, one of the malarial parasites. Those who are Fy negative thus do not bind the parasite and do not develop malaria. They have a considerably selective advantage over individuals with the other Fy alleles in malarial areas. Other associations between blood groups and diseases are known.

THE HLA SYSTEM

Characteristics and Inheritance

The HLA (H = human, L = leukocyte, A = antigen) system is the major histocompatibility complex (MHC) in humans. Major normal functions of the HLA system include acting as a marker of self and the presentation of antigen particularly to T-helper cells. There are three MHC regions located together on the short arm of chromosome 6 (6p): the class I and II HLA genes and the class III genes that code for non-HLA products that are often involved with immune function. The most clinically important antigen groups at this time are the class I loci—HLA-A, HLA-B, HLA-C—and the classical class II loci—HLA-DR, HLA-DP, and HLA-DQ. The roles of others are emerging. The HLA system is the most polymorphic system known. This allows for a tremendous amount of human variability, especially in ensuring resistance to a wide variety of pathogens.

The HLA system is defined either serologically or by nucleotide sequence analysis. An international committee determines and updates standardized nomenclature and accepts new designations. The older serologic definitions use the locus specificity, such as HLA-A, followed by a number, as in the following examples: HLA-A2, HLA-B27, HLA-DR4, and HLA-Cw2. Much of the classic work in this area defined HLA specificity in this way. Those defined by sequence analysis use the gene name followed by an asterisk and a four-digit number such as *B*2703* in which the locus is *HLA-B*, the first two numbers (27) are the specificity, and the last two numbers (03) are the unique nucleotide sequence for that specificity. Thus, *HLA-B*2701* through *HLA-B*2707* are related alleles that encode different HLA molecules, but all type serologically as HLA-B27. In the case of the class II antigens, some of which consist of one or more alpha and beta chains that are coded for by alpha and beta genes, there is a more precise designation. An example is *DRB1*0401* in which it is shown that the reference is to the HLA-DR locus, the first beta chain, with the specificity being 04 and the nucleotide sequence being 01. In discussing the antigens that are coded for by the HLA alleles, "w" has also been retained to distinguish HLA-Cw8. It also is used in T-cell-defined specificity, which is designated by Dw (for HLA-D-associated) followed by a number such as Dw13.

The major class I antigens—HLA-A, HLA-B, and HLA-C—are present on the cell membrane of almost all cells, although somewhat weakly on erythrocytes and spermatozoa. A small amount is in the serum. Class I antigens present antigenic peptide to CD8+ T cells and determine the response of natural killer cells.

Class II antigens—HLA-DQ, HLA-DP, and HLA-DR—are somewhat more restricted in their distribution because they are primarily expressed on the surfaces of immunocompetent cells such as B-lymphocytes, monocytes, endothelial cells, dendritic cells, activated T-lymphocytes, and macrophages. Class II molecules present antigenic peptide to CD4+ T cells.

The class III region includes certain complement components such as C2, Bf, C4A, and C4B, and other genes with immune-related as well as products unrelated to the immune system such as steroid 21-hydroxylase, the major heat shock protein, and tumor necrosis factors (TNF).

Because letters were assigned to the HLA loci in the order of their discovery, they do not reflect their order on the chromosome. Because of the close proximity of each locus to the other HLA loci on the chromosome, the genes are tightly linked and are usually inherited together, with infrequent (less than 1%) recombination occurring. The segment of each chromosome with its set of HLA genes is known as a *haplotype*, whereas the two haplotypes together comprise the HLA genotype. Thus, multiple HLA specificities are present in each individual. Inheritance is codominant, and the phenotypic expression of the genes as evidenced by the specific antigens they produce can be demonstrated by HLA typing procedures.

Linkage Disequilibrium and Population Distribution of HLA

The phenomenon of linkage disequilibrium occurs when two or more of the alleles in the HLA system occur together in a haplotype significantly more frequently than would be expected by chance alone. In European populations, HLA-A1 and HLA-B8 occur together with an observed frequency that far exceeds the expected frequency. The frequency of individual HLA antigens varies according to different populations; for example, HLA-A9 is present in 65% of Asian populations but only 17% of European Caucasian populations. HLA-B8 is common in White populations and rare in Asians.

Disease Associations

Intense interest in the HLA system was originally generated because of the realization of its role in grafts and transplant success. That interest now includes the relationship between specific HLA antigens and certain diseases. Some of the strongest associations have been with autoimmune diseases or disorders with an immunologic defect. This association has led to the search for an autoimmune or immunological association with disorders originally not known to be so associated, such as in type 1 diabetes mellitus and narcolepsy. Estimates of the strength of the association can be made. *Relative risk* refers to how much more frequently a specific disease develops in an individual carrying a specific HLA antigen compared to the frequency of disease in individuals who are not carrying the HLA antigen. In addition, not all who have a particular HLA type may develop a given disorder despite the strong association. The etiologic fraction for a positive association in which the relative risk exceeds one, in a broad sense, indicates how much of the disease is due to the HLA factor. Formulas for these calculations may be obtained. In addition to disease susceptibility, HLA-related protective effects have also been noted. For example, HLA-DR2 and the associated HLA-DQB allele are associated with resistance to type 1 diabetes mellitus, and *HLA-B*53* is protective against severe malaria in West Africa.

Two of the most striking and undisputed associations are between HLA-B27 and ankylosing spondylitis, an inflammatory joint disease often resulting in vertebral fusion, and of *HLA-DQB1*0602* and narcolepsy, a primary sleep disorder characterized by excessive daytime sleepiness and disturbances of rapid eye movement (REM) sleep due to deficiency of the neuropeptide hypocretin. HLA-B27 is found in 90–95% of patients with idiopathic ankylosing spondylitis regardless of ethnic group. In populations without the disorder, HLA-B27 is found in 6–8% of European and North American Whites, 2% of Chinese and Black Americans, and 0.2% of Japanese populations. It is estimated that a male with the B27 antigen has a relative risk of developing the disorder that is 90 to 100 times greater than a male not possessing this antigen. The chance for a person who has HLA-B27 to develop ankylosing spondylitis is estimated at 5% to 20%. Thus, not all those with HLA-B27 develop ankylosing spondylitis, although some may have subtle symptoms that never develop into disease and are thus overlooked unless carefully looked for. HLA-B27 is found in 75% of persons with Reiters disease, and up to 90% of persons who develop arthritis after enteric infection due to *Shigella*, *Salmonella*, and certain *Yersinia* species.

In narcolepsy, *HLA DQB1*0602* is present in 90–100% of persons with narcolepsy and cataplexy (present as part of the classic group of symptoms in narcolepsy in the majority of patients; it is a brief sudden episode of weakness in voluntary muscles that may be triggered by emotion such as laughing or anger). In contrast, HLA DQB1*0602 is present in 12–38% of the general population. Hypocretin genes are located in this HLA vicinity, although how they interact is not known. There has also been an association between HIV-1 disease and various HLA genotypes. For example both HLA-B27 and HLA-B57 have been associated with slow progression, while certain *HLA-B35* alleles (*HLA-B*3502*, *3503*, and *3504*) have been associated with rapid progression.

Clinical Uses of HLA

Currently the largest single use for HLA typing is in tissue and organ transplantation, including blood products. In some institutions, typing of the HLA-A, HLA-B, and HLA-C loci is used to screen donors for platelet and leukocyte transfusions because of the problem of sensitivity for those persons already having such multiple transfusions.

OTHER EXAMPLES OF HUMAN GENETIC VARIATION

Other interesting interactions between certain genes and environment exist for various blood components in addition to those already discussed and for lactase. In another study, women with nonsecretor Lewis phenotypes and the recessive phenotype were more prone to recurrent urinary tract infections, perhaps because they provide a specific receptor for uropathogenic organisms so they can attach to these cells. Haptoglobin polymorphisms of the Hp 2-2 type seem more frequently associated with autoimmune disorders than the others. Variations in bone mineral density are associated with polymorphisms at the Vitamin D receptor locus on chromosome 12.

In mammals, lactase activity is highest in the newborn and then declines; by adulthood, the recessive allele for lactase is "switched off" in most adults, but in some there is a hereditary persistence of lactase, and this does not occur. This may have conferred a selective advantage on societies that had cow's milk available for food. Individuals who lack lactase activity may experience gastrointestinal symptoms such as flatulence, abdominal pain, and diarrhea after ingesting small to moderate amounts of lactose in dairy products. Analysis indicates that groups in Northern Europe and certain nomadic groups in Africa and Southwest Asia who were milking societies dating back 7,000 years have a high frequency of hereditary persistence of lactase activity, while the Chinese, Arabs, Melanesians, Thais, American Blacks, and Native Americans do not. Others are intermediate. In the United States, persons with low lactase activity can adjust to their changed environment by consuming less lactose or taking supplements, and thus minimizing annoying symptoms.

Another interesting area has to do with inherited taste, which is genetically determined and reflected in taste buds. In regard to bitterness, there are nontasters, regular tasters, and supertasters that can be detected by 6-*n*-propylthiouracil. Supertasters have approximately 1,100 taste buds per square centimeter, whereas nontasters have as few as 11. Supertasters are sensitive to fats and strong tastes of fruit and vegetables. It has been suggested that those who are supertasters dislike bitter foods and avoid cruciferous vegetables such as broccoli, which confer some chemoprotection against cancer. Thus, the type of taster one is may confer an advantage or disadvantage. Some variation may be associated with sex differences. It appears that males and females may process pain signals differently in part because of sex differences in μ-opioid receptors, eventually leading to tailoring analgesic medications differently according to sex. And persons with variants of the melanocortin-1 receptor gene, as seen in women with red hair and fair skin, appear to have greater analgesia from pentazocine than other women or even men with red hair. Examples of some genetic variations resulting in susceptibility or resistance to infectious and other diseases are shown in Table 3.5.

DETERMINING GENETIC PARENTHOOD AND FORENSIC AND OTHER APPLICATIONS OF VARIATION

Paternity suits are the most frequent reason for the determination of genetic parenthood, but it may also be done to determine maternity, especially in

TABLE 3.5   Selected Examples of Susceptibility and Resistance Genes in Infectious and Other Diseases

Genes/Variants	Comments
ABO blood group O	Susceptibility to cholera observed.
CCR5 Δ32 homozygosity	In whites, resistance to HIV infection.
Cystic fibrosis transmembrane conductance regulator (CFTR) mutation	Results in cystic fibrosis and in defects in clearing. *Pseudomonas aeroginosa* from respiratory tract. Certain mutations may be associated with sinusitis.
Duffy blood group negative	Resistance to *Plasmodium vivax* malaria.
Fucosyltransferase (FUT2) mutation, nonsecretors	Susceptibility to recurrent urinary tract infections.
Galactose-1 phosphate-uridyltransferase (GALT) mutation	Susceptibility to neonatal Gram negative bacterial sepsis.
HLA-DRB1*1101	Associated with resistance to persistent hepatitis C infections in some European populations.
HLA-DRB1*1302	Associated with resistance to persistent hepatitis B infections in West African populations.
HLA-DQB1*0501	Susceptibility to *Onchocerca volvulus* infection which causes river blindness.
Human prion protein gene (PRPN) homozygous at position 129	Associated with greater susceptibility to Creutzfeldt-Jakob disease.
Interleukin 12 receptor, beta-1 (IL12Rβ1)	Homozygous mutations associated with both *Salmonella* and *Mycobacterium* infections.
Microsomal epoxide hydrolase deficiency	Associated with chronic hepatitis C liver disease severity and hepatocellular carcinoma risk.
NRAMP1 variants	Associated in West Africans with susceptibility to tuberculosis.
Plasminogene activator inhibitor-1 4G/4G genotype	Associated with poor outcome from sepsis in meningococcal disease.

cases in which infants may have been exchanged in the hospital, or to establish parenthood in inheritance cases. Applications of DNA technology also include forensic identification of victims in disasters such as the 9/11 site in New York, matching DNA from crime scenes from saliva left on a murder victim with a suspect's DNA or with DNA profiles in databases of known criminals, for example.

The usual approach to determine genetic parenthood is through DNA analysis. DNA testing may use blood or buccal cell samples from the inside of the mouth. Specific DNA regions are used from the mother, the child, and the potential fathers. Usually at least four specific regions of DNA from the child and each parent are analyzed through comparing fragments by RFLP testing, which takes sev-

eral weeks, or by using polymerase chain reaction (PCR) to amplify the genetic material used for analysis, which generally takes only a week or less. The test is capable of excluding between 99% and 99.9% of the random population from the possibility of being the biological father. An example is shown in Figure 3.2. Other factors such as circumstances, access, and timing are usually also taken into account. Some pitfalls in the determination of genetic parenthood have included the receiving of blood transfusions, cases in which the mother and putative (suspected) father or two putative fathers were relatives, and inaccurate laboratory determinations or errors.

Aside from parenthood determination, molecular techniques are also used in forensics. Saliva,

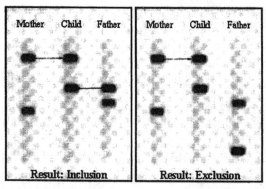

FIGURE 3.2   Paternity test showing two putative fathers, the mother, and the child in question. The father on the left has a marker that matches that of the child in question, whereas the father on the right does not. From ReliaGene Technolgies, Inc., New Orleans, LA. Design by Shantanu Sinha. Reprinted by permission.

blood, semen, and sweat all yield DNA that can be used for analysis. DNA databases are now being assembled in various states, although there is some controversy regarding who must submit to testing, criteria for maintenance in such databases, and who has access to the results. For example, in South Dakota, DNA samples are taken on arrest, and Virginia takes samples from all convicted felons. DNA samples from various suspects may be compared with a sample that was found on a victim. DNA profiling or fingerprinting techniques, which capitalize on variations such as STRs, may be used. Theoretically, though, two persons could have the same DNA profile for a particular DNA probe (remember that people have most of their DNA in common). This is why standard sets of specific highly variable regions are used. The greater the number of probes, the greater the odds are that the match is not coincidental, but the more time and expense are involved. Different agencies may use different techniques and different standard number of probes. The FBI tends to use STR analysis discussed earlier in a standard set of 13 STR regions on their CODIS software program with profiles from convicted offenders, evidence from the scenes of unsolved crimes, and missing persons. The odds that two persons will have the same 13 loci profile is approximately 1 in 1 billion. Other agencies use different techniques, including DNA chip technology. Opportunity is another consideration. For example, a

case that came to my attention several years ago involved the rape and murder of an 80-year-old woman. The defense attorney tried to claim that it was chance that a DNA match of his client was found in fluids in her vagina. However, in addition to this suspect's matching the DNA profile found (in addition to her own), the suspect was also in possession of the woman's TV set. The combination of evidence was enough to convince the jury to convict the suspect.

There are also anthropological applications of DNA analysis. The Y chromosome is passed from father to son, essentially retaining its integrity. Some researchers examined a cultural characteristic—the passing down of Jewish priesthood from father to son, originating with Aaron and reflected in certain last names such as Kohn or Cohen—and examined variation in the Y chromosome. In a sample of such men, two marker sites with variable DNA sequences on the Y chromosome were examined. Those who identified themselves as priests had different marker patterns from those who were not. Such a finding has potential implications. Men who come from this priestly lineage are not permitted to marry divorced women, and such testing might have a social effect if used for that purpose. The Y chromosome markers such as the *Alu* element have been used to study whether the Jomon or the Yayoi people were the origins of the modern Japanese.

Mitochondrial DNA (mtDNA) is passed from a woman to her children (see Chapter 4). The degree of similarity between humans can be quantitated by comparing the number of mutations in the mitochondrial genome. Theoretically, a human evolutionary tree could be developed. A group of investigators examined mtDNA from many diverse groups and used extensive RFLP mapping for comparative analysis. Their controversial finding, debated by many, was that all of the mtDNAs originated from one woman, nicknamed "mitochondrial Eve," who, they postulated, lived in Africa about 200,000 years ago. MtDNA has also been used to examine the evolution from Neanderthals. It is also used from older biological samples that lack nucleated cellular material such as hair, bones, and teeth to establish identity or in criminal cases. The Armed Services Institute of Pathology uses PCR mitochondrial sequence data to identify war remains.

Another application of DNA variation is in individual identification in times of war or disaster. In

he United States, storage of the DNA of armed
ervice personnel for such use has been the subject
•f controversy. This method has been used to iden-
ify remains and reunite families. In the aftermath
•f the terrorist attack on the World Trade Center in
New York City on September 11, 2001, DNA analy-
is was used in victim identification. In another application example, in some central and South
American countries, children of dissidents were
considered war booty and were often placed with
amilies connected to the military regime. Children
who were kidnapped by the Salvadoran military in
1982 were reunited with their families 13 years later
by use of DNA fingerprinting. DNA techniques
have also been used to identify human remains in
airline disasters and during combat by comparison
with DNA samples of the individual or comparison
with relatives. On a darker note, Germany was us-
ng saliva to screen Turkish and Iraqi visa applicants
who said they had relatives in Germany so as to ver-
ify the claim by DNA comparisons. Interestingly,
the National Football League used synthetic DNA
to tag all of the Super Bowl XXIV footballs to prevent fraud so that genuine ones could be identified
using a specially calibrated laser.

KEY POINTS

- Humans are remarkably alike. They are similar in 99.9% of their genes.
- Human variation is important in susceptibility and resistance to genetic and complex
  diseases.
- SNPs are important polymorphisms in
  humans.
- Knowledge about human genetic variation is
  being applied to forensic uses such as genetic
  parenthood, certain criminal acts, identification in times of war and disaster, and anthropological studies.
- Population genetics has provided information
  about the maintenance of certain variations
  and polymporphisms in specific groups.
- Genomic variation is applied to disease prevention and health promotion.
- ABO blood types are one of the most widespread polymorphisms.

4

Types of Genetic Disorders, Influences on Chromosome and Gene Action and Inheritance Modes

The term *genetic disorder* or *genetic disease* refers to diseases or disorders that result from deleterious or harmful changes in a person's genetic material. There are a variety of ways that genetic disorders can be classified:

- Chromosome abnormalities—due to quantitative or qualitative changes
- Inherited biochemical disorders—usually single gene disorders resulting from harmful alterations occurring in deoxyribonucleic acid (DNA) in the nucleus or mitochondria
- Multifactorial disorders—usually resulting from the interaction of mutations in multiple genes and environmental factors
- Environmental—due to exposure to a mutagenic agent; known as *teratogenic exposures* when the fetus is affected

This classification is somewhat of an oversimplification. For example, in observing an individual with a recessively inherited genetic disorder, submicroscopic chromosomal deletions of normal alleles can result in the expression of single or multiple gene disorders because the abnormal counterpart is not "countered" by the presence of a normal allele rather than in the inheritance of two mutant alleles. Each classification is described briefly below, followed by factors influencing gene action and expression and modes of inheritance. Environmental changes are discussed in Chapter 11.

CHROMOSOME ABNORMALITIES

The basic structure of chromosomes and their transmission have been discussed in Chapter 2. In this chapter, various abnormalities are discussed. Certain changes in chromosome number or structure can result in various disorders. An alteration in the number of chromosomes is called *aneuploidy*. Because most of these tend to become evident at birth or in childhood, these disorders are discussed in Chapter 8. Chromosome abnormalities result in alterations in DNA usually with multiple genes affected and can result in a proportion of congenital anomalies, developmental and intellectual disabilities, and behavioral difficulties. The majority of spontaneous abortions or miscarriages (about 50–60%) are the result of chromosomal abnormalities, particularly if they occur early. Numerical changes in chromosomes are summarized in Table 4.1. Structural changes in chromosomes are summarized in Table 4.2 and illustrated in Figure 4.1

Incidence

Large surveys of consecutive newborns have allowed the incidence of chromosome aberrations present at birth to be well established at 0.5–0.6%, although prenatal diagnosis and selective termination of pregnancy have had an impact on decreasing this. The incidence of the specific chromosome abnormalities found is summarized in Table 4.3.

TABLE 4.1   Changes in Chromosome Number (aneuploidy)

Change	Description	Example of Condition
Monosomy	1 chromosome is missing.	Turner syndrome. Cells in females contain 45 chromosomes with 1 X chromosome rather than 2.
Trisomy	1 extra chromosome is present.	Trisomy 21 (Down syndrome). Cells contain 47 chromosomes.
Tetrasomy	2 extra chromosomes are present.	Cells contain 48 chromosomes. Not compatible with life.
Triploidy	1 extra chromosome set of haploid genome are present.	Cells contain 69 chromosomes. Not compatible with life.
Tetraploidy	2 extra chromosome sets of haploid genome are present.	Cells contain 92 chromosomes. Not compatible with life.

Autosomal trisomies account for about 25%, sex chromosome abnormalities for about 35%, and structural rearrangements for about 40%. These figures represent only a small fraction of chromosomally abnormal conceptions. Nature exercises considerable selection, as only a small percentage of these abnormal conceptions survive to term. Between 10% and 20% of all recognized conceptions end in spontaneous abortion. Studies of the products of spontaneous abortion have indicated that, overall, between 50% and 60% have detectable chromosomal abnormalities. Approximately 95–99% of all Turner syndrome embryos are spontaneously aborted, as are about 95% of those with

TABLE 4.2   Major Changes in Chromosome Structure

Change	Description
Deletion (del)	Part of a chromosome is missing with the accompanying DNA. Can be at the end (terminal) or in the middle (interstitial). Example: del 5p, cri-du-chat syndrome.
Duplication (dup)	Part of a chromosome is duplicated along with the accompanying DNA so that an extra piece of chromosomal material is present. Example: In cat eye syndrome, there is duplication of a certain segment of chromosome 22 resulting in iris coloboma, anal atresia and various congenital malformations.
Inversion (inv)	Alterations in which a portion of the chromosome is rearranged by two breaks occurring, 180 degree rotation of the chromosome piece between them and its reinsertion. Example: About 40% are of chromosome 9. May or may not result in visible effects.
Ring chromosome (r)	Formed when a segment at the end(s) of one of a pair of chromosomes is lost and fuse to form a circular structure. Example: Ring chromosome 14 is associated with psychomotor delay, mental retardation, and dysmorphic craniofacial features. It is very rare.
Translocations (t)	Transfer of a chromosome segment to another chromosome after breakage has occurred. In reciprocal translocation, two chromosomes exchange pieces. A Robertsonian translocation usually involves two acrocentric chromosomes whose long arms fuse; often small fragments are lost. In a balanced translocation, no genetic material is added or lost. Balanced, reciprocal translocations usually do not cause problems. Example: Translocation trisomy 21 or Down syndrome may result from the presence of 46 chromosomes that includes a translocation chromosome such as t(14;21) or t(14q21q) so that the genetic material of 47 chromosomes with genetic material of 3 chromosome 21s is present. There is a normal chromosome 14, two normal chromosome 21s, and a translocation chromosome consisting of the second chromosome 14 and an extra chromosome 21.

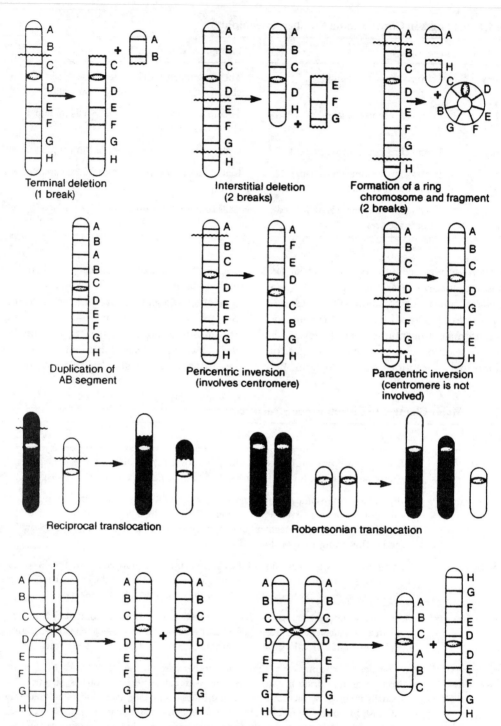

Terminal deletion
(1 break)

Interstitial deletion
(2 breaks)

Formation of a ring
chromosome and fragment
(2 breaks)

Duplication of
AB segment

Pericentric inversion
(involves centromere)

Paracentric inversion
(centromere is not
involved)

Reciprocal translocation

Robertsonian translocation

Normal division of centromere (*left*), and abnormal division (*right*) showing the formation of two isochromosomes

FIGURE 4.1   Diagrammatic representation of alteration in chromosome structure.

TABLE 4.3   Incidence of Selected Chromosome Abnormalities in Live-Born Infants

Abnormality	Incidence
Autosomal trisomies	
Trisomy 21 (Down syndrome)	1:650–1:1,000 live births
Trisomy 13 (Patau syndrome)	1:4,000–1:10,000 live births
Trisomy 18 (Edwards syndrome)	1:3,500–1:7,500 live births
Sex chromosome disorders	
45,X (Turner syndrome)	1:2,500–1:8,000 live female births
47,XXX (triple X)	1:850–1:1,250 live female births
47,XXY (Klinefelter syndrome)	1:500–1:1,000 live male births
47,XYY	1:840–1:1,000 live male births
Other sex chromosome abnormalities	
Males	~1:1,300 live male births
Females	~1:1,300 live female births
Structural	
Rearrangements (e.g., translocations, deletions)	~1:440 live births

Note: Based on statistics from surveys in different populations and not age adjusted. Data prior to use of prenatal diagnosis and selective termination of pregnancies became widespread.

trisomy 18 and 65–75% of those with trisomy 21. These data support the concept of not intervening therapeutically in cases of threatened spontaneous abortion. Chromosomal abnormalities account for 6–12% of stillbirths and perinatal deaths, respectively, about 7% of deaths between 28 days and one year of age, and slightly over 7% of later infant deaths. The different incidence figures reported from study to study reflect variety in gestational ages included, population differences, differences in chromosome preparation techniques, and different rates of culture failure, particularly in tissue obtained from autopsy material. Extrapolating from available data, it appears that chromosome abnormalities are present in 10–20% of all recognized conceptions. This may eventually be higher, as techniques for determining cytogenetic causes improve. More than 1,000 chromosome abnormalities have been described in live births.

SINGLE GENE INHERITED BIOCHEMICAL DISORDERS

The group of single gene errors, often called *inherited biochemical disorders*, includes a subgroup known as inborn errors of metabolism. Most inherited biochemical disorders are single gene defects, or Mendelian defects, and are caused by a heritable permanent change (mutation) occurring in the DNA, usually resulting in alteration of the gene product. Gene products are usually polypeptide chains composed of amino acid sequences that form an entire molecule or subunit of such entities as structural proteins, membrane receptors, transport proteins, hormones, immunoglobulins, regulatory proteins, coagulation factors, and enzymes. Thus, gene mutation results in defective, absent, or deficient function of these products (often known as *loss-of-function* mutations), or, in some cases, no discernable phenotypic effect. Mutations not showing a phenotypic effect are called *null mutations*. Mutations that result in new protein products with altered function are often called *gain-of-function* mutations. Mutations may also code for a protein that interferes with a normal one, sometimes by binding to it resulting in what is known as a *dominant negative* mutation. The consequences of altered function depend on

- The type of defect;
- The molecule affected;
- The usual metabolic reactions it participates in;
- Its usual sites of action;
- How much (if any) residual activity remains;
- Its interactions including those with other gene variants, the body milieu, external factors;
- The degree of adaptation that is possible.

Some proteins and enzymes are widely distributed in body cells, whereas others are confined to one type (e.g., hemoglobin is expressed only in red blood cells).

No official nomenclature currently exists for the inherited biochemical errors. Thus, great variation is seen in schemes used for classification and description. Such schemes may be based on mode of inheritance (e.g., autosomal recessive—citrullinemia), the chief organ system affected (e.g., nervous system—Huntington disease), the biochemical pathway affected (e.g., urea cycle—argininemia), the general type of substance metabolized (e.g., amino acid—phenylketonuria), the specific cell type or tissue affected (e.g., red blood cell—adenylate kinase deficiency), the specific substance metabolized (e.g., branched chain amino acid—maple syrup urine disease), on a functional basis (e.g., active transport disorder—cystinuria), or by gene location (nuclear or mitochondrial).

Difficulties arise with any of these methods because in some disorders, the basic defect is unknown; several organ systems can be involved (e.g., Holt-Oram syndrome, comprising limb and heart defects), or more than one type of inheritance has been identified for a disorder (e.g., retinitis pigmentosa), and so considerable overlap exists. For example, Tay-Sachs disease could be classified as a lysosomal storage disease, a neurologic disease, or an autosomal recessive disorder. Relatively common, such disorders include sickle cell anemia, cystic fibrosis, neurofibromatosis, and hemophilia A. These are discussed in detail in Chapter 9; examples of such disorders that typically are manifested in adulthood such as Huntington disease are discussed in Chapter 10.

MULTIFACTORIAL DISORDERS

Some disorders, often including a variety of congenital malformations, do not follow a single gene inheritance pattern and are not known to be due to a chromosomal abnormality. They result from mutations in more than one gene combined with environmental factors. Some relatively common birth defects such as neural tube defects, cleft lip, cleft palate, and some congenital heart defects are inherited in this manner. Some common or complex disorders such as cancer, diabetes mellitus, and heart disease are believed to fall in this category and are discussed in Chapter 10.

ENVIRONMENTAL DISORDERS

Certain substances in the environment are capable of causing damage and mutation, resulting in effects on genetic material and resultant disease. The developing embryo and fetus can be exposed to teratogens during pregnancy, especially in the first trimester, resulting in birth defects. A *teratogen* is an agent that acts on the embryo or fetus, prenatally altering morphology or function, or both. Teratogens can include infectious agents such as the rubella virus, alcohol, certain drugs and medications such as valproic acid used as an anticonvulsant, and chemicals such as lead and mercury.

FACTORS IN CHROMOSOME ERRORS

A number of influences and mechanisms may be associated with chromosome errors. Below, some of the most important, including maternal age and meiotic and mitotic nondisjunction, are discussed.

Parental Age

The increased risk for trisomy 21 (Down syndrome) and other trisomies, although to a lesser extent, with advancing maternal age has long been known. This effect begins to assume more importance at about age 35, and that is the reason for the inclusion of maternal age of 35 and older as one of the indications for amniocentesis. Prenatal screening and diagnosis with selective pregnancy termination has had a considerable impact in reducing the number of liveborn children with Down syndrome. Without accounting for prenatal diagnosis and selective pregnancy termination, the overall incidence of Down syndrome is about 1 in 800 live births, regardless of maternal age. The traditional risk figures for giving birth to a child with Down syndrome are widely used as follows:

Maternal Age in Years	Traditional Risk
20	1/1,667
25	1/1,250
30	1/952
35	1/385
40	1/106
45	1/30
49	1/11

These figures do not include conceptions that are not liveborn, or the risk of other trisomies (i.e., trisomy 13; trisomy 18; 47,XXX; 47,XXY). Thus, the risk for bearing a child with any of these trisomies may be as much as twice the age-specific risk for trisomy 21. Nurses should recognize the implications of these data for health teaching. Chromosomally speaking, both men and women should be encouraged to plan to complete their families before the age of 45 and 35 years, respectively, and women who plan to become, or are already pregnant, by that age should be referred for genetic counseling and amniocentesis.

Nondisjunction and Mosaicism

The basis for the association of increased maternal age with the increased risk of bearing a child with trisomy 21 has been thought to be caused by nondisjunction of chromosome 21 during oogenesis. When the extra chromosome is of paternal origin, nondisjunction in spermatogenesis is a possibility in older men. The precise reason for the nondisjunction remains to be found.

There are two types of cell division: mitosis and meiosis. In normal mitosis (somatic cell division for growth and repair), each daughter cell ends up with the same chromosome complement as the parent. During oogenesis and spermatogenesis, meiosis (reduction division of 2N germ cells) normally results in gametes with the haploid (N) chromosome number. Nondisjunction can occur in anaphase 1 or 2 of meiosis or in anaphase of mitosis.

If nondisjunction occurs in meiosis, the chromosomes fail to separate and migrate properly into the daughter cells, so that both chromosomes of a pair end up in the same daughter cell, leading to some gametes with 24 (N+1) chromosomes and some with 22 (N–1) chromosomes. When such gametes are fertilized by a normal gamete, trisomic or monosomic zygotes result, such as in trisomy 21 or in Turner syndrome (45,X), respectively. Offspring resulting from such fertilization generally have a single abnormal cell line. If nondisjunction occurs in the first meiotic division, only abnormal gametes result; if it occurs in the second division, half of the gametes will be normal. Nondisjunction during meiosis is shown in Figure 4.2. Anaphase lag, in

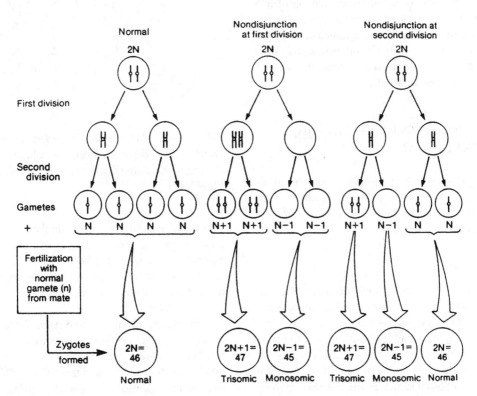

FIGURE 4.2   Mechanisms and consequences of meiotic nondisjunction at oogenesis and spermatogenesis.

which the chromosomes of a pair separate but one member "gets left behind" and is lost, leads to monosomy. If this occurs in meiosis, it affects the gamete. Variation in crossing over or recombination may be associated with nondisjunction in oocytes.

The occurrence of these errors during mitosis results in mosaicism in somatic cells except in the first zygotic division, which results in tetrasomy. An individual who is mosaic possesses two or more cell populations, each with a different chromosome constitution that (in contrast to a chimera) arises from a single zygote during somatic cell development. The number of cells that will have an abnormal chromosome make-up will depend on how early in the division of the zygote the error occurs. The earlier it occurs, the higher the percentage of abnormal cells there will be. The results of abnormal division in mitosis leading to mosaicism are shown in Figure 4.3. Chromosome abnormalities resulting from errors in mitosis are seen only in descendants of the initial cell with the error. Mosaicism is a common finding in chromosomal syndromes, and the degree to which a person is clinically affected depends on the percentage of cells with the abnormal chromosome make-up (Figure 4.3). Some persons with mild mosaicism show few or no phenotypic changes. Chromosome analysis of too few cells can miss mosaic persons with a small percentage of abnormal cells.

INFLUENCES ON GENE ACTION AND EXPRESSION

Because genes operate within an integrated body system, their expression can be affected by internal and external variables. The most important of these variables are discussed next.

Age of Onset

In many of the inherited genetic disorders, the mutant gene itself is present from fertilization onward; the appearance of its effects may not be seen immediately but can occur at different times in the lifespan (see Chapter 1). Such appearance may be caused or influenced by any of the factors discussed in this section or by factors in the external environment. A correct diagnosis, which is important not

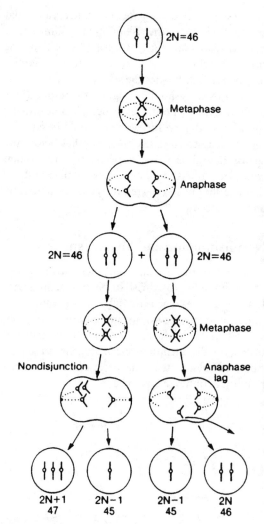

FIGURE 4.3   Mitotic division. (*Top*) Normal. (*Bottom*) Nondisjunction and anaphase lag producing mosaicism with three types of cell lines—(45/46/47).

only for treatment of the individual but also for genetic counseling, prenatal diagnosis, and life and reproductive planning for both the family and the affected person, is complicated by the fact that the same disorder may show different clinical pictures at different ages.

One of the most notorious diseases for late age of onset is Huntington disease. Less than 10% of affected individuals show any symptoms before age 30. By age 40, about 50% of those who will become affected have developed disease; by age 50, 75%; by age 60, 95%; and by age 70, almost 100%. It was not too long ago that there was no available method to distinguish individuals with the gene from those without it. Individuals with a family history of Huntington disease in a parent used to have no way of knowing whether they had inherited the mutant gene until symptoms occurred. By the time it was known if a parent in fact had Huntington disease, the children may already have had their own children. This situation is often true as a prototype for other late-onset inherited disorders such as autosomal dominant polycystic kidney disease, which is discussed in more detail in Chapter 10.

Heterogeneity, Allelism, and Phenocopies

The same or similar phenotype may result from:

- Different mutant alleles at the same locus (glucose-6-phosphate dehydrogenase (G6PD) deficiency variants);
- Mutant genes at different loci that affect the same product (Hb variants with mutations in different chains);
- Mutant alleles at different loci that affect different products (coagulation factor defects). For example, both a deficiency in factor VIII and one in factor IX produce coagulation defects and hemophilia, but biochemically and genetically they are different.

Different types of mutation within a gene may lead to dysfunction and disease. For example, cystic fibrosis can result from deletions, point mutation, and splicing errors within the *CFTR* gene. Different mutant alleles can lead to the same genetic disorder but may result in differences in severity or prognosis. Biochemical, genetic, molecular, and clinical analyses can all be used to demonstrate heterogeneity. If two persons with albinism (a condition lacking pigment) with the same mutation at the same gene locus have children, all of them also will be albino, but if the mutations are in genes at different loci, then none of their children will be affected (except possibly by a rare mutation).

Some genetic disorders may show the apparent same phenotype but different modes of inheritance. On close examination or detailed molecular analysis, they may actually be a similar group of disorders. Examples are Ehlers-Danlos syndrome (a group of connective tissue disorders) and Charcot-Marie-Tooth disease (a group of peripheral nervous system disorders) that can show autosomal dominant, autosomal recessive, or X-linked inheritance. It is important to determine the correct inheritance pattern within a given family in order to provide accurate genetic counseling.

Different mutant alleles at the same locus can cause different changes to occur in the resultant defective enzyme, causing differences in functioning (e.g., different degrees of stability and activity). This can result in different clinical pictures although the same enzyme is affected, as in the mucopolysaccharide disorders Hurler and Scheie syndromes. In each of these examples, the enzyme α-L-iduronidase is defective, but the clinical course of Scheie syndrome has a later onset and is different from and milder than Hurler (see Chapter 9). Some disorders caused in this way show different forms and degrees of severity at different points in the life cycle. Such disorders may show an acute, severe, progressive infantile form; a subacute juvenile form; and a milder chronic adult form. This may be because a less severe enzyme alteration may allow the person to function adequately for years unless he or she encounters a stressor such as infection, or even aging, or when a substance that has been accumulating finally reaches a toxic level. Notable examples of such disorders include Tay-Sachs disease (see Chapters 9 and 12), Niemann-Pick disease (see Chapter 9), citrullinemia (a urea cycle disorder due to deficiency of argininosuccinate synthase), and Gaucher disease (see Chapter 9).

Sometimes disorders resulting from environmental factors mimic those caused by single gene mutations. These are called *phenocopies*. An example is thalidomide, a teratogenic drug, in which the limb defects resulting closely resemble those of Robert syndrome or pseudothalidomide (SC) syndrome, which are inherited in an autosomal recessive manner.

Penetrance

In the case of a mutant gene, individuals either have it or they do not. *Penetrance* refers to the percentage of persons known to possess a certain mutant gene who actually show the trait. Incomplete or nonpenetrance occurs when a person is known to have a specific gene and shows no phenotypic manifestations of that gene. As an example, if in a specific family a person's parent and offspring both had tuberous sclerosis, the person would be assumed to have the gene even if he or she was clinically unaffected. Incomplete penetrance is a frequent finding in the autosomal dominant disorders. Estimates of penetrance have been calculated for certain autosomal dominant genes so that they can be used in calculating risks for genetic counseling. For example, the penetrance for otosclerosis is 40%; it is nearly 100% for achondroplasia (a type of autosomal dominantly inherited dwarfism; see Chapter 9). One of the effects of incomplete penetrance is that the gene appears to skip a generation. This characteristic can be responsible for errors in genetic counseling if care is not exercised, although the use of molecular diagnostic techniques allows greater precision. The risk for a person to manifest a specific disorder is equal to the risk for inheriting the gene multiplied by the penetrance.

Variable Expressivity or Expression

Variable expressivity occurs when an individual has the gene in question and is clinically affected, but the degree of severity of the manifestations of the mutant gene varies. As a simple example, in the case of polydactyly, the extra digit present may be full size or just a finger tag. Such variation may occur within a single family and may be caused by the influence of other factors on the major defective gene. It is most obvious in autosomal dominant disorders. Careful examination or testing is necessary before deciding that someone is free of the manifestations of a genetic disorder. The extent of severity of a disorder in one family member is not related to its severity in another. This means that the offspring of a parent who is mildly affected, with only minor manifestations of a disorder, could be severely, moderately, or mildly affected. The severity cannot be predicted reliably by the gene's expression in another family member.

New Mutation

If no other cases exist in a family and neither parent can be found to have any subclinical signs of the disorder, it may be caused by a new mutation. Such a case is often called *de novo* or *sporadic*. The affect-

ed person with the new mutation can transmit the disorder to his/her offspring in the same manner as an affected individual with an affected parent. When truly unaffected parents have had a child with a genetic disease caused by a new mutation, the risk of having another child with the same disorder is no greater than for that of the general population (except in rare cases of gonadal mosaicism, explained below). New mutations are most frequently seen immediately in the dominantly inherited syndromes, because only one mutant gene is necessary to produce a phenotypic effect. When a recessive single gene disorder appears in a person and both parents are not heterozygous, this should prompt cytogenetic analysis of the affected individual because a microdeletion of chromosomal material that includes the normal gene may be present that allows expression of a single recessive mutant gene without the countering effect of the normal gene that is missing. The more incapacitating the disorder is, the more likely it is for a large percentage to be due to new mutations because the affected person is less likely to reproduce. Disorders in which a high proportion of cases are caused by new mutations include Apert syndrome (an autosomal dominant disorder with craniostenosis, shallow ocular orbits, and syndactyly) and achondroplasia (a type of disproportionate dwarfism).

Genetic and Environmental Background

Genes function against the background of other genes and the internal and external environment. A mutant gene may interact differently with different genetic constitutions or within different tissue types. This helps to explain the varying degree of clinical severity seen in individuals with the same genetic disorder. The sex constitution of the individual is one part of the genetic background that regulates the internal environment through hormonal and other changes, and it can influence the expression of genes in varying degrees. An example of modifying genes is the milder disease seen in persons homozygous for the sickle cell gene who also have hereditary persistence of fetal hemoglobin. Thus, although mutation in one gene may be the major determinant, mutations at one or more other loci may be necessary for either pathogenesis or influencing severity.

A simple example of environmental influence is seen in classical phenylketonuria (PKU). The individual can have the mutant genes, but if dietary phenylalanine is restricted, the individual may not show any clinical manifestations such as severe mental retardation. He or she still has the gene mutations, but the environment has been manipulated so that substrate is limited and toxic products do not build up. Other environmental influences in various genetic conditions may include maternal nutrition, infection, noise, drugs, radiation, temperature, and amniotic fluid characteristics. Further, the way in which all proteins function together in cells, tissues and organs, and differential gene expression also influences ultimate functioning.

Epistasis

One way in which the genetic background can affect gene action is illustrated by *epistasis*. Epistasis is the masking of the effect of one set of genes by a different set of genes at another locus. As an example, if an individual is homozygous for alleles for albinism, then any alleles at another locus for brown hair would not be expressed and the person would have white hair. Thus, one can say that the albinism genes are epistatic to the genes for hair pigment.

X Chromosome Inactivation (the Lyon Hypothesis or Principle)

Because there are many genes known to be on the X chromosome and because females have two Xs whereas males have only one X, visible differences due to inequality in gene dosage would be expected. Normal females and males have been shown to have equivalent amounts of enzymes coded by X-linked genes, such as G6PD, hypoxanthine-guanine-phosphoribosyl1transferase (HPRT) (deficiency resulting in Lesch-Nyhan syndrome), clotting factor VIII (deficiency resulting in hemophilia A) (see Chapter 9), and others. Mary Lyon, in 1961, hypothesized that in female somatic cells, only one X is active, thus "compensating" for any male and female gene dosage difference. Although there are some deviations from it, the basic tenets of the now well-accepted Lyon hypothesis are as follows:

- In any female somatic cell, only one of the two Xs is active. In persons with several Xs, all but one X are inactivated.
- X chromosome inactivation occurs early in embryonic development, probably at the early blastocyst stage.
- The inactive X (or Xs) can be seen in interphase nuclei as sex chromatin, heterochromatin, or the Barr body.
- In any given cell it is generally random whether the maternal or paternal X chromosome is inactivated.
- Once it occurs, all descendants of the original cell will have the same X chromosome inactivated.
- Inactivation is irreversible (except perhaps in the oocyte).

A common, easily visible example of this principle is seen in calico cats. These females have a gene for black color on one X and one for yellow color on the other. X inactivation results in random patches of black and yellow fur, for a mottled appearance. Male calico cats are of an XXY constitution. The inactivation of one of the X chromosomes in the female essentially leads to a mosaic condition or two-cell populations in females who are heterozygous for X-linked recessive disorders.

Because X inactivation is generally a random occurrence, in the population at large, there is a 50-50 chance as to whether the maternal or paternal X is inactivated. But any given individual may have ratios that deviate. Occasionally the percentage of cells that have the X with the normal gene turned off is very high. This leads to a skewed population in which the preponderance of cells having the X bearing the mutant gene is the active one. This explains why hemophilia can clinically manifest itself in a female known to be a heterozygous carrier, although this can also result from chromosomal microdeletions of the normal gene. It also explains why traditional methods of carrier detection are difficult for X-linked recessive disorders, as the possible range for enzyme activity values can vary greatly, depending on the genetic constitution of the X chromosome inactivated. Some genes appear to escape inactivation, being expressed in both active and inactive X chromosomes. There are genes that control X inactivation. The gene *XIST* (X-inactivation-specific transcript) is one.

Nonrandom or skewed X inactivation can also result from (1) chance, (2) imprinting (discussed later), (3) monozygotic twinning with unequal distribution of the X with the mutant gene, (4) cytogenetic abnormalities, (5) gene expression differences, (6) clonal selection in which there is nonrandom inactivation of the X chromosome with the mutant allele, (7) preferential selection that is either positive or negative for the X chromosome with the abnormal gene, and (8) a specific gene mutation affecting X inactivation. Methylation (discussed in Chapter 2) maintains the X inactivation.

Sex-Limited Traits

Autosomal genes that are normally expressed phenotypically in either males or females but not in both are sex limited. The sex that does not express the gene may still possess and transmit it. Examples of such traits are milk production and menstruation in females and sperm production in males.

Sex-Influenced Traits

Sex-influenced genes act differently in males and females and are often frequent in one sex and rare in the other. Pattern baldness is an autosomal dominant trait in males, requiring only one copy of the gene. In females it appears to be recessive and expressed only when two copies are present, probably due to hormonal influences such as androgen levels. Rare homozygous females can thus manifest the trait. Sometimes it is not expressed until menopause.

Parental-Age Effect

The frequency of some gene mutations in offspring rises with parental age, especially that of the father, whereas some chromosome abnormalities are associated with advanced maternal age. Women over 34 years of age have an increased risk for children with certain chromosomal abnormalities such as trisomy 21. Information related to older fathers is clearest for autosomal dominant mutations because they need only one mutant allele for effects to be manifested, whereas recessive mutations need two and may therefore be unseen for several generations,

whereas dominants can be shown in the next generation. Mutation is an ongoing event in the human gene pool, but many mutations cause little noticeable effect individually, especially in recessive conditions. In the normal course of events, older individuals would have more exposure to mutagenic agents such as environmental radiation and chemical exposure than would younger individuals. In older males, the continuous production of sperm may result in errors in DNA replication or an inability to repair DNA damage.

Disorders that have an advanced paternal age association are shown in Table 4.4. The current population mean paternal age is about 27 years. The risk for sporadic autosomal dominant single gene mutations is four to five times greater for fathers aged 45 years and older than for fathers 20 to 25 years old. Most sperm banks will not accept the sperm of older men for artificial insemination and other assisted reproductive techniques for this reason. The American Society for Reproductive Medicine (2004) gives detailed guidelines for sperm donation, including that "the donor should be of legal age but younger than 40 years of age" (p. S10). The recommended age for oocyte donors by this group is between 21 and 34 years of age. Nurses can encourage male clients to complete their families after age 20 and before 40 years of age and to avoid unnecessary radiation and drug exposure. Males should avoid conception for a few months after exposure to radiation, cytotoxic drugs, or chemical mutagens. Women are at increased risk below age 15 as well as over age 35. In the younger age groups, this may be because of nutritional competition between a fetus and the mother's own growth or for some other reason.

Linkage and Synteny

Genes that are located on different chromosomes are said to assort independently and are unlinked. Genes that are located close together (50 or fewer map units) on the same chromosome are *linked*; those that are on the same chromosome but are more than 50 map units apart are *syntenic*. The closer together that two pairs of genes are, the more likely it is that the two alleles that are together on the same chromosome will remain together when gametes are formed without any exchange or re-

TABLE 4.4   Genetic Disorders Associated With Increased Parental Age

Disorder	Description of Major Features	Inheritance Mechanism
Achondroplasia	Short-limbed type of dwarfism with large head (see Chapter 9)	AD
Acrodysostosis	Intellectual disability, short limbs with deformities, especially in arms and hands; growth deficiency; small head, nose, and maxilla	AD
Apert syndrome	Craniofacial deformities such as craniostenosis; skeletal deformities, especially "sock" feet and syndactyly	AD
Basal cell nevus syndrome	Nevi that become malignant; rib and spine anomalies; variable degree of intellectual disability; eye abnormalities	AD
Crouzon craniofacial dysostosis	Hypoplasia and abnormalities of skull and face; craniosynostosis, premature suture closure; shallow eye orbits	AD
Marfan syndrome	Elongated thin extremities; cardiovascular complications, especially of aorta; ocular anomalies, especially of lens	AD
Oculodentodigital dysplasia	Digital anomalies such as incurved fifth finger (camptodactyly) or syndactyly; tooth enamel hypoplasia, other dental abnormalities; microphthalmos, glaucoma possible	AD
Treacher Collins syndrome (mandibulofacial dysostosis)	Malar and mandibular hypoplasia; conductive deafness; ear malformations; lower eyelid defects; limb abnormalities	AD
Waardenburg syndrome 1	Bilateral perception deafness; pigment disturbances of hair and eyes (e.g., white lock of hair and uniform light-colored irises or heterochromic irises); lateral displacement of inner canthus of eye; may have other anomalies	AD
Progeria	Thin skin; alopecia; growth deficiency; atherosclerosis; appearance of premature aging	AD AR(?)
Duchenne muscular dystrophy	Progressive degenerative muscle disease with weakness (see Chapter 9)	XR
Hemophilia A	Coagulation disorder with deficiency of factor VIII (see Chapter 9)	XR

Note: AD = autosomal dominant; AR = autosomal recessive; XR = X-linked recessive.

combination between them. This information can be used to study families that have a genetic disorder for which there is no means of detection and who also have a detectable trait linked to the mutant gene in question. For example, the ABO blood group locus is linked to that for the nail-patella syndrome (an autosomal dominant disorder including nail and eye abnormalities and absent or hypoplastic patella), the myotonic dystrophy locus is linked to the blood group secretor locus, and hemophilia is linked to the deutan locus for color blindness. For information to be applicable clinically, families must be large enough for accurate study and possess different allele combinations at the linked loci that allow for accurate genetic study and analysis. Linkage analysis today is often accomplished using various computer programs (see Chapter 2). Haplotype refers to several linked genes on a segment of chromosome, and is frequently used in relation to human leukocyte antigen (HLA) (see Chapter 3). The phenomenon of linkage disequilibrium occurs when two or more of alleles occur together in a haplotype significantly more frequently than would be expected by chance alone.

Consanguinity

Concern about consanguinity relates mostly to marriage between blood relatives. Although most individuals would be distantly related to their mate if one went back far enough in time, only relationships closer than first cousins are usually genetically important. Each individual carries from 5 to 10 harmful recessive genes that are not usually apparent. Individually, each of these is extremely rare (except for a few, like cystic fibrosis), so that the likelihood of selecting a mate with the same harmful recessive genes is remote. This chance becomes less remote if the two individuals are related to each other by blood or are from the same ethnic group or population isolate. The consequence of consanguineous mating results from the possible bringing together of two identical recessive alleles that are inherited by descent from a common ancestor, thus bringing out deleterious genes in the homozygous (aa) state. The resulting homozygous phenotypes that are deleterious are more obvious than those that are neutral or favorable. This effect may also operate for single-nucleotide variations in genes. Effects that determine one trait are more evident than those contributing to a complex trait, such as body size or intelligence.

Many cultures and groups have actively encouraged consanguineous marriages. These have included the ancient Egyptians, Incas, royalty, and many modern societies, such as Japan, various Hindu groups in India, Muslim groups especially in the eastern Mediterranean, and groups in which arranged marriages are an accepted custom. The frequency of consanguineous marriages depends on social custom, religious customs and laws, socioeconomic concerns, family ties and traditions, the degree of geographic isolation of a village, and the degree of isolation of a specific group within a community. It is estimated that in parts of Asia and Africa, consanguinous marriages account for about 20–50% of all marriages. Other groups oppose it. In South Korea, it is frowned upon to marry someone with the same family name, and same-clan marriages are barred. Every 10 years or so there is an amnesty period during which such marriages can occur. Among certain followers of the Koran, there are taboos against marriage between a boy and a girl who were breast-fed by the same woman more than a certain number of times during the first two years of life. Thus consanguinity may be perceived differently among different cultures. Consanguinity is further discussed in Chapter 5.

Anticipation

Anticipation is said to occur when the severity of a genetic disease increases with each generation, or the age at which the disorder manifests itself becomes earlier and earlier with each vertical generation. Anticipation is generally seen in autosomal dominant disorders. This phenomenon was observed in Huntington disease, and eventually the reason was found to be unstable triplet repeat expansion of the nucleotides cytosine, adenosine, and guanine (CAG). The expanding repeats accounted for the anticipation phenomenon, which is described in detail later in this chapter.

TYPES OF INHERITANCE AND PATTERNS

Genetic conditions can be inherited in various ways. Typical Mendelian patterns of inheritance of mutations in single genes are autosomal recessive, autosomal dominant, X-linked recessive, X-linked dominant, and Y. In addition to typical Mendelian patterns and multifactorial inheritance, recognition of mitochondrial disorders due to mitochondrial inheritance has been relatively recent. The traditional knowledge regarding transmission of genetic disorders is still basically correct. However, new knowledge of what are called nontraditional inheritance mechanisms have been identified. These include uniparental disomy, genomic imprinting, unstable or expanding triplet repeat mutations, and gonadal mosaicism. Aspects of gene action and expression influence the manifestation of genetic disorders as well. Transmission of chromosomes and pertinent abnormalities such as nondisjunction have been discussed earlier. Each major type of inheritance pattern, its characteristics, and examples are discussed in the following.

Autosomal Recessive (AR)

In AR inheritance, the mutant gene is located on an autosome rather than on a sex chromosome. Therefore, males and females are affected in equal proportions. The affected person usually inherits one copy of the same mutant gene from each heterozygous (Aa), or carrier, parent, and is thus homozygous (aa) at that locus, having two copies of the mutant gene. Parents who have had a child with an AR disease are sometimes referred to as "obligate heterozygotes," meaning that each must have one copy of the mutant gene, even if no test for detection exists. Occasionally a rare recessive disorder is manifested in a person when only one parent is a carrier. This can result in one of two ways:

1. Because of a small deletion of the chromosome segment involving the normal gene, thus allowing expression of the mutant gene on the other chromosome of the pair
2. Because the person inherits two copies of the same chromosome from the parent with the mutant gene (uniparental disomy)

Because normal gene function is dominant to the altered function of the mutant recessive gene, the heterozygote usually shows no obvious phenotypic manifestations but, depending on the disorder, may show biochemical differences that form the basis for heterozygote detection by biochemical testing, although DNA testing is now commonly used where possible. Enzyme defects and deficiencies are frequent.

In clinical practice, most situations involving AR inheritance come to attention in a variety of ways, as shown in Box 4.1. Therefore, such individuals may have different immediate and long-range needs, ranging from genetic testing and carrier detection to genetic counseling to prenatal diagnosis, and the nurse should refer such individuals to a professional providing these services.

If a couple has had a child with an AR disorder, the rest of the family history for the genetic disease may be completely negative, due in part to the trend to smaller family size and in part because two copies of a rare gene are needed in order to be affected. If there are other affected individuals, they are usually members of the same generation. If the parents of the affected child are related to each other by blood (consanguinity), this suggests but does not prove AR inheritance. The more common the disorder is in the general population, the less relevant is the presence of consanguinity.

BOX 4.1

Clinical Practice Situations Involving AR Inheritance

- Recent birth of an affected infant.
- Recent diagnosis usually of an affected child.
- Couples who have been identified as carriers of a specific disorder (e.g., Tay-Sachs disease) and are contemplating marriage or children.
- One member of a couple has a sibling or cousin known to have a genetic disorder and is concerned that he/she may be a carrier.
- Both members of a couple belong to a population group in which a specific genetic disorder is frequent (e.g., thalassemia in Mediterranean people).
- A couple is contemplating pregnancy after an earlier birth of an affected child, who may be either living or deceased.

The mechanics of transmission of autosomal recessively inherited genes are shown in Figure 4.4. The most common situation is when both parents are heterozygotes (carriers). The theoretical risks for their offspring, regardless of sex, are to be:

- Affected with the disorder (aa), 25%;
- Carriers like their parents (Aa), 50%;
- Normal, without inheriting the mutant gene (AA), 25%.

Of the phenotypically normal offspring (AA and Aa), two-thirds will be carriers. These risks hold true for each pregnancy. Because chance has no memory, each pregnancy is, in essence, a throw of the genetic dice; in other words, the outcome of the past pregnancy has no effect on a future one. These theoretical risks hold true with large numbers of families. Within an individual family at risk with two carrier parents, the actual number of affected children can, by chance, range from none who are affected to all who are affected. This does not change their risks for another pregnancy from those described previously. This is a point that clients

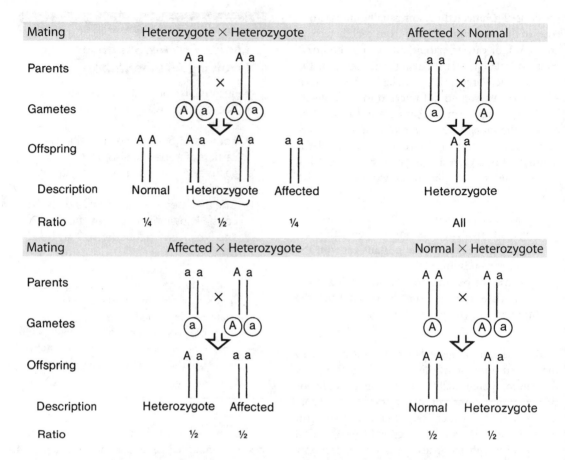

Mating	Heterozygote × Heterozygote				Affected × Normal	

Key: *AA* = normal, *Aa* = heterozygous carrier, *aa* = affected individual.

FIGURE 4.4   Mechanisms of autosomal recessive inheritance with one pair of chromosomes and one pair of genes.

often need clarified and reinforced. Nurses should therefore be able to understand it and explain it. If two carriers have had three unaffected children in three sequential pregnancies, it does not mean that their next child will be affected: each prior event has no bearing on the outcome of the next pregnancy in AR inheritance.

In general, most AR disorders tend to have an earlier, more severe onset than do diseases with other inheritance modes. Many are so severe that they are incompatible with a normal lifespan, and many affected individuals do not reach reproductive age. Due to recent advances in diagnosis and treatment in certain AR diseases, such as sickle cell anemia and cystic fibrosis, individuals who formerly died in childhood now are reaching young adulthood and

having their own children, creating obligatory transmission of the mutant gene to all of their offspring. If the affected person mates with someone who does not carry the same mutant gene, then all of their children, regardless of sex, will be carriers but none will be affected (see Figure. 4.4).

If the affected person mates with someone who is a carrier for the same recessive gene, then there is a 50% risk of having an affected child and a 50% risk of having a child who is a heterozygous carrier, regardless of sex for each pregnancy. This risk is most likely to materialize for a disorder such as cystic fibrosis in which the frequency of carriers in the White population is about 5%, or for sickle cell disease in which the frequency of carriers in the American Black population is 7–9%. If the mother is the one who has the genetic disease in question, there may be effects on the fetus that result from an altered maternal environment, as in PKU. The salient characteristics of autosomal recessive inheritance are summarized in Table 4.5 Examples of different genetic disorders inherited in this manner are given in Table 4.6, and many of these disorders are explained in greater detail in Chapters 8, 9, 10, and 12.

Autosomal Dominant (AD)

As in AR inheritance, the mutant gene is on an autosome, so males and females are equally affected. Only one copy of the dominant gene is necessary for the detrimental effects to be evident; the affected individual is heterozygous, and there is no carrier status. It is believed that in most AD disorders, homozygous individuals who have inherited two genes for an autosomal dominant disorder are so severely affected that they die in utero or in infancy. An example of an exception is familial hypercholesterolemia (see Chapter 10) in which the homozygote survives but shows the very early onset of severe effects. In contrast to AR inheritance, structural protein defects, rather than those involving enzymes are common. Autosomal dominant disorders are usually less life-threatening than AR ones, although they may have more evident physical malformations.

TABLE 4.5   Major Characteristics of Autosomal Recessive Inheritance and Disorders

- Gene is located on autosome.
- Two copies of the mutant gene are needed for phenotypic manifestations.
- Males and females are affected in equal numbers on average.
- No sex difference in clinical manifestations is usual.
- Family history is usually negative, especially for vertical transmission (in more than one generation).
- Other affected individuals in family in same generation (horizontal transmission) may be seen.
- Consanguinity or relatedness is more often present than in other types of inherited conditions.
- Fresh gene mutation is rare.
- Age of disease onset is usually early—newborn, infancy, early childhood.
- Greatest negative effect on reproductive fitness.

A later age of onset of symptoms and signs is frequent and may not become evident until adulthood. In practice, persons usually seek counseling or come to clinical attention for reasons shown in Box 4.2.

The recognition of an autosomal dominant disorder in a child may indicate the presence of that disorder in one of the parents as well. However, there are exceptions. When the parents appear normal, several possibilities exist:

- The gene can be present but nonpenetrant.
- The gene expression may be minimal and may not have been detected by the practitioner.
- The disorder can be caused by a new mutation.
- The child is not the natural offspring of both parents.

Careful examination of both parents is extremely important. In one case of a child brought for counseling with full-blown Waardenburg syndrome (deafness, heterochromic irises, partial albinism, and broad facial appearance), no evidence was at first seen in either parent. This case occurred before subgrouping of this syndrome was known. If the disorder was caused by a new mutation, then the risk for those parents to have this syndrome appear in another child would be negligible. If, however, one of the parents had the syndrome, then the risk for recurrence in another child would be 50%. It turned out that the only manifestation that the mildly affected mother had was a white forelock of hair, which she usually dyed. Thus, simply looking at the couple would not have revealed the situation.

> **BOX 4.2**
>
> ### Usual Clinical Practice Situations Involving Autosomal Dominant Inheritance
>
> - The person or his or her mate is affected with a particular AD disorder.
> - Someone in their family (often a parent, aunt or uncle, or sibling) has an AD disorder.
> - They have had a previous child with an AD disorder.

TABLE 4.6   Selected Genetic Disorders Showing Autosomal Recessive Inheritance

Disorder	Occurrence	Brief Description
Albinism (tyrosinase negative)	1:15,000–1:40,000 1:85–1:650 (Native Americans)	Melanin lacking in skin, hair, and eyes; nystagmus; photophobia; susceptible to neoplasia, strabismus, impaired vision
Argininosuccinic aciduria (ASA)	1:60,000–1:70,000	Urea cycle disorder; hyperammonemia, mild mental retardation; vomiting; seizures; coma; abnormal hair shaft
Cystic fibrosis	1:2,000–1:2,500 (Caucasians) 1:16,000 (American Blacks)	Pancreatic insufficiency and malabsorption; abnormal exocrine glands; chronic pulmonary disease (see Chapter 9)
Ellis–van Creveld syndrome	Rare, except among eastern Pennsylvania Amish	Short-limbed dwarfism; polydactyly; congenital heart disease; nail anomalies.
Glycogen storage disease Ia (von Gierke disease)	1:200,000	Glucose-6-phosphatase deficiency; bruising; hypoglycemia; enlarged liver; hyperlipidemia; hypertension; short stature
Glycogen storage disease II (Pompe disease)	3:100,000–4.5:100,000	Infant, juvenile, and adult form; Acid maltase deficiency. In infant form, cardiac enlargement, cardiomyopathy, hypotonia, respiratory insufficiency, developmental delay, macroglossia, death from cardiorespiratory failure by about 2 years of age.
Hemochromatosis	1:3,000 (Whites)	Iron storage and tissue damage can result in cirrhosis, diabetes, pancreatitis, and other diseases; skin pigmentation seen (see Chapter 12)
Homocystinuria	1:40,000–1:140,000	Mental retardation; skeletal defects; lens displacement; tall; risk for myocardial infarction; caused by cystathionine beta-synthase deficiency
Metachromatic leukodystrophy	1:40,000	Arylsulfatase A deficiency leading to disintegration of myelin and accumulation of lipids in white matter of brain; psychomotor degeneration; hypotonia; adult, juvenile, and infantile forms.
Sickle cell disease	1:400–1:600 (American Blacks)	Hemoglobinopathy with chronic hemolytic anemia; growth retardation; susceptibility to infection, painful crises, leg ulcers, dactylitis (see Chapter 5)
Tay-Sachs disease	1:3,600 (Ashkenazi Jews) 1:360,000 others	Progressive mental and motor retardation with onset at about 6 months; poor muscle tone; deafness; blindness; convulsions; decerebrate rigidity; death usual by 3 to 5 years of age (see Chapters 9 and 12)
Usher syndromes	Rare	A group of syndromes characterized by congenital sensori-neural deafness, visual loss due to retinitis pigmentosa, vestibular ataxia, occasionally mental retardation, speech problems; several subtypes.
Xeroderma pigmentosa (complementation groups A-G)	1:60,000–1:100,000	Defective DNA repair; sun sensitivity, freckling, atrophic skin lesions, skin cancer develops; photophobia and keratitis; death usually by adulthood. Some types have central nervous system involvement.

This is an example of variable expression in which the parent was only mildly affected but the child had severe manifestations. Such cases represent a challenge to the practitioner. In this case, the counselor, knowing the full constellation of the syndrome, specifically asked the mother if anyone in the family had premature white hair. If the mother had not been directly asked, she may not have volunteered this information because

- The relevance of it was not recognized by the client;
- Of guilt feelings when only one parent transmits a disorder;
- Of fear of stigmatization or being blamed for transmission of the disorder or
- Of other reasons.

The mechanisms of transmission of autosomal dominant traits are shown in Figure 4.5. In matings in which one partner is affected and one is normal, the risk for their child to inherit the gene, and therefore the disorder too (except in disorders with less than 100% penetrance), is 50%, regardless of sex. The chance for a normal child is also 50%. This holds true for each pregnancy regardless of the outcomes of prior pregnancies. Unless nonpenetrance has occurred, those truly unaffected individuals run no greater risk than the general population of having an affected child or grandchild of their own. Risk calculations that include the possibility of nonpenetrance can be made by the geneticist. If a woman were an affected heterozygote for a rare AD disorder with 60% penetrance and she was planning a family with a normal man, the risk for each child to both inherit the mutant gene and manifest the disorder is as follows: the risk to inherit the mutant gene from each parent (50% from the mother and the population mutation rate from the father, which in this case is disregarded because of rarity), multiplied by the penetrance (60%) or $(.5 \times .6 = .3)$. Therefore, the risk for the child to inherit the gene is 50% and to both inherit the gene and manifest the disorder is 30%.

If two individuals affected with the same AD disorder have children, as is frequently seen in some conditions such as achondroplasia (a type of dwarfism), then for each pregnancy, the chance is 25% for having a child who is an affected homozygote, 50% for having an affected heterozygote like the parents, and 25% for having a normal child without a mutant gene (see Figure 4.5). The homozygote is usually so severely affected that the condition is lethal in utero.

In many AD disorders, the primary defect is still unknown, so that diagnosis of the individual who is known to be at risk for having the disorder before symptoms become clinically evident or prenatal

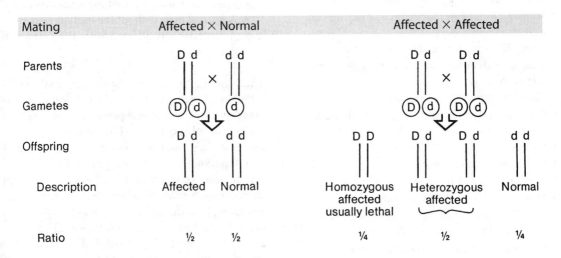

Mating	Affected × Normal		Affected × Affected		
Parents	D d × d d		D d × D d		
Gametes	ⒹⒹ Ⓓ		ⒹⒹ ⒹⒹ		
Offspring	D d	d d	D D	D d D d	d d
Description	Affected	Normal	Homozygous affected usually lethal	Heterozygous affected	Normal
Ratio	½	½	¼	½	¼

Key: *DD* = homozygous affected, *Dd* = heterozygous affected, *dd* = normal.

FIGURE 4.5   Mechanisms of autosomal dominant inheritance with one pair of chromosomes and one pair of genes

diagnosis for their offspring may not be possible, although gene mapping and DNA technology are making this situation less common. In disorders in which the onset is characteristically late and diagnosis is not available, individuals with a family history of such a disorder have difficulty in making reproductive and life plans because they may not know whether they have inherited the mutant gene. Some choose alternate reproductive options such as artificial insemination, in vitro fertilization, embryo transfer and implantation, or adoption rather than run a possible 50-50 risk, but others become aware of the hereditary nature of the disease only after they have had children. Some choose to "take a chance." Nurses should encourage individuals to talk with their partners about the options, and, if possible, both should also talk with a counselor to clarify their feelings and options. Such supportive counseling may need to be ongoing.

A summary of the major characteristics of autosomal dominant inheritance is given in Table 4.7. Examples of disorders inherited in an AD manner are shown in Table 4.8.

TABLE 4.7   Major Characteristics of Autosomal Dominant Inheritance and Disorders

- Gene is on autosome.
- One copy of the mutant gene is needed for effects.
- Males and females are affected in equal numbers on average.
- No sex difference in clinical manifestations.
- Vertical family history through several generations may be seen.
- There is wide variability in expression.
- Penetrance may be incomplete (gene can appear to skip a generation).
- Increased paternal age effect may be seen.
- Fresh gene mutation is frequent.
- Later age of onset is frequent.
- Male-to-male transmission is possible.
- Normal offspring of an affected person will have normal children and grandchildren.
- Least negative effect on reproductive fitness.
- Structural protein defect is often involved.
- In general, disorder tends to be less severe than the recessive disorders.

X-Linked Inheritance

In both dominant and recessive X-linked disorders, the mutant gene is located on the X chromosome. Males have only one X chromosome. There is no counterpart for its genes. In males, therefore, any gene located on the X chromosome is expressed when present in one copy regardless of whether it is dominant or recessive in females. Males cannot be carriers; they will show the effects of the gene in question and are said to be *hemizygous*. A female receives one X chromosome from each of her parents for a normal sex constitution of XX. A male receives his single X chromosome from his mother and his Y chromosome from his father for a normal sex constitution of XY. Whether it is the X chromosome that a woman gets from her father or the X she gets from her mother that is passed to her sons and daughters is random. Figure 4.6 illustrates X and Y chromosome transmission.

X-Linked Recessive (XR)

The most common pattern of X-linked recessive transmission is that in which the female partner is a heterozygous carrier for the mutant gene (see Figure 4.7). If her partner is normal, then for each pregnancy, the couple runs a 25% chance for the offspring to be one of the following:

- A female carrier like the mother
- A normal female without the mutant gene
- A normal male without the mutant gene
- A male who is affected with the disease in question

Thus, the risk for a male offspring to be affected is 50%. As in the other types of single gene inheritance, the outcome of one pregnancy does not influence the others; these odds remain the same. The carrier female usually shows no obvious clinical manifestations of the mutant gene unless X inactivation is skewed (see the earlier discussion). In such an instance, she may be a *manifesting heterozygote.* For example, if the mutant gene was for Duchenne muscular dystrophy, a carrier female might demonstrate muscle weakness, enlarged calves, and moderately elevated serum creatine kinase levels. If the mutant gene were for hemophilia A, she might demonstrate prolonged bleeding times. Females with X chromosome abnormalities, even submicroscopic

TABLE 4.8 Selected Genetic Disorders Showing Autosomal Dominant Inheritance

Disorder	Occurrence	Brief Description
Aniridia	1:100,000–1:200,000	Absence of the iris of the eye to varying degrees; glaucoma may develop; may be associated with other abnormalities in different syndromes.
Achondroplasia	1:10,000–1:12,000	Short-limbed dwarfism; large head; narrowing of spinal canal
Adult polycystic kidney disease	1:250–1:1,250	Enlarged kidneys, hematuria, proteinuria, renal cysts, abdominal mass; eventual renal failure; may be associated (adult) with hypertension, hepatic cysts, diverticula; cerebral hemorrhage may occur; cystic kidneys seen on X-ray films (see also Chapter 10).
Facioscapulohumeral muscular dystrophy 1A	1:100,000–5:100,000	Facial weakness; atrophy in facial, upper limb and shoulder girdle, and pelvic girdle muscles; speech may become indistinct; much variability in progression and age of onset
Familial hypercholesterolemia (type IIa)	1:200–1:500	Low-density lipoprotein (LDL) receptor mutation resulting in elevated LDL, xanthomas, arcus lipoides corneae, and coronary disease (see Chapter 10)
Hereditary spherocytosis	1:4,500–1:5,000	Red cell membrane defect leading to abnormal shape, impaired survival, and hemolytic anemia
Huntington disease	1:18,000–1:25,000 (United States), 1:333,000 (Japan)	Progressive neurologic disease due to trinucleotide repeat expansion of CAG. Involuntary muscle movements with jerkiness, gait changes, lack of coordination, mental deterioration with memory loss, speech problems, personality changes, confusion, and decreased mental capacity. Usually begins in mid-adulthood (see Chapter 10).
Nail-patella syndrome	1:50,000	Nail abnormalities, hypoplasia or absent patella, and iliac horns; elbow dysplasia; renal lesions and disease; iris and other eye abnormalities; glaucoma; gastrointestinal problems
Neurofibromatosis 1	1:3,000–1:3,300	Café-au-lait spots, neurofibromas, and malignant progression are common; complications include hypertension. Variable expression.
Osteogenesis imperfecta type I	1:30,000	Blue sclera; fragile bones with multiple fractures; mitral valve prolapse; short stature in some cases; progressive hearing loss; wormian bones (see Chapter 9)
Polydactyly	1:100–1:300 (Blacks), 1:630–1:3,300 (Caucasians)	Extra (supernumerary) digit on hands or feet
Tuberous sclerosis-1	About 1:10,000	White leaf-shaped macules; seizures; intellectual delay; facial angiofibromas; erythemic nodular rash in butterfly pattern on face; learning and behavior disorders; shagreen patches; may develop retinal pathology and rhabdomyoma of the heart
van der Woude syndrome	1:80,000–1:100,000	Cleft lip and/or palate with lower lip pits, missing premolars
von Willebrand disease	1:1,000–30:1,000	Deficiency or defect in plasma protein called von Willebrand factor, leading to prolonged bleeding time; bleeding from mucous membranes

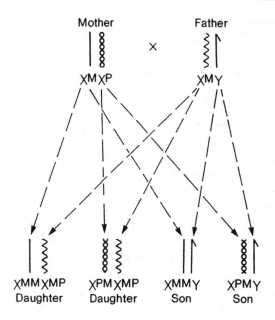

Key

X^M = maternally derived X

X^P = paternally derived X

X^{MM} = X derived from maternal grandmother and mother

X^{PM} = X derived from maternal grandfather and mother

X^{MP} = X derived from paternal grandmother and father

FIGURE 4.6   Transmission of the X and Y chromosomes.

deletions, may also manifest X-linked recessive (XR) disorders if the normal gene on the counterpart chromosome was deleted. Such individuals should have cytogenetic analysis. In practice, individuals at risk for X-linked recessive disorders usually seek genetic counseling for the reasons shown in Box 4.3.

Because better treatment has increased the lifespan for many XR disorders such as hemophilia, affected males are now reproducing. If the female is normal in such a mating, all of their female children will be carriers and all the males will be normal; stated otherwise, the theoretical risk for each pregnancy is that there is a 50% chance that the offspring will be carrier females and a 50% chance that they will be normal males. If the male is affected and the female is a carrier for the same disorder, as may occur in the very common XR disorders such as G6PD deficiency and color blindness, then with each pregnancy, there will be a theoretical risk of 25% for the birth of each of the following offspring:

an affected female, a carrier female, a normal male, or an affected male (see Figure 4.7).

A much rarer mating is that of an affected female and normal male in which with each pregnancy, there is a 50% chance that the child will be a female carrier and a 50% chance that the child will be an affected male.

In the past, little could be accomplished in the way of prenatal detection for X-linked recessive disorders except to determine the sex of the fetus. For the more common types of matings, this often resulted in the loss of normal, as well as affected, male offspring due to termination of those pregnancies in which the fetus was a male. It is now possible to provide more accurate prenatal diagnosis for many of the XR disorders by using molecular technology, so the nurse should be sure to refer such couples to a genetic counselor for the latest information and not rely on older printed material. A summary of the characteristics of XR disorders is given in Table 4.9, and examples of these disorders are in Table 4.10.

X-Linked Dominant (XD)

This type is less frequently seen than the other modes of inheritance discussed. Because the mutant gene is dominant, only one copy is necessary for its effects to be manifested phenotypically. Both males and females can be affected, and both can transmit the gene. Because of the gene's location on the X chromosome, there are several differences between this type of inheritance and AD inheritance:

- An affected male (except in cases of new mutation) has an affected mother because males inherit their X chromosome from their mother, not their father.

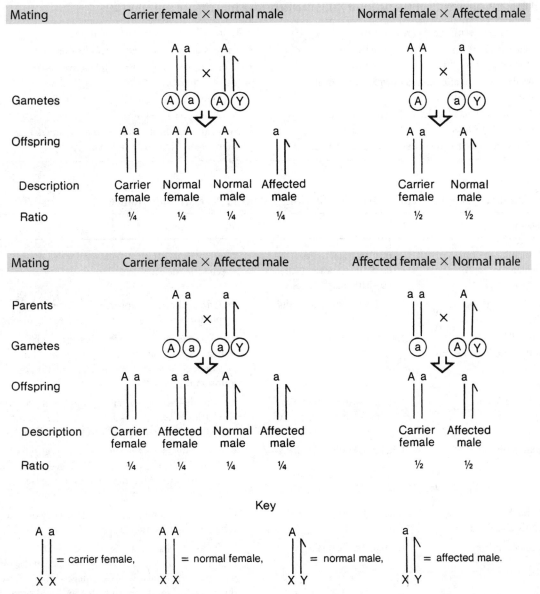

FIGURE 4.7   **Mechanisms of X-linked recessive inheritance with one pair of chromosomes and one pair of genes.**

- Male-to-male transmission is not seen because males transmit their X chromosome only to their daughters, not to their sons. Thus, an affected male would transmit the disorder to all of his daughters and none of his sons.
- There may be an excess of female offspring in the family tree or pedigree, as some X-linked dominant genes are lethal in the male.
- Some affected females may be less severely affected than males because of X inactivation.

Affected females are more likely to transmit the gene to their offspring because the gene is less severe in females due to X inactivation. If her mate is not affected, the theoretical risk for each pregnancy to her offspring is a 25% chance for each of the following:

- An affected female
- An affected male
- A normal female
- A normal male

TABLE 4.9   Major Characteristics of X-Linked Recessive Inheritance and Disorders

- Mutant gene is on the X chromosome.
- One copy of the mutant gene is needed for phenotypic effect in males (hemizygous).
- All daughters of affected males will be carriers if the mother is normal.
- All sons of affected males will be normal if the mother is normal.
- Males are more frequently affected than females.

- There are some fresh gene mutations.
- There is no male-to-male transmission.
- Transmission is often through heterozygous (carrier) females.
- Two copies of the mutant gene are usually needed for phenotypic effect in females.
- Unequal X inactivation can lead to "manifesting heterozygote" in female carriers.

TABLE 4.10   Selected Genetic Disorders Showing X-Linked Recessive Inheritance

Disorder	Occurrence	Brief Description
Color blindness (deutan)	8:100 Caucasian males 4:100–5:100 Caucasian females 2:100–4:100 Black males	Normal visual acuity; defective color vision with green series defect
Duchenne muscular dystrophy	1:3,000–1:5,000 male births	Muscle weakness with progression; eventual respiratory insufficiency and death (see Chapter 9)
Fabry disease (diffuse angiokeratoma)	1:40,000 males	Lipid storage disorder; ceramide trihexosidase deficiency, α-galactosidase deficiency; onset in adolescence to adulthood; angina, pain attacks, autonomic dysfunction, angiokeratoma
G6PD deficiency	1:10 Black American males 1:50 Black American females	Enzyme deficiency with subtypes shows effects in RBC; usually asymptomatic unless under stress or exposed to certain drugs or infection (see Chapter 6)
Hemophilia A	1:2,500–1:4,000 male births	Coagulation disorder due to deficiency of factor VIII. Severity varies with factor VIII levels; in severe cases, spontaneous bleeding in deep tissue (see Chapter 9)
Hemophilia B (Christmas disease)	1:4,000–1:7,000 male births	Coagulation disorder caused by deficiency of factor IX; similar to hemophilia A
Hunter syndrome	1:100,000 male births	Mucopolysaccharide storage disorder with iduronate 2-sulfatase deficiency; intellectual disability usual; hepatomegaly; splenomegaly; coarse facies; dwarfing; stiff joints; hearing loss; mild and severe forms (see Chapter 6)
Lesch-Nyhan syndrome	Rare	Deficiency of purine metabolism enzyme HPRT; hyperuricemia, spasticity, athetosis, self-mutilation, developmental delay (see Chapter 9)
Menkes disease	1:200,000 male births	Copper deficiency caused by defective transport; short stature; seizures; spasticity; hypothermia; kinky, sparse hair (pili torti); intellectual disability
X-linked ichthyosis	1:5,000–1:6,000	Symptoms usual by 3 months; may be born with sheets of scales (collodion babies); dry scaling skin, often appears as if unwashed; developmental delay; bone changes; vascular complications; corneal opacities; steroid sulfatase deficiency

Put a different way, there is a 50% chance that the offspring of each pregnancy will be affected without considering the sex of the offspring.

The gene is often lethal in males because males have no normal gene counterpart. Therefore, the mating of an affected male and normal female is uncommon. For each pregnancy, there is a 50% risk for an affected female and a 50% risk for a normal male. Thus, all female children would be affected, although severity might differ, and all male children would be normal (see Figure 4.8). In such cases, prenatal determination of fetal sex would be all that

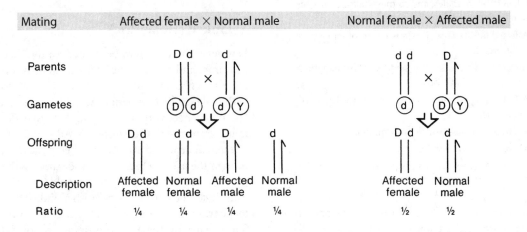

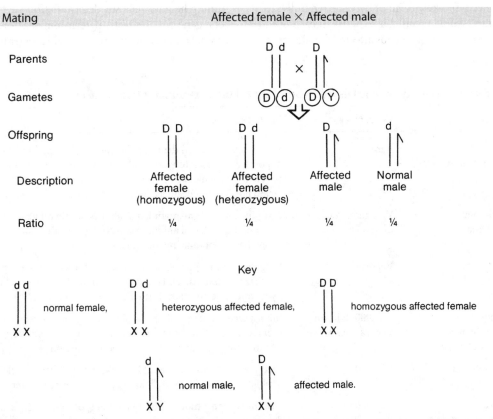

FIGURE 4.8   Mechanisms of X-linked dominant inheritance with one pair of chromosomes and one pair of genes.

TABLE 4.11   Major Characteristics of X-Linked Dominant Inheritance and Disorders

- Mutant gene is located on X chromosome.
- One copy of the mutant gene is needed for phenotype manifestation.
- X inactivation modifies the gene effect in females.
- Often lethal in males, and so may see transmission only in the female line.
- Affected families usually show excess of female offspring (2:1).
- Affected male transmits gene to all of his daughters and to none of his sons.
- Affected males have affected mothers (unless new mutation).
- There is no male-to-male transmission.
- There is no carrier state.
- Disorders are relatively uncommon.

would be necessary in order to allow the parents to make reproductive choices.

The very unlikely event of two affected individuals mating would result in a 25% risk of each of the following: (1) a homozygous affected female (prob-ably lethal in utero), (2) a heterozygous female, (3) an affected male, and (4) a normal male. The fragile X syndrome is considered to be inherited in an XD fashion with incomplete penetrance. The features of X-linked dominant inheritance are summarized in Table 4.11, and a list of some disorders inherited in this way is given in Table 4.12.

Y-Linked (Holandric)

Few genes are known to be located on the Y chromosome, and so this type of inheritance has little clinical significance. Most Y-linked genes have to do with male sex determination. Y-linked genes manifest their effect with one copy and show male-to-male transmission exclusively. All sons of an affected male would eventually develop the trait, although the age at which they do so varies. None of the affected male's daughters would inherit the trait. It can be hard to distinguish Y-linked inheritance from AD disorders that are male sex limited. Some genes on the Y chromosome are for determining height, male sex determination such as the *SRY* gene for the testis-determining factor, tooth enamel and size, hairy ears and a zinc finger protein.

TABLE 4.12   Selected Genetic Disorders Showing X-Linked Dominant Inheritance

Disorder	Occurrence	Brief Description
Albright osteodystrophy	Rare	Short stature; delayed dentition; brachydactyly; hereditary hypocalcemia; pseudohypoparathyroidism; many endocrine problems; muscular atrophy; mineralization of skeleton; round facies; possible intellectual disability; hypertension
Focal dermal hypoplasia	Very rare, exact unknown	Atrophy; linear pigmentation; papillomas of skin on lips, axilla, and umbilicus; digital anomalies; hypoplastic teeth; ocular anomalies (coloboma, microphthalmia)
Incontinentia pigmenti	Very rare	Irregular swirling pigmentation of skin (whorled look), progressing to other skin lesions; dental anomalies; alopecia; intellectual disability common; seizures; uveitis; retinal abnormalities
Ornithine transcarbamylase (OTC) deficiency	1:80,000 in Japan Very rare elsewhere	Inborn error in urea cycle metabolism; failure to thrive; hyperammonemia; vomiting; headache; confusion; rigidity; lethargy; seizures; coma; many males die in neonatal period
Orofaciodigital syndrome type I	1:50,000	Cleft palate, tongue, jaw, and/or lip; facial hypoplasia; intellectual disability; syndactyly; short digits; polycystic kidneys with renal failure
X-linked hypophosphatemia or vitamin D resistant	1:25,000	Disorder of renal tubular phosphate transport; bowed legs; growth deficiency rickets with ultimate short stature; possible hearing loss

MITOCHONDRIAL INHERITANCE

Genes are also present in the mitochondria of cells. Mitochondria (mt) are cell organelles that use oxygen in the process of energy production. MtDNA can replicate in postmitotic cells. Mitochondria are transmitted along maternal lines (matrilinearity). Paternal mitochondria may be transferred to the egg during fertilization but are lost very early in embryogenesis. Therefore, virtually all mitochondria that are passed along to the fetus are maternally derived. An mtDNA mutation can be present in all mtDNA copies (homoplasmy) or in some (heteroplasmy). The percentage of mtDNA mutations necessary to cause dysfunction is believed to vary depending on the type of tissue affected and even among cells in the same tissue. Cells with high energy demands such as nerve and muscle have many more mitochondria present than others. Mutation may be present in mtDNA somewhere in the cell, but disease will not be evident until the mutation is present in a sufficient number of the mitochondria. Mitochondrial genes encode subunits of enzyme complexes of the respiratory chain and oxidative phosphorylation system, while some subunits are encoded by nuclear genes. Thus, mutations in either or both can affect ultimate enzyme function. Most nuclear gene defects resulting in mitochondrial disorders are associated with abnormalities of oxidative phosphorylation (OXPHOS). Diseases due to mtDNA mutations often involve tissues dependent on large amounts of adenosine triphosphate (ATP), such as the skeletal and heart muscles, central nervous system, kidney, liver, pancreas, and retina; sensorineural hearing loss is frequent.

Mitochondrial diseases can result from

- Mutations in the mtDNA,
- Defects in nuclear DNA that affect mitochondrial function such as defects of the Krebs cycle (these are becoming better understood and defined),
- Defects in communication between mtDNA and nuclear DNA,
- Nonhereditary defects of mtDNA such as those resulting from zidovudine (an antiretroviral drug).

During the division of cells containing both mutant and normal mtDNAs, individual cells can ac-

cumulate varying proportions of each. A mother with a homoplasmic mtDNA mutation can transmit only that mutant mtDNA to her offspring, while a mother with varying levels of mutated mtDNA may not always transmit mutated mtDNA, depending on the percentage of mutated mtDNA present. However, above a certain level, it is likely that all children will receive some mutated mtDNA. Susceptibility of specific tissue types to impaired mitochondrial function as a result of an mtDNA mutation, the proportion of mutated mtDNA in a given cell or tissue type, and the severity of the specific mutation determine the phenotype. This may explain why some disorders show a childhood form with early onset, rapid progression, and multiple organ effects, while others lead to an adult form with late onset, slower progression, and effects mainly confined to the nervous and muscular systems.

Accumulating damage to mtDNA in somatic tissues over time appears important in aging and in Parkinson's disease development. External influences are known to have effects, some of which are reversible. For example, zidovudine, which is used in the treatment of human immunodeficiency virus (HIV) infection, can inhibit mtDNA replication and cause mtDNA depletion, resulting in mitochondrial myopathy that is usually reversible when it is discontinued.

Like mutations in nuclear DNA, those in mtDNA may be sporadic or inherited. Because mtDNA mutations are inherited through the female, a mother would potentially transmit the mutation to all of her offspring, while an affected father would not transmit it to any of his offspring. Some disorders due to mitochondrial mutation include Leber hereditary optic neuropathy, Leigh syndrome, mitochondrial myopathy with encephalopathy, lactic acidosis and stroke-like episodes (MELAS syndrome), and myoclonic epilepsy with ragged red fibres (MERRF). Mutations in certain nuclear genes may predispose to mtDNA aberrations and thus result in mitochondrial disorders. Characteristics of mitochondrial inheritance are summarized in Table 4.13. Empiric recurrence risk figures for true mitochondrial diseases are about 3% for siblings and 6% for offspring, but in some families, in which a mother is known to have a point mutation for a mitochondrial disorder or more than one child has been affected, the risk is estimated at 1 in 2. These figures should be interpreted cautiously. As researchers

TABLE 4.13   Major Characteristics of Mitochondrial Inheritance and Disorders

- Mutant gene is located in the mitochondrial DNA.
- Each mitochondrion contains multiple DNA molecules.
- Cells contain multiple mitochondria.
- Normal and mutant mitochondrial DNA for the same trait can be in the same cell (heteroplasmy).
- Inheritance is through the maternal line.
- Males and females are affected in equal numbers on average.
- Variability in clinical expression is common.
- There is no transmission from a father to his children.
- Disorders are relatively uncommon.

learn more about these disorders, more precise information will become available.

The number of known mitochondrial disorders has increased rapidly. Gene mutations in the nucleus can also influence mitochondrial function and expression of mitochondrial mutations. Most nuclear gene defects resulting in mitochondrial disorders are associated with OXPHOS abnormalities. In mitochondrial disease, every body tissue can be affected by mutations in mtDNA, and so diseases may be multisystemic. The major signs and symptoms traditionally involved skeletal muscle, the heart muscle, and the brain and nervous system, but systemic manifestations may be seen, and certain constellations of features may occur. Unexplained hearing loss may be an early feature. Some symptoms that might alert the clinician to consider mitochondrial disorders are ataxia, weakness, seizures, respiratory insufficiency, failure to thrive, ophthalmoplegia, retinopathy, strokelike episodes, short stature, episodic vomiting, and sensorineural hearing loss. Phenotypic manifestation is wide ranging, and some patients exhibit isolated deafness or diabetes. Symptoms may show wide clinical variability among patients and even within a family, and may worsen after exercise. In adults, exercise intolerance and generalized fatigue may be early indications. The athlete Greg Le Mond announced retirement from competitive cycling in December 1994 because of a mitochondrial myopathy. Laboratory results include abnormalities in serum lactate or pyruvate after exercise and ragged red fibers seen on muscle biopsy in certain disorders such as MERFF. Friedreich ataxia, a progressive neurodegenerative disease, is now known to be the result of mutation of a nuclear-encoded mitochondrial protein known as frataxin that functions in some way to affect iron homeostasis in mitochondria and respiratory chain deficiency. The 1555A–>G mitochondrial mutation results in susceptibility to deafness after taking the aminoglycosides. Testing is available for this mutation, which then has a very practical application in that another antibiotic can be used in treatment. Maternal transmission may be ascertained by family history. Selected mitochondrial diseases are shown in Table 4.14.

NONTRADITIONAL INHERITANCE

A number of assumptions underlie the basic tenets of patterns of inheritance. While these are correct in the majority of instances, there are exceptions to those assumptions that have been elucidated relatively recently. These include differential gene expression, uniparental disomy, imprinting, gonadal mosaicism, and unstable mutations involving expanding repeats that often include the phenomenon of anticipation.

Uniparental Disomy

In the normal course of events, a child inherits one of each pair of genes and chromosomes from the mother and one from the father. In uniparental disomy, both chromosomal homologues are inherited from the same parent instead of inheriting one copy of each chromosome pair from the mother and the father (e.g., two paternal chromosome 9 homologues and no maternal chromosome 9 homologues). The child has a normal total number of chromosomes. This is illustrated in Figure 4.9. Uniparental disomy (UPD) may apply to all or part of a chromosome. If all the genes involved are normal, then this may occur without being recognized, although sometimes growth restriction and other effects may result. However, if a mutant allele for an AR disorder was present on one parental chromosome and this is the one inherited, then it now will be present in two copies and be manifested. UPD

TABLE 4.14   Selected Mitochondrial Diseases

Condition	Comment
Kearns-Sayre syndrome	Onset usual in later childhood or adolescence; manifestations include progressive external ophthalmoplegia, pimentary retinopathy, and cardiac conduction defects such as heart block
Leigh syndrome	Typical onset in infancy usually before 6 months; developmental delay, failure to thrive, poor sucking, vomiting, anorexia, irritability, seizures; if presents in childhood, may see ataxia, dysarthria, cognitive decline, respiratory disturbances, and ocular manifestations such as nystagmus or gaze palsy
Leber hereditary optic neuropathy (LHON)	Typical onset in early adulthood; may present with sudden painless central visual loss, headache on onset, cardiac conduction defects, and dystonia; may be incomplete penetrance and male bias in expression; pediatric-onset form.
Mitochondrial myopathy with encephalo-pathy, lactic acidosis, and stroke-like episodes (MELAS)	Usually begins with migraine-like headache, seizures, dementia, nausea and vomiting, and stroke-like episodes leading to neurological deficits, aphasia, hemianopia
Myclonic epilepsy with ragged red fibers (MERFF)	Presents in childhood or young adulthood with myoclonic epilepsy, ataxia, and other signs and symptoms such as dementia, optic atrophy, and deafness

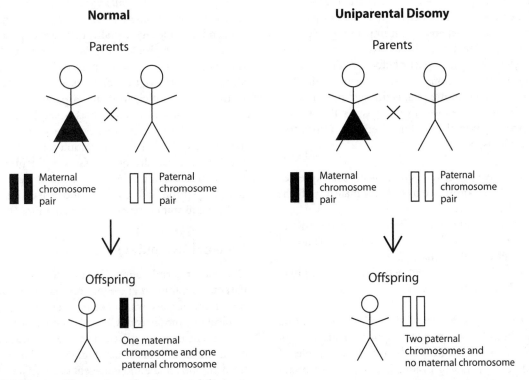

FIGURE 4.9   Illustration of uniparental disomy.

was first recognized in a person who had inherited two maternal copies of chromosome 7 and came to attention with cystic fibrosis, short stature, and growth hormone deficiency. Uniparental maternal disomy for chromosome 7 may be responsible for up to 10% of cases of Silver-Russell syndrome (growth restriction, asymmetric limbs, small triangular facies), as well as some cases of intrauterine growth restriction.

Genomic Imprinting

Another nontraditional inheritance mechanism is genomic imprinting, also called *parental imprinting* and *genetic imprinting*. Normally, one of an identical pair of alleles from one parent is expressed in the same way as the other of the pair from the other parent. In imprinting, the alleles of a given pair of genes are not expressed in an equivalent manner depending on the parent of origin. A gene is said to be maternally imprinted if the allele derived from the mother is the one that is silenced, turned off, repressed, or inactivated, and paternally imprinted if it is the allele contributed by the father that is turned off or inactivated. Thus, certain genes may be expressed from either the maternal or paternal chromosome, depending on imprinting. Methylation (see Chapter 2) is involved in imprinting, which is thought to occur before fertilization and confers transcriptional silencing for that gene. Imprinting is transmitted stably through mitosis in somatic cells and is reversible on passage through the opposite parental germline. Genomic imprinting may be suspected when

- A given genetic disorder is always expressed when transmitted by only the male or only the female parent;
- The sex of persons affected by the disorder in a pedigree will be approximately equal and not show a differentiation;
- A disorder is present in one monozygous twin but not the other.

Clinically, uniparental disomy and imprinting have been predominantly recognized in disorders of growth and behavior. The best-known examples of differential gene expression, due to parent-of-origin effects of uniparental disomy and imprinting, are Prader-Willi and Angelman syndromes. Prader-Willi syndrome (PWS) is a disorder that includes uncontrolled overeating, early obesity, hypotonia, hypopigmentation, small hands and feet, and intellectual disability ranging in degree (see Chapter 9). Angelman syndrome (AS) is marked by severe intellectual disability, inappropriate laughter, decreased pigmentation, speech impairments, ataxia, and jerky arm movements, and seizures. In both disorders, UPD and imprinting errors involving genes on the long arm of chromosome 15 can be a cause. Beckwith-Wiedemann syndrome (an overgrowth disorder with macroglossia, omphalocele, and/or hypoglycemia) is associated with uniparental paternal disomy for the short arm of chromosome 11p, and imprinting abnormalities including insulin-like growth factor 2 (IGF2).

Unstable Repeat Expansions

Present throughout the human genome are short repeated segments usually in tandem that contribute to polymorphism and thus are useful as markers. The most common repeats associated with disease to date are repeated units of three nucleotides that are arrayed contiguously and known as *triplet repeats* or *trinucleotide repeats*. The nucleotides are cytosine (C), guanine (G), thymine (T), and adenine (A). Usually, there are fewer than 20 to 40 of any given repeat. When these nucleotides become unstable and expand or lengthen, usually during meiosis, they may cause disease. Many of these show anticipation and a parent-of-origin effect, and some have a length associated with premutation. Some of the diseases so far known to be associated with this type of mutation at specific sites are fragile X syndrome (CCG; see Chapter 9), Huntington disease (CAG; see Chapter 10), myotonic dystrophy (CTG); Machado-Joseph disease (CAG); and spinocerebellar ataxia type 1 (CAG).

Gonadal (Germline) Mosaicism

Gonadal or germline mosaicism occurs when one parent has a mutant allele that results from mutation in the gonads, which occurs after fertilization, resulting in mosaicism. Clinical manifestations in that parent may not be seen because the mutation occurs in the cells of the developing gonad in either the male and female and is present in few, if any, somatic cells. Thus, some germ cells may be normal, and others may carry the specific mutation. Gonadal mosaicism may occur in both autosomal dominant and X-linked inheritance. One example is the case in which a clinically normal father had two children with osteogenesis imperfecta by two different women. The children both had the same point mutation in type I collagen, and it could be detected in their hair root bulbs, lymphocytes, and sperm. In this case, gonadal mosaicism was detected in the father. It has also occurred in the apparent sporadic occurrence of a male with Duchenne muscular dystrophy in which the apparent noncarrier mother may have had gonadal mosaicism. Gonadal mosaicism is important because if it is present, there is a risk of a second affected child following a first affected child who is thought to have a sporadic or new mutation. Genetic counseling and evaluation for apparent new or sporadic mutations should take the possibility of gonadal mosaicism into account.

MULTIFACTORIAL INHERITANCE

Multifactorial refers to the interaction of several genes (often with additive effects) with environmental factors. Some have used the terms *multifactorial* and *polygenic* synonymously, but the latter does not imply any environmental component. Many morphologic features and developmental processes are believed to be under multifactorial control, with minor differences determining variability in the characteristic they determine. The spectrum ranges from different degrees of normal to abnormal outcomes. The concept of this gene-environment interaction is well illustrated by the interruption of the development of the palate, leading to a cleft.

CASE EXAMPLE

Allen was an eight-month-old boy whose parents brought him to the cleft palate clinic. The referral was based on a finding of an "isolated cleft palate." The family history was negative for clefting in other blood relatives over three generations. During the initial physical assessment at the clinic, the alert health practitioner noted that Allen also had small depressions on his lower lip. Further examination revealed that these were lip pits. Although presumed by the clinical findings, analysis of genomic DNA from a buccal swab was done. Allen was diagnosed with van der Woude syndrome. This is a mutation in a gene, IRF 6 (interferon regulatory factor 6), and is inherited in an autosomal dominant manner. The family was referred for genetic counseling. Allen would have a 50% risk of having a child with van der Woude syndrome, and this might be clinically manifested as a cleft lip, cleft palate, or lip pits in any combination or degree of severity. Because his parents were shown ultimately to be free of this gene mutation, their risk for another child with van der Woude syndrome was that of the general population. A boy with van der Woude syndrome is shown in Figure 4.10.

Some of the more common congenital anomalies that are inherited in a multifactorial manner are listed in Table 9.1. One must, however, be careful to exclude specific identifiable causes before counseling on this basis. One way to accomplish

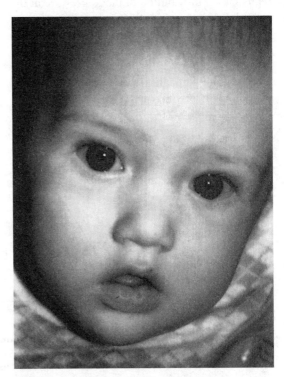

FIGURE 4.10   Child with Van der Woude syndrome. Note the lip pits. Courtesy of Dr. A. Carbonell.

this is to always seek diagnosis in an infant with congenital anomalies, especially if they are multiple. This includes chromosome analysis that should include high-resolution studies, detailed histories, a complete physical examination, and possibly DNA analysis.

An example of a normal trait inherited in a multifactorial manner is stature, in which ultimate height may be constrained within a range by genetic factors, but environmental factors (especially nutrition) play an important role in the final achievement of the genetic potential. This has been demonstrated in studies of immigrant families coming to the United States in which the height of the first generation of offspring is above the mean height of the first generation of the offspring of siblings who remained behind.

Mathematical calculations of additive multiple gene effects show a normal bell curve distribution within the population. To arrive at the concept of the presence or absence of a birth defect, one needs only to postulate a threshold beyond which the abnormal trait is manifested (Figure 4.11). In the case of some types of hypertension, the bell curve may represent the distribution of blood pressure in the general population, with the upper end of the continuous distribution representing hypertension, the exact threshold depending on the definition of "hypertension" used.

When each parent has several unfavorable alleles with minor effects that never encounter an unfa-

vorable environment, they themselves may fall below the threshold. But when one of their children by chance inherits a genetic constitution with a large number of these unfavorable alleles from each parent and also encounters some environmental insult that someone without that particular genetic susceptibility could handle, a malformation results. Because relatives share a certain number of their genes in common, depending on their degree of relationship, they are at greater risk for the same defect than are others in the general population.

A theoretical example to help conceptualize the process is given in Figure 4.12. Consider 5 gene pairs with 10 possible alleles per person that are responsible for the determination of a certain developmental process. In our example, each parent has 4 abnormal alleles out of the 10. Theoretically, the way the example is composed, their offspring could inherit from 0 to 8 of the abnormal alleles. Two offspring are shown in Figure 4.12 (top). People in the general population might have from 0 to 10 abnormal alleles and be distributed in the bell curve as shown in Figure 4.12 (bottom). Perhaps this hypothetical developmental process can function without apparent problems to result in a normal organ or part as long as a certain minimal normal number is retained or, conversely, until 8 unfavorable alleles are present. Then liability is too great, the threshold is passed and a defect is manifested.

An analogy (although not an exact one) often used to explain this type of inheritance to the lay-

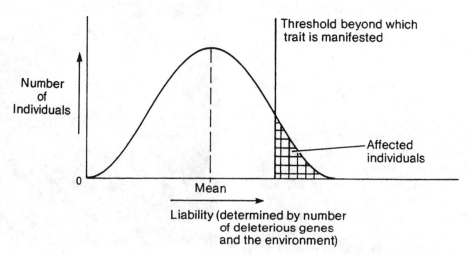

FIGURE 4.11   Distribution of individuals in a population according to liability for a specific multifactorial trait.

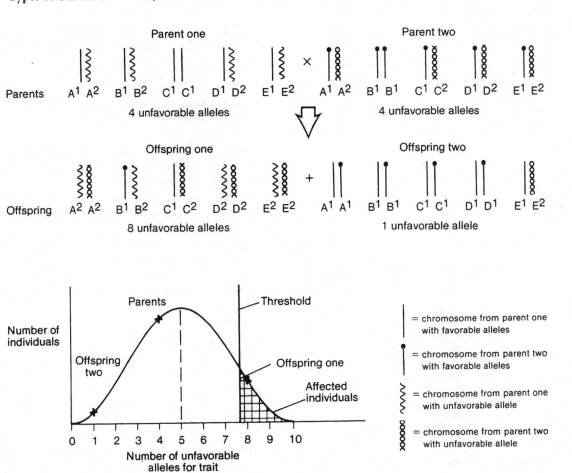

FIGURE 4.12   (*Top*) **Theoretical example of transmission of unfavorable alleles from normal parents demonstrating chance assortment of normal and unfavorable alleles in two possible combinations in offspring. (*Bottom*) Position of parents and offspring from the example above is shown for a specific theoretical multifactorial trait.**

person is to ask the person to imagine two glasses of water, each of which is three-fourths full. These represent the unfavorable genes of the parents, whereas the airspace represents the favorable genes for the trait. They are below the threshold, which is the rim of the glass. When the water is poured into a glass (representing the child) that has an ice cube in it (representing unfavorable environmental factors), the water overflows, thus exceeding the threshold (Figure 4.13). It must be emphasized that this is what occurred with this pregnancy and that the genetic factors may be combined differently next time, and the unfavorable environmental factors may not be present. The actual recurrence risk fig-

ures for their specific trait should be presented along with this.

The characteristics of multifactorial inheritance are summarized in Table 4.15. For the most part, only empiric (observed) recurrence risk figures are available for use in counseling. In contrast to the single gene disorders, in which the recurrence risk for subsequent pregnancies remains the same regardless of the number of affected offspring, in multifactorial inheritance, the risks increases with the number of affected individuals. For example, for some types of congenital heart disease, if one child is affected, the risk to the next is 2–4%, and if two siblings are affected (or one parent and one sibling),

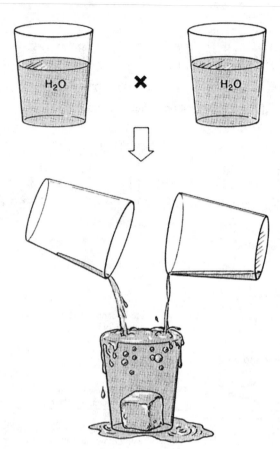

FIGURE 4.13   Water glass analogy for explaining multifactorial inheritance. In the top illustration, the water represents the parents' unfavorable alleles. The rim of the glass is the threshold. In the bottom illustration, the child inherits a large number of unfavorable alleles, plus unfavorable environmental factors (represented by the ice cube), and therefore "overflows" the threshold and manifests the anomaly.

TABLE 4.15   Major Characteristics of Multifactoral Inheritance Assuming a Threshold

- The genetic component is assumed to be polygenic, quantitative, and additive in nature.
- The more severe the defect in the proband (index patient), the greater the recurrence risk in first-degree relatives.
- When the person with a congenital anomaly is of the less commonly affected sex, the greater the recurrence risk is in first-degree relatives.
- The more affected individuals in a family there are, the greater the recurrence risk is for additional members.
- The frequency of the defect in first-degree relatives is approximately equal to the square root of the frequency in the general population.
- There is a sharp drop in the frequency of affected persons between first- and second-degree relatives and a less sharp one between second- and third-degree relatives.
- The consanguinity rate is often higher in affected families than in the general population.
- The risk for recurrence is higher if consanguinity is present.
- The risk for an affected parent to have an affected child is similar to the risk for unaffected parents with one affected child to have another affected child.
- If concordance for the defect in monozygotic twins is more than four times higher than that in dizygotic twins, the defect is likely to be multifactoral.

this rises to 8%. The risk for recurrence after one affected child is higher if the population incidence is higher. For example, neural tube defects are especially prevalent in Northern Ireland. Thus, the risk for a child with a neural tube defect is higher for one affected child born in Northern Ireland than it is for one born in the United States.

For defects in which one sex is affected more frequently than others, the risk to the relatives is greater when the defect occurs in the less frequent-ly affected sex. This is because it is assumed that the threshold is higher for that sex and that it takes a greater number of unfavorable factors to exceed it (see Figure 4.14). The biological basis for the sex difference seen has not yet been identified.

The extent of the severity of the disease also influences the recurrence risk estimates. The more severely the child is affected, the more unfavorable factors are presumed to be operating and the higher will be the risk for recurrence. Another characteristic is that the frequency of the defect in first-degree relatives (parents, siblings, offspring) is approximately equal to the square root of the frequency in the general population. Thus, if the population frequency for a specific defect was 1:10,000, it would be 1:100 among first-degree relatives. In addition, there is a sharp drop in the frequency of

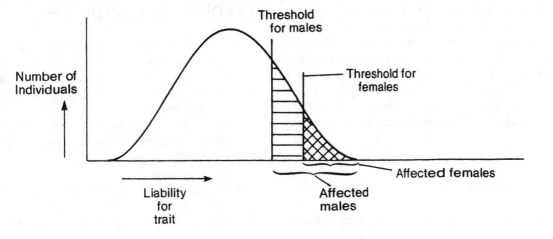

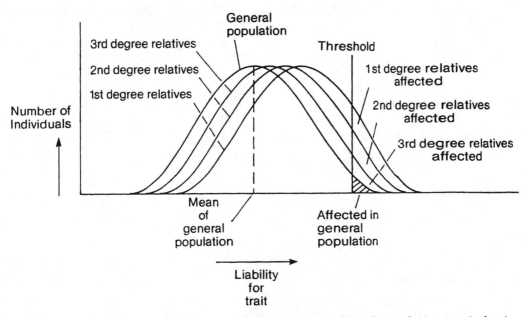

FIGURE 4.14   (*Top*) Distribution of the population for an anomaly such as pyloric stenosis that is more frequent in males than females. Note the difference in the position of the thresholds. The threshold for males is lower than that for females. (*Bottom*) Differences in the distribution of liability for a multifactorial trait is due to the degree of relatedness after birth of an affected infant.

affected persons between first- and second-degree relatives and less between second- and third-degree relatives (Figure 4.14). For example, for cleft lip, the expected risks for first-, second- (aunts, uncles, nephews, nieces), and third-degree (first cousins) relatives are, respectively, 40, 7, and 3 times that of the 1:1,000 incidence in the general population.

Risks for relatives less closely related are essentially the same as for the rest of the population.

The usual risk for recurrence of a multifactorial defect after one affected child is often cited as between 2% and 6%. However, those figures do not take into consideration all of the factors above, and thus, it is not as accurate as it should be. Each family should be individually evaluated and counseled.

END NOTES

Knowledge of mechanisms of gene inheritance continues to expand. Complexities of epigenetic and other mechanisms that influence the regulation of gene expression and the influence of the modifying effects of other genes in the genome as well as environmental factors add to knowledge and understanding.

KEY QUESTIONS FOR DISCUSSION

- Since normal males and females have one and 2 X chromosomes respectively, why don these females have greater quantities of som of the gene products produced by genes on th X chromosome?
- You note that the sister of a boy with Du chenne muscular dystrophy has enlarge calves. What might that suggest? What action would be appropriate?
- A family who has received genetic counselin for an autosomal recessive disorder for the affected child tells the nurse, "We are so re lieved. There is a one in four chance for this t happen again. We can plan for three mor children without worrying!" What would b some things for the nurse to think about? Wha would be appropriate responses from th nurse, and why?

5

Prevention, Genetic Testing, and Treatment of Genetic Disease

In regard to genetic disorders, prevention is the ideal goal. If total prevention is not possible, the effects of morbidity and mortality as well as the burden on the family and community may be reduced. There are various ways of achieving this, but to date prevention is not absolute. Treatment is also a way to prevent some of the morbidity and mortality engendered by genetic disease. This chapter reviews prevention, including genetic counseling. Genetic testing for diagnosis as opposed to screening is discussed (screening is covered in Chapter 12) followed by treatment of genetic disease

PREVENTION

Methods of prevention begin with education of the public and health care professionals and identification of those at risk are listed below:

- Education of the public and professionals at the appropriate educational level and considering and respecting cultural, social, and religious practices
- Family history over three generations and preparation of pedigree as part of risk assessment
- Identification of those at risk because of genetic constitution through history, screening, or targeted testing
- Follow-up with genetic counseling
- Research

- Access to and delivery of health care services, both preventive and therapeutic; includes cancer surveillance and preventive activities in those at risk for familial cancers as discussed in Chapter 10
- Identification and avoidance of environmental hazards
- Preconception counseling, discussed in detail in Chapter 8, including stabilization of any maternal diseases, avoiding agents harmful to the fetus, vaccinations, folic acid supplementation, adequate nutrition, and discussion of potential risks based on ethnic origin.
- Newborn screening
- Carrier screening
- Predictive screening
- Genetic testing
- Prenatal detection and screening
- Prenatal diagnosis
- Identification of alternative reproductive options
- Selective pregnancy termination

Major preventive measures include genetic testing and screening followed by genetic counseling, discussed below. An area of prevention includes surveillance and prophylaxis after diagnosis with, for example, a mutant gene that confers susceptibility to cancer. Examples include *BRCA1* and *BRCA2* mutations that confer a susceptibility to breast cancer (discussed in Chapter 10) and the *APC* gene mutation confering susceptibility to colon cancer.

In the breast cancer examples, if the person possesses the gene mutation that indicates he/she has increased susceptibility, he/she can embark on a program of surveillance and prevention as discussed in Chapter 10.

Genetic Counseling

In response to increased demand for genetic counseling and the realization that little was known about the best ways to offer such services, a committee of the American Society of Human Genetics developed the definition shown in Box 5.1.

Genetic services are often offered by a team of professionals that may include any of the following as core individuals: physician, geneticist, genetic counselor, genetic associate, nurse, nurse practitioner, social worker, psychologist, or pastoral counselor. Any persons with the referral indications given in Chapter 7 are candidates for genetic counseling referral. Those persons most commonly referred for genetic counseling are the following:

- Persons or couples who have had a child with a birth defect or known genetic disorder
- Persons or couples who are known to be heterozygous carriers of a specific genetic disease
- Persons affected by a trait or disorder known or suspected to be inherited
- Persons who have a known or suspected inherited disorder in the family and are contemplating marriage or starting a family
- Persons who are experiencing reproductive problems such as infertility, multiple miscarriages, or stillbirths or are considering artificial reproductive techniques
- Persons who are contemplating marriage to a relative or entering an interracial marriage
- Members of ethnic groups with a high frequency of specific known genetic disorders to detect carrier status
- Those with possible exposure to toxic agents, illnesses, or mutagens during pregnancy
- Women 35 years of age and older who are considering prenatal diagnosis
- Persons seeking risk assessment prior to genetic testing or interpretation of genetic tests for certain complex disorders, such as cancer or heart disease

---

BOX 5.1

Definition of Genetic Counseling

"Genetic counseling is a communication process which deals with the human problems associated with the occurrence, or the risk of occurrence, of a genetic disorder in a family. This process involves an attempt by one or more appropriately trained persons to help the individual or family (1) comprehend the medical facts, including the diagnosis, the probable course of the disorder and the available management; (2) appreciate the way heredity contributes to the disorder, and the risk of recurrence in specified relatives; (3) understand the options for dealing with the risk of recurrence; (4) choose the course of action which seems appropriate to them in view of their risk and their family goals and act in accordance with that decision; and (5) make the best possible adjustment to the disorder in an affected family member and/or to the risk of recurrence of that disorder" (Genetic counseling, pp. 240–241).

The person who is seeking genetic counseling may be called the *counselee* or *consultand*. The term *proband* or *propositus* refers to the index case or to the person who first brought the family to the attention of the geneticist, for example, the affected child. In practice the actual counselee may be more than one person—for example, mother, father, and child. Genetic counseling is also offered in conjunction with testing and screening programs and for those considering adoption or various reproductive technologies. About 90% of those who should be so referred are not. Indications that nurses can use as guides for referral are given in Chapter 7. If a formal referral is initiated, the counselees should bring all relevant records, family data, and even photographs with them or send this material before their first appointment. The genetic counselor should be notified of the referral by phone or letter. The nurse or the referring professional should also check with the counselee to see that follow-through has occurred.

Some clients are very self-directed and motivated to seek counseling. Others may be there because "the doctor told me I should come." Elements of the Health Belief Model are relevant here in that the client must perceive that a serious situation exists, there is some personal vulnerability, and the benefits derived from the indicated action will outweigh the barriers or risks. Other factors such as denial and guilt are also operative.

Because many emotions are involved in a genetic disorder, it is not always helpful to provide genetic counseling immediately after the birth of an affected child or the unexpected diagnosis of a genetic disease in an adult. These events can precipitate a family crisis. Genetic disease is often perceived as permanent and untreatable. Shock followed by denial often is the first part of the coping process. When counselees are seen in this phase, which may be present three to six months after the crisis, they do not know what they want to know, and they may not hear what is said to them. Anxiety and anger follow, and this may be directed outward as hostility or inward as guilt. At this point, the counselee may be ready to intellectually understand and adjust only on an intellectual level. Depression occurs next, and if the counselee can achieve behavioral adjustment, successful accommodation can occur. Obviously, counselees may cycle between phases. Covert anger and avoidance behavior may lead to clients' canceling, not keeping, or arriving late for their appointments. Staff who do not understand the basis for this behavior may demonstrate anger and hostility toward the client, which will act to negate efforts to establish a good client-counselor relationship.

An initial early interview can be used to assess the degree of negative feelings and to use intervention techniques or provide support services for ongoing counseling if it appears indicated. Usually a family history can be obtained and may provide the clients with the feeling that they are taking some positive action. A second appointment is then scheduled.

Components of Genetic Counseling

As the setting, the professionals providing services, and the reasons for seeking counseling vary, so too does the counseling process. Nevertheless, all genetic counseling has some common elements. The usual components of the genetic counseling process are shown in Table 5.1. Their application and sequence also vary because the geneticist does not always know what additional information is needed until after the assessment process, the interview, and the histories are completed (e.g., chromosome analysis may need to be done, past records obtained, an illness in another family member confirmed). Usually there is more than one session anticipated, with information gathered and a relationship established first, and plans made to collect other needed data on which to formulate diagnoses or recurrence risks.

TABLE 5.1   Components of Genetic Counseling

Initial interview

Family history, pedigree preparation and analysis, other histories

Assessment of counselee (e.g., physical examination)

Considering potential diagnoses

Confirmatory or supplementary tests or procedures such as:

Chromosome analysis	Linkage analysis
Biochemical tests	Developmental testing
Molecular DNA testing or analysis	Dermatoglyphics
	Electromyography
X-ray films	Prenatal diagnosis
Biopsy	Immunological tests

Establishment of an accurate diagnosis

Literature search and review

Use of resources and registries on the Web

Consultation with other experts

Compiling of information and determination of recurrence risk

Communication of the results and risks to the counselee and family if appropriate

Discussion of natural history, current treatment options, and anticipatory guidance if relevant

Discussion of options

Review and questions

Assessment of understanding and clarification

Referrals—for example, prenatal diagnosis and specialists

Support of decisions made by counselee

Follow-up

Evaluation

Note: Order may vary depending on the reason for the initial referral: Psychosocial support should be provided throughout the process. All explanations should be culturally appropriate for counselees and appropriate to their educational level.

Obtaining a History and Preparing a Pedigree

Recently there has been increased attention in the health care community regarding the importance of the family history over three generations. Most information regarding the taking of the history is discussed in Chapter 7. There are, however, some points that should be considered here. The taking of the family history also gives the counselor a chance to observe family interactions, and it can provide clues for effective approaches when discussing risks and options. It is very helpful to have both members of a couple present when the history is taken because one person rarely has the precise information necessary about both sides of the family or, if they have attempted to gather it beforehand, they may not have asked the relevant questions indicated by the suspected genetic disorder (e.g., in neurofibromatosis 1 in the family, it may be helpful to know if axillary freckling is present in any relatives who cannot be personally examined). If all agree, it may be helpful to have an older relative present for part of the information gathering because that person may have detailed information about the family. Taking the history is time-consuming because one cannot just ask a general question such as: "Does anyone in your family have a birth defect, intellectual disability, or genetic disease?" The concepts of disease, disability, and retardation may be culturally defined. Many counselees do not know what constitutes a genetic disease, and they may not equate "slowness" with intellectual disability. Thus, questions must be specifically tailored for the individuals, at their level of understanding, and within their sociocultural context. The history taking must result in the preparation of a pedigree, which may be helpful in determining the mode of transmission operating in a given family, even in the absence of a definite diagnosis, that will allow a basis for counseling (see Chapter 7).

Anyone who has done such a history is aware of some of the problems and pitfalls that may be encountered. An issue for one couple who came for counseling was whether the disorder, which had incomplete penetrance, was a sporadic event or was caused by an autosomal dominant gene in that family. I was told that "Aunt Mary had something wrong with her. She was never allowed to marry, and they mostly kept her in her room." This could

or could not be relevant to the situation at hand and needed to be further explored and documented. Sometimes this is difficult because people are reluctant to talk about defects and intellectual disability in their families.

Often additional family information needs to be obtained and sent to the counselor. Some families do not wish to let other members know that they are seeking counseling, and this greatly complicates the obtaining of accurate information. A negative family history can have several meanings. If a couple has come for counseling, it is important to talk to the mother alone at some point in the interview. In such privacy, it is possible to ascertain, for example, situations involving the possibility of nonpaternity of the present mate, of sperm donation, or of adoption that has not yet been revealed to the child who may be accompanying his/her parents. Thus, a negative family history may mean that this mutation is a sporadic or a new one or may be due to other reasons (see Chapter 7 for a complete list), including failure of the interviewer to ask the critical questions or conduct a thorough assessment or the withholding of information by the client.

Another sensitive area is that of consanguinity. By asking the names of all the relatives in the family history, the counselor can inquire further about those with the same last name on both sides of the family. Another way to ascertain this is by determining where both families have lived at various points in time, what their ethnic origin is, and what other countries the family originated from. Occasionally couples who did not realize they were related discover that they indeed have a common ancestor. A counselee whose child had Ellis–van Creveld syndrome (dwarfism with polydactyly and heart disease, which is common in the Pennsylvania Dutch) turned out to be married to a cousin. Both had Pennsylvania Dutch ancestors. The counselor can also lead into the subject by asking if there is any chance at all that the two partners are related. I have had several genetic counseling clients who were contemplating cousin marriages. Myths abound about such matings, particularly those between first cousins. One client reported that he had been told by a health professional that all of their children would be crazy or retarded. In fact, the risks are associated with the chance of bringing together the same recessive gene possessed by each

e of them in their offspring. If no known genetic
ease exists in the family and the persons do not
long to an ethnic group with a genetic disease that
above the usual population frequency, then the
k for homozygosity at a gene locus is 1/16 for first
usins. In the absence of a positive family history
d under good economic conditions, empiric risk
imates for a genetic disease, malformation, or
rly mortality among the offspring of first cousin
arriages are about 3–4% over the general popula-
n risk. For first cousins once removed and sec-
d cousins, the observed risk is about 1–1.5% over
at of the general population. An uncle-niece mat-
g would carry about a 10% risk. Individuals may
related to one another in more than one way.

Confusion about exact familial relationships is
mmon to many people. Accurate risk estimates
nnot be made unless the correct relationship is
own, and so it may be up to the nurse to clarify it.
r example, "first cousins once removed" refers to
e relationship between the grandchild of one sib-
ng and the child of another sibling, whereas "sec-
d cousins" refers to the relationship between the
andchildren of two siblings. These relationships
e illustrated in Figure 5.1.

Incest in the legal sense refers to matings be-
ween related individuals who cannot be legally
arried; in the genetic sense, it refers to matings be-
ween persons more closely related by blood than
uble first cousins (those who have both sets of
andparents in common). All states prohibit parent-
ild, grandparent-grandchild, and brother-sister
arriages, and the vast majority prohibit uncle-
iece and aunt-nephew marriages. The most fre-
ent form of genetic incest is father-daughter,
llowed by brother-sister. The degree of genetic
sk for an infant born of an incestuous mating be-
ween first-degree relatives is an important concern
 adoption agencies and prospective adoptive parts. The risk is approximately one-third for serious
onormality or early death, with an added risk of
tellectual disability. Most abnormalities become
vident within the first year of life, and a reasonable
ggestion is that the finalization of adoption wait
ntil this time.

Deaths of siblings or stillbirths should be pur-
ed. A parent may initially say that a child died of
eart disease and not think it relevant to mention
at the child had Holt-Oram syndrome. It is par-

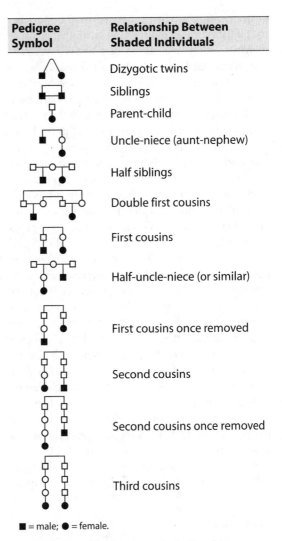

Pedigree Symbol	Relationship Between Shaded Individuals
	Dizygotic twins
	Siblings
	Parent-child
	Uncle-niece (aunt-nephew)
	Half siblings
	Double first cousins
	First cousins
	Half-uncle-niece (or similar)
	First cousins once removed
	Second cousins
	Second cousins once removed
	Third cousins

■ = male; ● = female.

FIGURE 5.1   Illustration of relationship
patterns by pedigree. Adapted from Harper, P.S.,
Practical genetic counseling (4th ed.), Oxford:
Butterworth Heinemann, 1993.

ticularly important, especially in the case of parents
who have had a child with a visible malformation,
that in concluding the history of the pregnancy, the
counselor raise issues that the couple may otherwise
leave unspoken but not necessarily unthought, such
as, "Many times, parents who have had a baby with
anencephaly feel that some event in their pregnancy [like a long car trip taken against advice] caused
or contributed to it." It is important to get them to
verbalize any feelings on this issue so that they can

be dealt with. The clients may feel that they are being punished for an indiscretion or sin that is real or imagined. They may, aloud or silently, ask, "Why me? What did I do to be punished like this?" In many cultures (e.g., Italian and other Mediterranean, some African, Middle Eastern, Caribbean and Latin), there may be the belief that the malformation was the result of a curse or of the "evil eye" (*el mal ojo*). Thus, the counselor must adjust the tone and content of the counseling toward the cultural group of the counselee. It is also important to know how the culture views not only the occurrence of a genetic condition but also beliefs about healing and the body. Who are the authority figures in the culture? How can they be included in facilitating adjustment? What is the decision-making power of the individual and couple, or are there others who will have a major influence? What are the concepts of privacy and stigma or shame in this culture? The occurrence of a genetic disorder can also be used to accentuate family difficulties that may have been latently present before the event, such as, "I told you not to marry her; her family is no good." The history taking can be concluded by asking, "Is there anything else you think I should know about you or your family or that you would like to tell me?" It is not infrequent that even after a long initial counseling session, a counselee has telephoned to supply information that he or she "forgot" to tell me and that turns out to be quite relevant.

Establishing a Diagnosis

The family history is a first step in the establishment of a diagnosis if it has not been made before the client seeks genetic counseling. Diagnoses should be confirmed where possible. When no diagnosis has been established, then one of the roles of the geneticist is to recommend appropriate testing in order that one can be made. This may include chromosome analysis, molecular testing, or biochemical testing that is appropriate to the possible disorder, symptomatology, or ethnic group of the counselee; X-ray films; skin or muscle biopsy; electromyography; or others. Carrier status should be established if it is relevant and possible. If the syndrome is unknown, then referral to specialists may be indicated. For example, photographs, laboratory records, histories, physical examination data, and specimens may all need to be sent to an expert in a rare disor-

der or entered into a computerized system for opinion. Sometimes the establishment of a diagnosis is not possible. The affected person may be deceased, and essential information or autopsy results were not obtained, all testing and examination results are inconclusive, or a syndrome may not have been previously identified. This points up the need for the nurse to be alert for the need to obtain pictures, specialized measurements, and tissue specimens in cases of spontaneous abortions and stillbirths.

The genetic counselor should know his or her own limitations in diagnosis and be able to provide referral to get answers. For example, the client's eye may need examination by an expert in ophthalmology. The affected persons should be carefully examined if feasible. Family members who are at a risk for the disorder should be meticulously examined especially when they are asymptomatic, in order to detect minimal signs of disease. An example is the case of a 30-year-old man who was at risk for facioscapulohumeral muscular dystrophy IA (an autosomal dominant disorder with muscle weakness and retinal anomalies) and showed no obvious symptoms of muscle dysfunction. But when a neurologist examined him, he was found to have "forme fruste" or minimal manifestation of the disorder, a finding that considerably changed the risk for his transmitting the gene.

Sometimes despite the best of efforts and for a variety of reasons, no diagnosis can be established. In one case a woman in her mid-20s was contemplating having children. She had a 22-year-old brother who had a muscle disorder, and she sought counseling to determine the risk of one of her children having the disorder. Her brother's diagnosis had been made years before, when all muscle weaknesses of that variety were lumped into a single category and named accordingly. In more recent years they had been found to be heterogenous and transmitted by different modes of inheritance. Her brother was severely physically incapacitated but unaffected as far as intelligence was concerned; he had graduated from college. The counselor suggested that he be rediagnosed in order to accurately determine her risk, as the family history was unhelpful in this regard. The counselee felt very strongly that she did not want him to know she was concerned about a child of hers having the disorder, but after all the years she had watched him grow and devep, she felt that she could not assume this responsibility in her own child. She therefore refused any communication with him in regard to diagnosis by herself, another family member, a physician, or the counselor. The only options at that time were to review with her the risks for the two types of inheritance then known to be involved and refer her for some psychological counseling in the hope that she might modify her feelings. She subsequently moved out of state, so follow-up was not achieved.

Sometimes when a precise diagnosis cannot be made, the history and pedigree clearly reveals the mode of inheritance operating in that particular family, and counseling can proceed on that basis. Searches of the literature may be valuable in locating case reports with similar features and contacting the author or in locating experts who are using new techniques for rare disorders.

Inaccurate diagnosis can result from failure to recognize mild expression of a disorder. In another situation, young adults who learned that their institutionalized sibling had tuberous sclerosis and that this could be inherited sought counseling. Examination included using a Woods lamp to look at the skin for white, leaf-shaped macules and expert ophthalmological evaluation. Neither sibling had intellectual disability or seizures, which are often part of the disorder. One was ultimately found to have characteristic skin lesions and therefore could be presumed to be affected. Counseling could proceed on the basis of the risk of transmitting this autosomal dominant disorder and the unpredictability of its severity in any children he might have. Sometimes the counselee may deliberately conceal stigmata of a disorder. In Chapter 4, a woman with Waardenburg syndrome I who had only the white forelock of hair was described. When speaking to the counselor privately, she revealed that she dyed her hair to conceal it. However, she did not want the counselor to tell her husband (this was a second marriage) that she in fact had the gene that was present in its full-blown form in her child, because she felt that she could not handle the guilt or blame she believed would be forthcoming.

Another type of diagnostic problem is exemplified by the case of a couple who was referred to a counselor for infertility. A chromosome analysis was done that revealed that the wife had a male karyotype of 46,XY. She had testicular feminization syndrome. It is important to emphasize that she was not a male in nongenetic ways. She was raised as a female, believed she was a female, and looked phenotypically like a female, but she could not conceive. She was married to a normal man. Some counselors believe that the counselor should not give them a specific diagnosis, but just tell them generally that there is a chromosome problem causing the infertility and recommend adoption. Others believe that full disclosure is necessary and can be accomplished if handled in a sensitive way, with provision for backup ongoing psychological counseling. No matter which course of action is chosen, there will certainly be many problems to be faced.

Determining and Communicating Recurrence Risks and Discussing the Disorder

After the initial visit there may be a considerable lapse of time during which all of the information is assembled. If the counselee is not aware that this is a usual occurrence, there may be considerable concern generated, so this information should be included at the conclusion of the initial visit. When the process of information gathering is completed, the geneticist must use all of the information collected to determine the risk of recurrence of a disorder for a child of the counselee, or for the counselees themselves, to be either a carrier or to develop the disorder in question. When planning the process of sharing the acquired information with the counselee, the geneticist takes into account the educational level and the ethnic, socioeconomic, and cultural background of the couple. Many counselees are reluctant to acknowledge that they do not understand the counselor, and so they may come away from the session with misinformation and confusion. Therefore, the counselor must take care to explain things in simple terms and repeat the content in different ways. The use of pictures, videotapes, computer programs, audiotapes, charts, photographs, and diagrams is helpful. In some Native American cultures, storytelling is an appropriate way to communicate the information. Understanding may also be assessed by asking the client to repeat the information in his/her own words as the session proceeds. Clients can also be asked to discuss the meaning of this information to them so that misconceptions can be addressed. Most counselees already have formed an idea about recurrence risks before genetic counseling, which is usually higher than the real risks. Some counselors also form ideas about risks in which they arbitrarily label those above 10% as high and below 10% as low. This pre-interpretation of material in order to present material simply is unacceptable.

Recurrence risks can be presented in different ways. The meaning of probability or odds can sometimes be clarified by the use of special color-coded dice appropriate to the mode of inheritance. Coin flipping is another method used. Risks can be phrased in more than one way, and the manner of their presentation is important. For example, one can say, "For each pregnancy, there is a one in four chance that the infant will have Hurler disease," or, "For each pregnancy, there is a three in four chance that the baby will *not* have Hurler disease." In the Mendelian disorders, it is important to clarify that this risk is true for each pregnancy—that "chance has no memory"—and so although they may have one affected child already, this does not influence the outcome of future pregnancies (aside from the possibility of gonadal mosaicism). In any case, the counselee must process the information relative to the risk of recurrence and make it personally meaningful as each views it in terms of his/her own life experience. The meaning of a high risk of having male children with a genetic disease may be different to a Mexican-American couple, because of a higher cultural value placed on a male infant, than to one of different ethnic origin. For some Bedouin populations, among whom about 60% of marriages are consanguineous, childbearing has a very high value. Women attain a higher status when they become mothers. Therefore, for example, some families prefer to take a 25% risk of a child affected with an autosomal recessive disorder and have the child die soon after birth, than not have children, or practice selective pregnancy termination.

Sometimes the counselee's perception of the risk is quite different from that of the counselor's. Some see a risk of 50% for an affected child as "having a chance to break even" and do not view it as high. Others find a 2% risk unacceptable. Risks are also seen in the light of what they are for. Some can accept a high risk for a child to be born with a cleft lip, whereas for others, even a minimal risk of intellectual disability cannot be borne. Sometimes the counselor can be surprised by the client's response. A couple who both have achondroplasia were told their chances of conceiving a child of normal stature are only one in four. This was good news to them, as they believed they would have difficulty in

adjusting to raising a child of normal stature. In an opposite example, woman who had two children with celiac disease was given a risk of 10% for the next pregnancy to be similarly affected. This estimate was too low for her because she believed that the adjustment of the whole family to a gluten-free diet would be compromised by the birth of a normal child. Sometimes it is difficult for the counselor to remain neutral when parents with a genetic disorder choose to have a child who has a high risk for having the same disorder; however, most believe that genetic counselors need to support their clients in their decisions or refer them to someone who can. Risk figures may also be looked at by the client in terms of what else is going on in their lives. For example, women who are illegal immigrants, in an abusive relationship, struggling with poverty, living in dangerous or unsanitary conditions, and other issues may not regard genetic risks for a pregnancy as a pressing life issue regardless of the extent of that risk.

Along with risk figures, the natural history and impact of the disorder in question should be discussed, as the burden may not be appreciated or else it may be exaggerated. Then options appropriate to the individual counselee's problem can be discussed. These include prenatal diagnosis, a treatment plan, and other reproductive options. Alternatives such as "taking a chance," adoption, sterilization, sperm and egg donation, in vitro fertilization, preimplantation diagnosis, and selective embryo transfer can be presented if they are relevant. Although the couple should make the ultimate decision for options, the counselor may encourage them to think over the possibilities for a period of time if time is not a critical factor in their situation. In some cultures, the counselees may need to consult the entire family or certain respected members such as elders. Then the counselor should support their decision and help to make arrangements to facilitate that decision regardless of the personal opinion of the counselor. If that is not possible, they should be sure that another staff member meets with the clients to do that. If the family has sought genetic services because of the need to ascertain what the problem is in a family member, then decision making centers around the need to plan for the resources necessary for coping. To do this, they must have some ideas of what types of problems and what degree of disability and deterioration may be realistically expected, what treatments and reources are available, what living adjustments need to be made, and what kinds of ultimate outcomes are possible.

What is considered a disability varies from culture to culture. Arrangements may be made with persons who have made various types of decisions in this regard. In the case of deciding on reproductive alternatives, it may be useful to have them meet with parents of a child with the disorder in question, and perhaps with both parents who have chosen pregnancy termination and those who have not. Long-term help with coping may be provided by the same genetic group during the counseling sessions or referrals, and arrangements may be made by the coordinator for comprehensive ongoing care. The counselees may need to have their self-worth affirmed and perhaps mourn the loss of their "normal" child if they have not already done so.

In the case of some disorders, it is desirable to notify extended family members that they are at risk for a detrimental gene, chromosomal aberration, or an adverse outcome because of their possible condition. The counselee's permission for this and for a release of information should be obtained, preferably before any testing or counseling. This issue is discussed further in Chapter 12. The siblings of an affected person may need to be tested or examined, and the extent of this could depend on their age. If a couple is seeking counseling after birth of an affected infant, it may be appropriate to inform the parents that genetic counseling would be important in the future for other family members, such as other children in the family at the appropriate age. In Japanese and some other cultures, privacy may be quite valued.

After risks and options have been discussed, understanding can be assessed. Counselees should be able to tell the counselor in their own words what they understand about the disorder, how it was caused, what the risk is for recurrence, and what kinds of options are available and should be considered. Counselees should always be asked if there is anything else they want to know or if there are any other questions they have. Clients should always be supported in the decisions that they reach.

The traditional approach to genetic counseling was nondirective. The use of a directive approach without modifiers may reflect traditional paternalistic or maternalistic views of counseling. An approach reflecting an omnipotent or a one-sided relationship can be accentuated by the sometimes intimidating physical setting of a hospital or clinic, particularly if the genetic counseling is taking place in the context of a clinical trial. The use of a nondirective approach implies that both decision making and chosen courses of action become primarily the responsibility of the counselees, and not the counselor. This allows the counselee to maintain autonomy and control and to play an active role in decision making. It also provides some feelings of security for the counselor by relieving him/her of any decision-making burden. Another reason for using a value-neutral nondirective approach in genetic counseling is that the counselor often does not know the client well or does not have an ongoing relationship with the client because the counselor is usually not the regular health caregiver. Therefore, the counselor may not be aware of the counselee's resources, coping abilities, family and financial circumstances, or values or belief systems or understand the impact of the genetic problem at hand on this particular counselee. The counselees possess some information that is not necessarily shared with the counselor but contributes to their ultimate decision.

The nondirective approach contrasts with traditional medical practice. Therefore, some counselees expect to be told what to do as one counseling outcome, and they are confused when expected to make their own decisions. Clients may expect that the counselor should give expert advice because of his/her professional skills and knowledge. They may expect that as part of duty fulfillment and "getting their money's worth." Can any counselor be value neutral? For example, does an offer for prenatal diagnosis imply a recommendation to accept that offer or a tacit recommendation to terminate an abnormal pregnancy? Does respect for a client's decisions and autonomy ever conflict with the principle of avoiding harm?

Probably few genetic counselors can always use a completely directive or nondirective approach. For one thing, it can be almost impossible for counselors not to communicate some of their own feelings and opinions by nonverbal cues or voice tones. Probably most genetic counselors today believe that their role lies chiefly in the clarification of issues and options once the material necessary has been presented in a way that clients can understand. When counselees have reached a decision, every effort should be made to facilitate and support that decision.

Follow-Up

After counseling is completed, a postcounseling follow-up letter should be sent to the counselee and the referring professional, reiterating the essential information covered in the counseling session. This gives them something tangible to refer to when needed. A follow-up phone call is used to see if there are any additional questions. A home visit can be arranged through the community health nurse or genetic clinic nurse to assess coping, identify problems, and answer questions.

The Nurse in the Genetic Counseling Process

Nurses may play a variety of roles in genetic counseling that reflect their preparation, area of practice, primary functions, and setting. These roles will involve collaboration with other disciplines. One of the prime ways in which the nurse who is not involved in the offering of direct genetic services can help is by recognizing and referring clients and families in need of such services to the appropriate professionals. If the nurse is not sure about appropriate professionals, he or she should find out from another knowledgeable person. It may be a reasonable standard of practice to know which patients to refer to genetic specialists or counselors. Whether genetic counseling has been offered to hospitalized patients and their families for whom it would be appropriate can be noted on the chart and discharge summary, along with the results. Nurses also need to assess clients' understanding of any treatments to be carried out, such as for prophylactic penicillin in children with sickle cell anemia to prevent infection, and help the clients plan how they will implement the therapy, especially over the long term.

In addition to providing direct counseling or education, nurses may assist clients or families with genetic or potential genetic problems in many other ways:

- Become familiar with terminology and concepts used in genetics.
- Become involved with public education about genetic disorders and their prevention.
- Help increase public awareness of availability of genetic services.
- After providing a referral or information about genetic counseling, follow up on the action that was taken.
- May tell clients what they can expect from the genetic counseling session.

- May accompany clients to the session if, for example, the nurse has a close professional relationship with them, and all parties involved agree.
- Identify the meaning of the genetic problem involved for this client and family.
- Clarify misinterpretations and misunderstandings, including information about presymptomatic or cancer risk assessment.
- Reinforce the information given by the geneticist.
- Help in alleviating any family guilt.
- Encourage the family or client to voice fears about issues such as acceptance, stigmatization, dependency, and uncertainties.
- Assess the coping mechanisms of the client or family and build on strengths.
- Be able to explain meanings of results of commonly used genetic tests in the practice area of the nurse.
- Help in identifying and getting external support from the family's friends, agencies, financial aid sources, equipment resources, and others.
- Help the family identify ways to cope with the reactions of family, relatives, friends, and others.
- Refer the client or family to community resources, schools, parent groups, and other supportive groups.
- Act as a liaison between the client or family and the resources and sources they will need.
- Notify the geneticist immediately if the family shows significant misunderstanding or misinterpretation so he or she can recontact the family.
- Assess the client's and family's ability to carry out the treatment plan or long-range goals.
- Be sensitive to common potential problems such as strains within the mate relationship and problems arising with siblings.
- Help the individual or family to reaffirm self-worth and value.
- Refer the family for further psychotherapeutic counseling if it appears necessary.
- Assist the family in decision making by clarifying and identifying viable options.
- Clarify the options related to reproductive planning, and assist clients in obtaining necessary information.
- Be alert for crises in parenting if it is the child who has a genetic disorder.

- If none exists in the area, found and lead a group of parents facing similar issues.
- Support the client's or family's decisions.
- Maintain contact and followup.
- Apprise the counselor of any special information about the counselee (e.g., cultural beliefs of the community) that may assist him or her.
- Assist in placing the genetic counseling information in the client's cultural context.
- Act as an advocate for the family.

cial, Legal, and Ethical Issues in netic Counseling

me of the issues in this area overlap with those ncerning genetic screening, prenatal diagnosis, d others because counseling is a component of her programs. These include the issues of privacy; nfidentiality; disclosure; sharing results with oth-, including family members, spouse, and outside rsons such as insurance companies or employers; ether the counselor has a major responsibility the counselee, others, or society; access to infor-ation; handling sensitive information such as un-vering misattributed parenthood; and duty to contact. These issues are discussed in Chapters 12 d 13.

ENETIC TESTING

though genetic screening and testing have ele-ents in common, there are also differences. *Ge-tic testing* tends to be diagnostic, while *genetic reening* is the first level of detection. Genetic test-g may be offered or conducted within the context ` general or targeted population screening pro-ams or be offered to specific at-risk individuals d families, but the term *genetic testing* commonly fers to the use of specific tests for individuals who e believed to be at increased risk for a specific ge-tic condition because of their family history or mptom manifestations. The Task Force on Ge-tic Testing has defined a genetic test as "the alysis of human DNA, RNA, chromosomes, pro-ins and certain metabolites in order to detect ritable disease-related genotypes, mutations, phe-types, or karyotypes for clinical purposes" (Holtz-an & Watson, 1997, p. 6). This can be a very clusive definition; others look toward a narrower ne. They subdivide predictive testing performed in

apparently healthy people into presymptomatic tests (for someone who has the mutant gene usual-ly resulting in disease but is asymptomatic) and pre-dispositional tests (for someone who has a gene mutation that may confer susceptibility for a given disease).

Genetic testing includes laboratory assays and other tests performed on blood, urine, fibroblasts, amniotic fluid or cells, chorionic villi, hair bulbs, squamous cells from the buccal mucosa, or other tissue samples. These include deoxyribonucleic acid (DNA) sequencing; gene expression assays; bio-chemical tests for enzymes, hormones, and the like; chromosome analysis and karyotyping; immuno-logical testing; and protein array analysis. Genetic screening involves testing of populations or groups that is independent of a positive family history or symptom manifestations and includes some predictive genetic testing. Screening may include population-based programs that are commonly sponsored by hospitals, health centers, community groups, or governmental agencies such as heterozy-gote (carrier) and newborn screening, those aimed at all pregnant women for detection of fetal anom-alies such as maternal serum screening for alpha-fetoprotein and other markers, or those conducted in the context of a specific industry or workplace for predictive screening. Screening is discussed in Chap-ter 12.

The concept of testing is aimed at individuals or families for specific reasons such as family history that may include carrier, presymptomatic, or predictive testing for traditional genetic disorders or for diseases such as certain breast cancers that may be called *cascade screening* when offered to ex-tended family members. Genetic tests in the context of screening or testing related to disease or suscep-tibility may be done for:

- Confirmatory diagnosis of a present disease state,
- Determining carrier status,
- Detecting disease susceptibility,
- Detecting abnormalities in the fetus,
- Predicting diseases in usually asymptomatic persons that may include late-onset or adult disorders.

Information that should be provided by the health care provider to the client considering genetic test-ing is given in Box 5.2.

BOX 5.2

Information for the Client Considering Genetic Testing

- The reason that testing is appropriate for this person or family.
- What is being tested for.
- What estimation of risk and for surveillance can be done without genetic testing.
- What the procedure being considered entails, including description, cost, length of time, and where it is to be done.
- What can and cannot be tested. If relevant, this should include the information that while some mutations will be looked for and detected, other rare ones might not be, and that negative result refer only to whatever was being tested and not to every genetic disorder. If one is testing for cystic fibrosis, the most common mutations in that population group will be looked for, but not every very rare mutation will be tested for. Usually within the context of an affected family, however, if a specific mutation has already been identified in a blood relative, it will be specificall looked for when another family member is undergoing genetic testing.
- What both positive and negative results mean, including that negative results do not necessarily translate to a zero risk and that a positive test may result in fear and anxiety, whereas negative results can also have emotional and relationship impact.
- The accuracy, validity, and reliability of the test including the likelihood of false-negative or false-positive results and the suitability of this test for the information the client is seeking.
- The possibility that testing will not yield additional risk information.
- The length of time between the procedure and when the results are obtained.
- How the results will be communicated to the client.
- What will be analyzed.
- Whether the actual test result will be revealed. For example, in Huntington disease, in some cases there may be some correlation between the number of CAG repeats and the predicted age of onset but there is a gray area, so some centers do not disclose the actual number although such disclosure is generally recommended.
- What happens to the sample used for testing—who owns it, what uses are possible.
- A discussion of the possible risks of life and health insurance coverage or employment discrimination after testing results are done, although there may be benefits such as if a person is free of a certain mutation, better insurance rates or coverage might result.
- The level of confidentiality of results and what this means (who can know or find out the results).
- Risks of psychological distress and negative impact on not only the individual but also the family, including stigmatization and altered self-image.
- Risk of passing on the mutation in the disorder being tested for to offspring and the meaning of the risks.
- What disclosure the client might consider for other family members and those he or she will tell (i anyone) about the test results; what obligation the health provider might feel to inform other family members.
- Provision for referral for periodic surveillance, further testing, lifestyle changes, or treatment after testing if needed.
- What these mean in the context of both positive and negative tests. As in other genetic testing, a negative test can have several meanings: that the individual is truly free of the disease, that the result is false negative due to laboratory error, or that the person possesses alternate alleles other than what could be or what was tested for.

Detecting and Diagnosing
Chromosome Changes and Disorders

Many advances have been made in the performance of chromosome studies to identify changes. Detecting chromosome changes allows for

- Diagnosis of chromosome disorders,
- Determining the parental origin in some chromosome errors,
- Prenatal diagnosis,
- Relating specific chromosome changes to diagnosis, treatment, and prognosis in certain conditions, such as in a type of leukemia

There are various ways of performing chromosome analysis. The sample for such studies from the person or persons of interest may be white blood cells, epithelial cells from the buccal mucosa, hair bulbs, skin fibroblasts, amniotic cells, or other tissue. Red blood cells are not used because they do not have a nucleus. A variety of staining methods can be used, depending on the information needed from the chromosome analysis. Each chromosome has its own individual unique banding pattern and therefore can be identified with certainty. In the United States, the most frequent routine banding method used is Giemsa (G) banding, which produces light and dark bands on each chromosome in a unique manner. Other more specialized techniques are available for specific purposes.

Another technique is fluorescent in situ hybridization (FISH), a variation of in situ hybridization techniques using fluorescent dyes instead of labeled isotopes. Basically, a standard cytogenetic preparation is treated to remove excess ribonucleic acid (RNA) and protein, a fluorescent-labeled single-stranded DNA probe is hybridized to these denatured chromosomes if there is a complementary sequence, and a signal results at the site of hybridization that can be visualized using fluorescence contrast microscopy. FISH is used to detect aneuploidy (this has made it useful for rapid screening of uncultured amniotic fluid cells in only 24 to 48 hours), the origin of marker chromosomes, detection of microdeletions, small translocations, and other small aberrations, and can be used prenatally to detect fetal cells in maternal serum.

Describing and Interpreting
the Karyotype

Karyotypes are arranged in a standardized way according to international agreement: first, on the basis of chromosome size from the largest to smallest, and second, according to the location of the centromere (the constricted portion of the chromosome). The only exception is that chromosome 22 is longer than chromosome 21, but it was agreed to retain this order and nomenclature because chromosome 21 was already too well associated with Down syndrome to make such a change realistic. Chromosomes are classified according to the position of the centromere as follows: metacentric (the centromere is in the center of the chromosome), submetacentric (the centromere is slightly off center, resulting in one longer and one shorter arm), acrocentric (the centromere is very near one end of the chromosome with one very short and one very long arm), and telocentric (the centromere is at one end but these are not seen in humans). In 1960, cytogeneticists at the first international conference on nomenclature designated the groups and the chromosome pairs belonging to each group (see Figure 5.2) as follows:

Group A	Chromosomes 1 to 3	Large metacentrics
Group B	Chromosomes 4 to 5	Large submetacentrics
Group C	Chromosomes 6 to 12, the X	Medium-sized metacentrics and submetacentrics
Group D	Chromosomes 13 to 15	Medium and large acrocentrics with satellites
Group E	Chromosomes 16 to 18	Relatively short metacentrics or submetacentrics
Group F	Chromosomes 19 to 20	Short metacentrics
Group G	Chromosomes 21 to 22, the Y	Small acrocentrics with satellites except for the Y

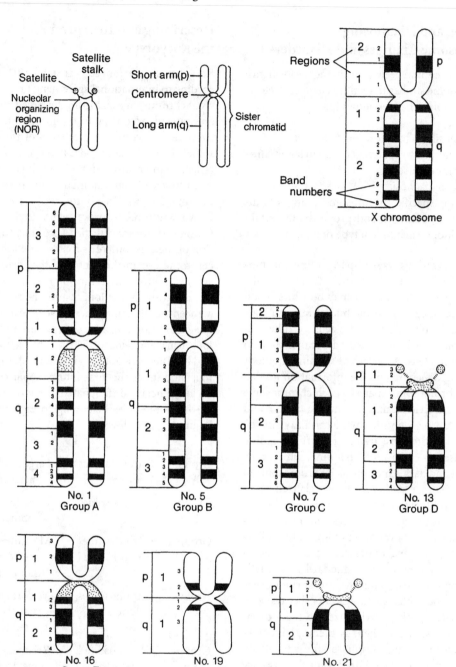

FIGURE 5.2 (*Top*) **Diagrammatic representation of chromosome structure at mitotic metaphase.** (*Bottom*) **Diagrammatic representation of chromosome bands as observed with Q, S, and R stating methods.**

(The bottom figure is redrawn from Paris Conference 1971, Supplement 1975: Standardization in Human Cytogenetics. In D. Bergsma (Ed.): White Plains: The National Foundation—March of Dimes, BD: OAS, XI(9), 1975. Used with permission.

To facilitate communication and prevent confu-sion, a kind of shorthand system for describing the chromosome constitution of a karyotype was devised. Because these symbols are in international usage to describe the chromosome constitution of an individual, nurses should be able to interpret the meaning of at least the most commonly used symbols. These are illustrated in Table 5.2, and their use is explained below. For some conditions, both simple and complex symbolism may be used according to the audience to which the communication is geared or to the necessity of clarifying a precise point. For more detail, the reader is referred to ISCN Shaffer & Tommerup (2005). An international system for human cytogenic nomenclature, which is the accepted standard.

Through laboratory procedures depending on what tissue sample is used, in the most common analysis, chromosomes can be visualized in a spread under the microscope, analyzed, photographed, and arranged in a karyotype. A karyotype is the arrangement of chromosomes by size, from largest to smallest, and morphology, according to the location of the centromere by an international classification system. Each chromosome with its bands can thus be identified. A chromosome spread is shown in Figure 5.3. It is conventional to place the sex chromosomes together at the bottom of the karyotype as shown in the karyotype of a normal male (Figure 5.4).

TABLE 5.2   Symbols and Nomenclature Used to Describe Karyotypes

Symbol	Karyotype	Symbol	Karyotype
A–G	Chromosome group	dup	Duplication
1–22	Autosome numbers	e	Exchange
X,Y	Sex chromosome	f	Fragment
diagonal (/)	Separates cell lines in describing mosaicism	g	Gap
		h	Secondary constriction or negatively staining region
plus sign (+) or minus sign (−)	Placed immediately before the autosome number indicates that the chromosome is extra or missing; placed immediately after the arm, structural, or other designation indicates an increase or decrease in length	i	Isochromosome
		inv	Inversion
		inv ins	Inverted insertion
		inv (p–q+) or inv (p+q–)	Pericentric inversion
(?)	Questionable identification of chromosome or structure	mar	Marker chromosome, unknown origin
		mat	Maternal origin
(*)	Chromosome or structure explained in text or footnote	mn	Modal number
		mos	Mosaic
	Break—no reunion, as in terminal deletion	p	Short arm or chromosome (pter: end of short arm)
:	Break and join	pat	Paternal origin
→	from-to	prx	Proximal
( )	Used to enclose altered chromosomes	q	Long arm of chromosome (qter: end of long arm)
ace	Acentric		
cen	Centromere	r	Ring chromosome
chi	Chimera	s	Satellite
cs	Chromosome	sce	Sister chromatid exchange
del	Deletion	t	Translocation
der	Derivative chromosome	rcp	Reciprocal translocation
dic	Dicentric	rob	Robertsonian translocation
dis	Distal	ter	Terminal or end

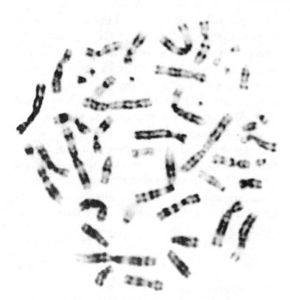

FIGURE 5.3   Giemsa banded chromosome spread.

Rules and Examples for Interpreting and Describing Karyotypes

Both general rules and examples of their use are given below:

1. The total number of chromosomes present is always given first, followed by the designation of the sex chromosome complement. Thus, the normal female is designated at 46,XX and the normal male as 46,XY.

    Example 1:   A triploid cell—69,XXY

    Example 2:   A tetraploid cell—92,XXYY

2. After the sex chromosome designation, it is customary to indicate chromosomes that are missing (–), extra (+), or structurally altered. The short arm of the chromosome is designated as p and the long arm as q. If (+) or (–) is placed before the chromosome number, this indicates extra or missing whole chromosomes (e.g., +21 or –4). A (+) or (–) placed after the arm designation indicates a change in that arm length (e.g., p– is a decrease in the length of the short arm; q+ is an increase in length of the long arm).

    Example 3:   Trisomy 13 (Patau syndrome) in a female—47,XX+13

Example 4:   Cri-du-chat or deletion of part o the short arm of chromosome in a male—46,XY,5p–

Example 5:   A male with an extra chromo some 15, which has an abnormal ly large long arm—47,XY,+15q

Example 6:   A male with 46 chromosomes tha includes a ring chromosome 9— 46,XY,r(9)

Example 7:   A balanced translocation be tween the long arms of chromo somes 13 and 14 in a male may b written as 45,XY,t(13q14q). Thi person has 45 chromosomes in cluding one chromosome 13, on chromosome 14, and one trans location chromosome composec of chromosomes 13 and 14 in stead of the usual two of each.

3. Different cell lines in the same individual ar separated by a slash.

    Example 8:   A male who is mosaic for trisomy 21—46,XY/47,XY,+21 or mos 46,XY/47,XY,+21

    Example 9:   A female mosaic who has three cell lines—45,X/46,XX/47,XXX or mos 45,X/46,XX/47,XXX

4. If one wishes to indicate a specific point on a chromosome, this is done by giving, in the following order; the number of the chromosome the chromosome arm (q or p), the region number, the band number, and, in some cases, if a band is subdivided, a sub-band. If sub-bands are subdivided further, there may be an additional digit but no period (see Figure 5.2). An example of both a short and detailed way to indicate the same terminal deletion of chromosome 3 in a male with 46 chromosomes is as follows:

    Example 10: 46,XY,del(3)(q22) or 46,XY,del (3)(pter→q22:) The single colon indicates a break in the long arm of chromosome 3 with deletion of the rest of the segment, and the retention in the cell of all of the short arm of chromosome 3 and the portion of the long arm be-

Male Karyotype

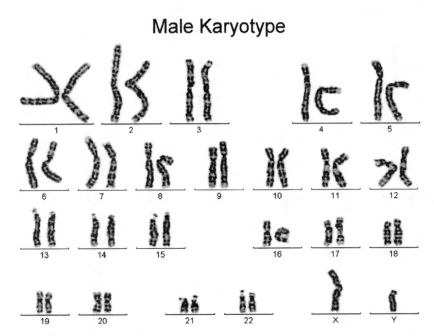

FIGURE 5.4   Normal male karyotype, 46,XY. Courtesy of Dr. Hana Aviv, Robert Wood Johnson University Hospital, New Brunswick, NJ.

tween the centromere and region 2, band 2.

Example 11: For three subbands in the short arm of chromosome 1, one would write 1p31.1, 1p31.2, 1p31.3 (sub-band 1p31.1 is closest or proximal to the centromere and 1p31.3 is distal). An example of further subdivision of sub-band 1p31.2 would be 1p31.21, 1p31.22, and so on.

5. Sometimes shorthand forms are used in nontechnical literature.

Example 12: Cri-du-chat can be referred to as 5p– without any other designation, and a translocation between chromosomes 8 and 22 is written as t(8;22) with no further designation. A semicolon is used to separate the chromosomes involved in the translocation.

New methods of banding have made it possible to detect abnormalities such as microdeletions or small insertions, additions, and those rearrangements that do not alter the size of the chromosome; detect normal variants (polymorphisms) that occur within the population; and identify fragments of chromosomes to determine their origin. High-resolution banding of prophase and prometaphase chromosomes allows a greater number of bands to be identified than the usual number (850 as opposed to 300, 400, or 550). A karyotype with high-resolution banding is shown in Figure 5.5.

Reasons for Chromosome Studies

Chromosome studies may be needed at any age depending on the indication. Reasons to recommend prenatal chromosome diagnosis are discussed in Chapter 8. Current indications for other age groups are summarized in Table 5.3. Some of these reasons are discussed in more detail next. Although the nurse may or may not be responsible for directly ordering chromosome studies, he or she should be able to identify individuals who may benefit from such studies and refer them to the geneticist or recommend such a course of action to the physician.

Some indications are most likely to be noticed at certain ages (e.g., dysmorphic features should be

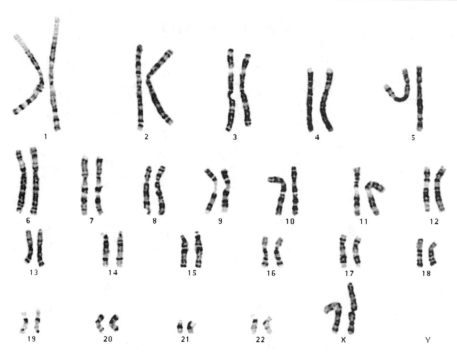

FIGURE 5.5   Karyotype showing high resolution chromosome banding. Courtesy of Dr. Douglas Chapman, Cytogenetics Laboratory, University of Washington Medical Center, Seattle, Washington.

noticed and accounted for before adulthood), but they should not be ignored if present later in life, as sometimes individuals slip through the cracks. General reasons for undertaking chromosome study common to all indications listed below are for genetic counseling of the individual and/or family members, reproductive planning, prenatal diagnosis, initiation of early treatment if needed, and realistic life planning including anticipatory guidance, and goal setting for the affected individual and family. In addition, specific reasons are added where salient.

Suspicion of a Known Syndrome or Presence of a Known Chromosome Variant in Family Member, Parent, or Sibling)

No one anomaly is exclusive to any one chromosome syndrome, and many abnormalities such as growth retardation and intellectual disability are common to most of the chromosomal syndromes. Therefore, even a suspected classic chromosome disorder such as Down syndrome must always be confirmed by chromosome diagnosis. The same disorder can arise from different chromosomal mechanisms, (an example is translocation Down syndrome as opposed to trisomy 21) or from non-

genetic mechanisms. It is important to distinguish among these in order to provide accurate genetic counseling and opportunity for prenatal diagnosis. For these same reasons, parents who have had a previous child or family member with an error or persons who have a family member with a chromosome error should have chromosome analysis for the reasons just given.

Unexpected Appearance of an Autosomal Recessive Disorder or an X-linked Recessive Disorder in a Female

The unexpected appearance of an autosomal recessive disorder in cases in which both parents are not carriers suggests the possibility of a chromosomal explanation. Sometimes these disorders appear because the affected individual has one mutant gene for the recessive disorder and a microdeletion involving the normal copy of that gene on another chromosome. Thus, one copy of the mutant gene is expressed and seen in the phenotype. The same can happen in an X-linked recessive disorder in which there is a small deletion of the chromosome section with the normal gene, allowing the carrier female to express the disorder because the mutant gene has

TABLE 5.3   Current Indications for Chromosome Analysis in Different Phases of the Lifespan

Indication	Antenatal	Newborn/ Infant	Child	Adolescent	Adult
Two or more dysmorphic features or anomalies		X	X	†	†
Intellectual disability		X	X	†	†
Infertility or premature menopause					X
History of two or more spontaneous abortions or stillbirths					X
Neonatal death		X			
Stillbirth or spontaneous abortion	X				
Confirmation of a suspected syndrome	X	X	X	X	X
Ambiguous genitalia		X	X	X	†
Inguinal masses/hernia in female		X	X		
Failure to thrive		X			
Short stature (especially female)			X	X	†
Low birth weight (small-for-date)		X			
Developmental delay		X	X		
Amenorrhea (female)				X	
Failure to develop secondary sex characteristics				X	†
Structural chromosome error in family member			X	X	X
Small genitalia (males)				X	†
Cancer (varies with type)		X	X	X	X
Hydatidiform mole	X	X			
Gynecomastia (male)				X	
Cryptorchidism (male)			X	†	
Lymphedema (female)		X			
Unexplained appearance of an autosomal or X-linked recessive disorder (female)		X	X	X	X

Note: Prenatal indications are discussed in Chapter 8.
X = primary indication; † = If not previously investigated and explained.

in effect, no opposition. Another explanation may be uniparental disomy. In this case, both chromosomal homologues are inherited from the same parent instead of inheriting one copy of each chromosome pair from the mother and the father (e.g., two maternal chromosome 7 homologues, and no paternal chromosome 7). This is further explained in Chapter 4.

Ambiguous Genitalia

Most ambiguous genitalia are detected at birth or in early infancy. Traditionally it has been considered a medical emergency because the sex in which to raise the child is seen as needing to be determined as quickly and early as possible and because of psychological reasons for the parents and family. The establishment of chro*mosomal sex constitution is one component of this process that also may involve reconstructive surgery, psychological counseling, and ongoing support by the nurse.

Two or More Dysmorphic Features or Anomalies

Because it is unusual for two defects to occur in the same person, small abnormalities may go undiagnosed if chromosome analysis is not undertaken. This analysis is needed to differentiate a defect related to a chromosome abnormality from one caused by intrauterine infection, teratogen exposure, a single gene disorder, or another cause for counseling and prognostic purposes. One cannot conclude that such anomalies are isolated defects unless a chromosome error is excluded as one possibility.

Spontaneous Abortion, Stillbirth, or Neonatal Death

In cases of spontaneous abortion, stillbirth, or neonatal death, material should be obtained for chromosome study as quickly as possible. This should be done whether or not external malformations are visible. The rate of failure for tissue culture is higher than usual in these situations, so several samples from different tissues should be obtained since there will not be an opportunity for a second specimen. A specific protocol should be developed for the medical unit, inpatient or outpatient, with all equipment available. Photographs of the head, face, body, and especially of any unusual features should also be obtained; physical measurements, a detailed written description of the physical findings, and a complete pathologist's report are essential. Often radiology also needs to be done, and if there is doubt, then it should be carried out. An inadequate study at this time leads to the inability of the genetic counselor to discuss the couple's chance for a future affected child or another stillbirth or spontaneous abortion.

Infertility or Premature Menopause

Although chromosome disorders do not account for the majority of infertile couples, it has been determined that 10–15% have a chromosome anomaly present in one member, ranging from an undiscovered sex chromosome disorder to chromosome rearrangements such as balanced translocations.

History of Two or More Spontaneous Abortions, Stillbirths, or Neonatal Deaths

The incidence of chromosome abnormalities in these was discussed earlier. About 10% of couples with recurrent abortion have a chromosome anomaly in one member. Among couples who have recurrent abortions plus a previous stillborn infant, the incidence of chromosome abnormalities has been estimated at 15–25%. The risk of another spontaneous abortion is about 25% after one, and greater if the couple has no live-born offspring. The risk is also greater if the embryo had a normal chromosome complement. About 2–3% of normal couples have two spontaneous abortions by chance alone.

Hernia or Inguinal Mass in the Female

It is possible that this may represent a Y-bearing gonad or testis as in testicular feminization syndrome. The phenotype is female, but the chromosome constitution is male. Some believe the mass should be removed to prevent the common sequelae of neoplastic development, whereas others prefer to leave it in place until after puberty.

Hydatidiform Mole

Pregancies resulting in hydatidiform moles (no fetus, placental tissue present) may be of normal or abnormal chromosome constitutions such as triploidy. Those with diploid chromosome constitutions have a risk for malignant transformation into choriocarcinomas. There is a recurrence risk of about 1% following a molar pregnancy.

Failure to Develop Secondary Sexual Characteristics, Amenorrhea (Females), Proportional Short Stature (Females), Gynecomastia (Males), Lymphedema or Webbed Neck (Female Infant), Cryptorchidism (Males), and Small Genitalia (Males)

These findings are very common in a variety of chromosome abnormalities, particularly of the sex chromosomes and therefore should be explored as soon as possible for optimal management (e.g., maximum height attainment in Turner syndrome) and in order to provide genetic counseling, treatment, and life planning.

Cancer

More than 90% of persons with chronic myeloid leukemia have a characteristic translocation [t{9;22}] in their bone marrow. Other cancers also show distinct cytogenetic abnormalities. Such studies are useful for diagnosis, treatment choice, and prognosis.

Intellectual Disability, Failure to Thrive, Developmental Delay, and Low Birth Weight

These are found with such great frequency in so many of the chromosome disorders that they are an indication for chromosome analysis. An individual feature such as developmental delay is not itself diagnostic, but the reason needs to be determined.

Presymptomatic and Predictive Testing

In presymptomatic or predictive testing, the person is tested for the mutant gene for the disease itself—for example, in the case of Huntington disease

HD) or familial monogenic Alzheimer disease—or or susceptibility to disease—such as in the case of *BRCA1* mutations and susceptibility to ovarian and breast cancer (discussed in Chapter 10). Various other disorders in this category could be screened or tested for, including hemochromatosis, familial hypercholesterolemia (both homozygous and heterozygous), neuroblastoma, and autosomal dominant polycystic kidney disease. Because of the availability of testing asymptomatic persons for mutations that can detect if they have certain gene mutations that might predispose them to the development of cancers, genetic testing is becoming more commonplace after risk assessment. This aspect is covered in detail in Chapter 10 under the discussion of cancer.

HD is an autosomal dominant incurable degenerative disorder most frequently manifesting itself in middle to late adulthood. It is caused by expansion of CAG repeats in the HD gene. Its symptoms are discussed in Chapter 10. Direct presymptomatic diagnosis is possible through ascertaining the number of the CAG repeat length. Since HD is not currently treatable, the benefits of testing relate to life and reproductive planning and psychological parameters.

CASE EXAMPLE

Huntington disease, an autosomal dominant disorder, usually becomes clinically evident in adulthood; it is progressive and eventually fatal. A woman, Brandi, age twenty-two, comes to the clinic because she believes that her paternal grandmother died of Huntington disease. She provided care for this grandmother until she was no longer able to do so and the grandmother was transferred to a skilled nursing facility. Brandi is about to be married, and before she does so, she is considering whether she would want natural children if she carries the mutant gene for Huntington disease. Her father, who is forty years old, does not want to know whether he has the mutant gene. One consideration would be to have verification of the diagnosis in her grandmother if possible. What other issues are there to consider in this case example?

A variety of studies have looked at why people decided to have testing or not. Some of the most frequent reasons for taking testing are "wanting to know" and for planning, putting affairs in order, and decision making. Reasons for not choosing to be tested were because of the potential psychological burden of a positive test and fear of not being able to cope, because the risk to their children would increase, lack of treatment, potential loss of or increased cost for health and life insurance, no plan to have more children, cost of testing, not being able to "undo" the knowledge, and others. Some of those who were not found to have the gene experienced survival guilt and emotional numbness and had difficulty coping with the impact on the family. Many had lived for years struggling with the fear of developing HD and the adjustment to the fact that these emotional struggles were unnecessary was difficult. Others believed they were ostracized by family members who had the HD gene. Partners of those who did not have HD were uniformly relieved. Some who have found that they have the HD gene have experienced hopelessness, depression, and suicide ideation. Others have not reported long-term significant problems. Reported adverse effects have been fewer than anticipated. Many feel that HD testing should be available only to those who have reached the age of majority in whatever country they reside; others do not.

Another issue has to do with whether to reveal the actual CAG length. This result is being increasingly requested because the longer repeat length in the abnormal area may be related to the age of onset prediction. To not reveal it is paternalistic and may not be consistent with the right to know. Discrimination has occurred in those who have been shown to have the HD gene. In one case, it was reported that a person was denied entrance to medical school on the basis that the educational efforts would be "wasted." This points to the importance of guaranteeing confidential results and of legislating nondiscrimination for genetic susceptibility or actual disease. Anonymous testing has been suggested for HD and other conditions similar to that done in human immunodeficiency virus (HIV) testing and has been done in a limited way. Preserving anonymity, however, may limit support and counseling. When a pregnant woman requests prenatal diagnosis for her fetus for Huntington disease if the father is at risk, providing this information to her, depending on the outcome and her actions, may reveal the gene status of her partner, resulting in violation of his right not to know.

Genetic Testing and Screening of Children and Adolescents

Should children or adolescents be tested for susceptibility to genetic disease, presence of the genes for late-onset diseases, or carrier status? The issue of genetic testing and screening of children and adolescents has been an area of great controversy. Some centers and groups have condemned such testing and refused to provide such services to children or adolescents even with parental consent, while others are more liberal. Newborn screening already tests infants for some disorders that do not have a direct therapeutic benefit. To be considered are personal issues such as medical, psychosocial, reproductive issues, and issues with a broader impact such as those affecting insurance, career, and future employment.

Reasons for considering testing in children commonly evolve from the diagnosis of a genetic disorder within a family, particularly one that has onset in late childhood, adolescence, or adulthood rather than the necessity for diagnosis of a genetic disorder because of the presentation of symptoms or because of an immediate health implication. Some reasons for such testing include:

- The institution of preventive measures or therapy that can treat or ameliorate the severity or influence the natural history of the disease in question. A direct, timely medical benefit or evidenced-based risk-reduction program are the most compelling reasons for testing.
- Sparing the child the unpleasantness and trauma of continued testing for disorders such as familial cancer when the child may not possess the gene in question.
- Knowledge for the parent in terms of their own financial and reproductive planning given the future outlook for their existing children.
- The elimination of the uncertainty of knowing whether they possess a gene for a serious disorder such as Huntington disease or adult polycystic kidney disease.
- The psychological benefit of a negative test— the chance for parents to adjust to a diagnosis and plan ways to disclose and cope with the news at the appropriate time for their child

- The opportunity for life planning based on this information, including choices related to education, career, lifestyle, and reproductive decisions. For example, a child at risk for retinitis pigmentosa could choose a career that does not require visual acuity or a child with familial hypertophic cardiomyopathy could receive early drug therapy for arrhythmia prevention.

Some reasons given for not performing such testing include:

- The child may not be able to understand the ramifications of testing such as future insurability risks and possible effects on education and employability.
- The child may not be able to give informed consent or even assent, thus taking away the child's right to decide.
- The potential psychological consequences of learning that one has a genetic disorder or is a carrier, such as lowered self-esteem, changes in family dynamics and in parent-child bonding, and loss of confidentiality of the child's condition since the parents will know the status.
- Stigmatization and labeling.
- The potential negative psychological consequences of learning that one does not have a disorder and developing "survivor guilt" or feeling alienated from an affected sibling or family member.

Several legal principles are important to the issue, including the scope and limits of parental authority, the "mature minor rule," emancipated minor status, and recognition of the age of 7 years to assent to participate in human subject research. Competence to make decisions includes the ability to understand and communicate, to reason and deliberate, and to develop and sustain moral values, and the child's developmental level. The Working Party of the Clinical Genetics Society (1994) believes that predictive genetic testing in children is appropriate when onset occurs in childhood or if there are medical interventions such as diet, medication, or surveillance for complications that can be offered; it does not believe such testing should be undertaken in a healthy child for an dult-onset disorder if there are no useful medical nterventions that can be offered. In regard to genetic testing for cancer susceptibility (see Chapter l0), the American Society of Clinical Oncology 2003) recommended that when cancer develops luring childhood and there are evidence-based isk-reduction strategies, the scope of parental authority includes deciding for the child participation or nonparticipation in such testing, and that if there s not an increased risk of childhood cancer that esting be delayed until the person is of an age to nake an informed decision. It is also important to note that children may have limited options to refuse if they wish to do so.

Decisions of both children and adolescents and their parents are also influenced by personal experiences with the illness being tested for. The provider needs to be able to discuss issues with families and help them to consider the risks and benefits in a nonadversarial, reasoned manner. As part of this, the capacity of the child to understand and make decisions should be considered, and not based solely on age. While parents are generally considered to act in the best interests of their children, many believe that the provider should be the advocate for the child's best interest and that if the provider believes that it is not in the best interest of the child, the provider is not obligated to perform testing. Others believe that the decision rests with the family. The joint statement by the American Society of Human Genetics Board and the American College of Medical Genetics Board of Directors (1995) states that "a request by a competent adolescent for the results of a genetic test should be given priority over parents' requests to conceal information" (p. 1234). The Task Force on Genetic Testing stated that "Genetic testing of children for adult onset diseases should not be undertaken unless direct medical benefit will accrue to the child and this benefit would be lost by waiting until the child has reached adulthood" (Holtzman & Watson, 1997, p. 13). In general, there is support for testing children in childhood when they are symptomatic, when a genetic disorder generally appears in childhood, and presymptomatically when there is a benefit to preventive treatment. Testing children for the carrier status is even more complex. Commercial testing companies often do not ascertain the age of a person submitting a sample for testing through the mail.

Ethical, Social, and Legal Issues

A variety of ethical issues including risks and benefits arise when considering genetic testing. Risks and benefits are presented in Table 12.6. Issues relating to testing in pregnancy are discussed in Chapter 8. Direct-to-consumer ordering of genetic tests via the computer is available, and a consumer alert has been issued by the Federal Trade Commission on July 27, 2006 to address a number of concerns including adequate information and privacy (Wolfberg, 2006). Ethical issues that overlap screening and testing are discussed in Chapters 8, 10 and 12.

THERAPEUTIC STRATEGIES EMPLOYED IN GENETIC DISORDERS

Although various types of therapeutic management are available, such management approaches depend on

- The nature of the defect;
- How well it is understood at the genetic and biochemical levels;
- The practical feasibility of correction.

In some conditions, certain management is tailored to the specific genotype. The client being treated may be the fetus, the infant, the child, or the adult. Treatment methods used in genetic disorders may involve surgical, cognitive/behavioral, pharmacologic, dietary, environmental avoidance, transfusion, plasma exchange, enzyme, behavioral, cell, or gene therapy (see Table 5.4). Some have been developed on the basis of knowledge of the defect in the gene and its product whereas others are empirical or are aimed at controlling or mediating signs and symptoms without cure. Different rationales thus underlie the previously described methods (see Table 5.5). They are basically aimed at

- Limiting the intake of a substrate or its precursor,
- Depleting the accumulation or promoting the excretion of a substrate, precursor, or product,
- Directly or indirectly replacing or stimulating production of the enzyme, or gene product,
- Replacing, repairing, or reprogramming the gene itself.

TABLE 5.4　Treatment Methods Used in Selected Genetic Disorders

Method	Examples
Surgical	Reconstructive surgery in cleft lip and palate; portacaval shunt in glycogen storage diseases I and III to limit deposition of glycogen. Liver transplant to provide missing enzymes in Wilson disease and hereditary tyrosinemia by replacing defective tissue. Bone marrow transplant to supply missing enzyme in severe combined immune deficiency caused by adenosine deaminase deficiency. Stem cell transplant in β-thalassemia. Correct defect in congenital heart disease.
Pharmacologic	Danazol (an androgen) in angioedema to prevent acute attacks. Tigason (synthetic retinoid) in Darier disease (autosomal dominant skin disorder). Growth hormone in pituitary dwarfism. Insulin in type 1 diabetes mellitus. Zinc in acrodermatitis enteropathica (an autosomal-recessive disorder) to ameliorate zinc deficiency and bring clinical improvement. Clofibrate in hyperlipoproteinemia III to decrease blood lipids.
Dietary	Limitation of phenylalanine in PKU for substrate restriction. Limitation of lactose and galactose in galactosemia for substrate restriction and prevention of accumulation. Administering uridine in orotic aciduria to inhibit the first enzyme in the metabolic pathway and decrease orotic acid.
Environmental avoidance	Avoiding mechanical stress to prevent fractures in osteogenesis imperfecta. Avoiding halothane and related anesthetics in malignant hyperthermia. Not eating fava (broad) bean in G6PD deficiency to prevent hemolytic anemia. Avoiding sulfonamides in unstable hemoglobins to prevent hemolysis. Avoiding alcohol consumption in acute intermittent porphyria. Avoiding ultraviolet light in xeroderma pigmentosa to minimize skin lesions.
Transfusion	Administration of factor VIII in hemophilia A as a replacement for the lacking circulating serum protein.
Behavioral	Infant stimulation program to maximize potential in Down syndrome and other syndromes that include developmental delay.
Plasmapheresis	In Refsum disease to remove high blood levels of phytanic acid due to defective metabolism.
Enzyme	By administering cofactor such as biotin to allow increased propionyl-CoA carboxylase activity in propionic acidemia. Intravenous administration of α-galactosidase A in Fabry disease.
Gene	Direct gene transfer of β hemoglobin gene copies into bone marrow cells of patients with β-thalassemia. Use of recombinant DNA to produce insulin. Use of ribozymes to inactivate expression of mutant gene.
Preventive	Genetic counseling. Genetic testing and screening. Prenatal detection and diagnosis. Newborn screening.

TABLE 5.5   Selected Approaches to Treatment of Genetic Disorders

Approach	Examples
Restricting or eliminating intake of substrate or precursor	
Diet therapy	Restricting intake of the branched chain amino acids in maple syrup urine disease (MSUD), or phenylalanine in PKU, to prevent the accumulation of these substances and subsequent consequences.
Environmental avoidance	Nonuse of barbiturates in hepatic porphyrias.
Depleting the accumulation or promoting the excretion of a substrate, precursor, or unwanted product	
Chelation	Using D-penicillamine as a chelating agent to deplete copper in Wilson disease. Using deferoxamine as a chelating agent to promote excretion of ferritin secondary to iron overload in β-thalassemia
Surgical bypass	Surgical bypass procedures such as portacaval shunt in glycogen storage diseases I and III, and ileal jejunal bypass in hyperlipoproteinemia II a to decrease cholesterol absorption from the gut.
Enhanced excretion	Enhancing excretion of bile salts to reduce serum cholesterol by giving cholestyramine in familial hypercholesterolemia. Promoting waste nitrogen excretion by giving arginine as a dietary supplement in patients with argininosuccinate synthetase deficiency.
Plasmapheresis (mechanical)	Plasmapheresis in Refsum disease for elimination of phytanic acid.
Metabolic inhibition	Clofibrate in hyperlipoprotenemia III to inhibit glyceride and decrease blood lipid levels.
Replacing or stimulating production of enzyme, gene product, or gene	
Enzyme induction	Use of phenobarbital in Gilbert and Crigler-Najjar syndromes results in increased glucuronyl transferase.
Cofactor administration (in vitamin-responsive forms)	Thiamine (B1) administration in pyruvic acidemia for pyruvate decarboxylase; in MSUD for branched chain ketoacid decarboxylase. Ascorbate administration in Ehler-Danlos syndrome VI for collagen lysyl hydroxylase. Pyridoxine (B6) in gyrate atrophy for ornithine ketoacid aminotransferase; in homocystinuria for cystathionine synthetase; in infantile convulsions caused by glutamic acid decarboxylase. Biotin in propionic acidemia for propionyl CoA carboxylase; in mixed carboxylase synthetase. Cobalamin (B12) for methylmalonicaciduria from adenosylcobalamin synthesis and methylmalonic CoA mutase. Folate for homocystinuria caused by methylenetetrahydrofolate reductase.
Enzyme administration (surgical and non-surgical approaches)	Organ and tissue transplantation as in the kidney for Fabry disease and cystinosis; Islet cell transplantation for diabetes; liver for hereditary tryrosinemia; fibroblasts in mucopolysaccharide disorders. Transfusion of placental glucocerebrosidase in Gaucher disease (experimental). Intravenous infusion of alpha-galactosidase A in Fabry disease. Oral pancreatic enzyme supplementation in cystic fibrosis.
Direct administration of gene product	Factor VIII in classic hemophilia. Cortisol in congenital adrenogenital syndrome Thyroxine in congenital hypothyroidism.
Direct gene transfer	Factor IX in hemophilia B (experimental)
Blocking production of a protein	
Antisense oligonucleotide	Blocks translation of mRNA into protein; for example, in blocking conversion of therapy angiotensinogen to angiotensin to control hypertension (experimental)

For example, diet therapy may be based on the principle of limiting the amount of a specific substrate that cannot be adequately metabolized by the appropriate enzyme, as in phenylketonuria, or it might be aimed at providing a product needed in order to circumvent a metabolic pathway, as in the provision of uridine in orotic aciduria. Gene product replacement might involve the administration of the product directly (e.g., insulin in type 1 diabetes mellitus) or indirectly by means of bone marrow transplantation (e.g., in severe combined immunodeficiency caused by adenosine deaminase deficiency). Toxic substances can be removed by chelation with drugs, plasmapheresis, or surgical bypass procedures. The administration of pharmacologic doses of vitamins supplies the needed cofactor for holoenzyme function in certain vitamin-responsive disorders.

For some disorders, multiple combinations of therapies are necessary. In Refsum disease (an autosomal recessive disorder with retinitis pigmentosa, ataxia, peripheral neurophathy, and accumulation of phytanic acid), for example, both dietary restriction of phytanic acid and plasmapheresis at weekly intervals are usual. Correction of birth defects such as craniofacial anomalies or limb anomalies usually involves multiple phases of surgical treatment at various stages of the development of the individual, along with the use of prosthetic devices and a long rehabilitation. Such interventions require a skilled treatment group that is prepared to deal not only with the physical correction by surgery, but with the nursing, psychological, speech, hearing, and rehabilitative measures needed to achieve optimum results. Thus, therapeutic approaches may range from a one-time surgical correction of a birth defect to a long-term special diet, to an infant stimulation program to improve maximum potential, to experimental gene replacement. This chapter concentrates on therapeutic modalities that are unique to, or especially important in, genetic disorders, and those requiring understanding and manipulation of the genetic problem at a biochemical level or at the level of the gene itself.

Diet Manipulation

One of the most common therapeutic modalities likely to be encountered by the nurse is diet manipulation. Diet manipulation may be used to restrict or eliminate a specific substrate from the diet in or-

der to prevent buildup of the substrate itself, its product in a specific metabolic pathway, or a metabolic by-product. Such diet manipulations have been applied to several inherited biochemical disorders. Because of the rarity and complexity of these disorders, specialized and expert team management is required and may be available only in specialized centers. After therapy is initiated, continued management can be accomplished in the person's home community. Often the community health or school nurse becomes the link between the family and a host of other professionals involved in the care. Because PKU is the most frequent among these, this will be discussed in detail as a prototype; others are briefly discussed. Principles that nurses can apply generally to patients on these long-term substrate restricted diets are given later.

Nursing Pointers

- Parents, and the child when old enough, need to understand the relationship of the basic defect in the disorder to the dietary restrictions. This should be explained in simple terms, and all information should be culturally congruent at a level the client can understand. The shock accompanying initial diagnosis may result in the nonretention of factual material that is presented at such a time, and so the information should be repeated again later.
- Parents should be told orally and also in written form the equipment that is necessary to have in the home to implement the diet and where it can be obtained. Some centers provide all necessary equipment.
- Parents must understand the dietary prescription and be able to use it with common household measurements. The importance of accurate measurement should be stressed.
- The dietary prescription should be given in written form and gone over verbally. All information should be in easily understood terms.
- Parents should be able to plan a sample day's diet from a given dietary prescription. The nurse can ask to have them do this while visiting the home.
- The meaning of the specific disorder in the family's cultural context should be determined and used in teaching and long-range planning.
- Consider ways for the dietary implementation and maintenance in the context of different

cultural, ethnic, religious, and social eating patterns, so that they can be applied to families in appropriate ways.

- Help may be needed for the mother to get used to the time-consuming routine of a special diet. The nurse may be able to help her organize a schedule.
- Financial needs should be recognized. Some states provide free formula, food, or financial assistance for metabolic disorders.
- Stress the importance of reading labels in all commercial foods or requesting such ingredient lists from commercial manufacturers if they are not listed on the label.
- Parents should understand the importance of not running out of special necessary foods or formula. They should have an emergency stockpile at all times.
- Essential products and formulas should be taken with the family on trips and vacations.
- Parents should know what to do in case of illness, refusal to eat prescribed foods, failure to stay on the prescribed diet, or appetite fluctuations. These should be in written form and verbally reviewed.
- Parents should have a telephone number to call in which a response is always available whenever they have specific diet-related questions.
- When possible, parents should be encouraged to use foods that are acceptable in the special diet for all family members, provided that a dietary imbalance would not result (e.g., everyone could have fruit ices for dessert instead of just the child with galactosemia, where lactose is restricted, while others ate ice cream).
- Neighbors, friends, relatives, babysitters, and teachers should have a clear explanation of foods that the child can and cannot have. If the child is likely to have a snack at a particular friend's house, specially prepared or acceptable snacks could be kept there. For example, home-baked cookies from a recipe that is low in phenylalanine can be enjoyed by all.
- Open communication and involvement of school officials and teachers so that the child is treated as one that is normal, healthy, and on a special diet is essential. The nurse may help initiate contacts or give a program to teachers to alleviate their concerns.
- Parents may be helped to plan the diet by using some foods from the school lunch menu if it is possible to minimize differences.
- Involving the child in his or her own food choices from approved foods can be done by the age of 3 years or when developmentally appropriate for that child.
- Parent groups are useful for support and sharing coping measures.

Intrauterine and Fetal Therapy

The widespread use of prenatal detection and diagnosis has allowed the early identification of fetuses with biochemical errors and congenital defects. Prenatal diagnosis of genetic disease in the fetus now expands the list of choices for the pregnancy:

- Selective termination of the pregnancy
- Choice of a different mode of delivery (e.g., cesarean section in a fetus with osteogenesis imperfecta)
- Altering the geographic site of delivery for highly specialized management
- Specific prevention of premature labor
- Induced preterm delivery for the earliest possible correction or to prevent further damage (e.g., amniotic band syndrome)
- Preparation for immediate postnatal treatment at the normal delivery time
- Direct fetal therapy such as placement of a shunt in the fetus for correction of obstructive hydrocephalus
- Fetal surgery involving direct fetal exposure
- Indirect fetal therapy or intrauterine treatment, for example, in the case of administration of intravenous and oral digoxin to the mother for intrauterine treatment of fetal paroxysmal tachycardia as well as direct injection to the fetus

These procedures have had various degrees of success and risk. Experimental techniques such as in utero surgery to correct certain craniofacial anomalies have been suggested. In utero hematopoetic stem cell transplantation has been accomplished in a few cases and may be particularly useful for immunodeficiency disorders such as X-linked agammaglobulinemia, hemoglobinopathies such as beta-thalassemia, and inborn errors of metabolism such as Gaucher disease.

Experience with many of the specific modalities used in intrauterine therapy has been limited due to the rarity of many of the individual disorders, technical difficulties, and the hazards that may be involved. For example, in fetal surgery, some of the possible undesirable outcomes are hemorrhage, infection, spontaneous abortion, premature labor, serious injury or death to the fetus or mother, the possibility of the need for future cesarean section due to the hysterotomy necessary for surgery, unsuccessful surgery, successful surgery but an unsuccessful outcome, the presence of other undetected defects in the fetus, and untoward effects from the anesthesia used.

As opportunities for fetal therapy grow, ethical and moral dilemmas are becoming more apparent. In addition to implications from the risks noted, others include divergent societal views of the fetus, conflicts between the rights and desires of the parents and of the fetus, the weighing of risks and benefits between the mother and the fetus, the lack of information on the chances for successful outcomes, the fact that the mother becomes a patient with the fetus and may possibly be an unwilling participant in fetal therapy, whether the right of a treatable defective fetus is the same as the right of a fetus with an untreatable defect, whether a fetus can be considered truly a patient, and the interests of the researchers in advancing expertise and knowledge. Dilemmas are increased when twins are present and one is normal and the other has a defect. Nurses should make sure that as much information is available to parents involved in such a decision as is available, help to clarify choices, make sure that the information presented is in terms that they understand, provide an environment that is free from coercion and pressure, and support whatever decision the couple makes. There are concerns by some that fetal treatment can become too aggressive when alternative methods are available. For example, how much advantage is attained by fetal bone marrow transplant as opposed to performing this procedure after birth?

Gene Product Replacement

The replacement of the normal gene product may be accomplished in several ways—by simply ad-ministering the missing substance (e.g., thyroxin for hypothyroidism or factor VIII for classical hemophilia or pancreatic supplementation below 10,000 units of lipase per kg in cystic fibrosis) on a periodic basis, manipulating the defective enzyme by cofactor or coenzyme therapy, organ or tissue transplantation, or directly replacing the deficient or defective enzyme. Several years ago, it appeared that enzyme replacement therapy would be relatively simple in those disorders in which the enzyme defect was identified at the molecular level. In practice, the administration of enzymes in conventional ways was not effective. A major reason was that most enzymes are not normally circulating serum components like factor VIII (a blood-clotting factor deficient in hemophilia A). They need to gain access to cell interiors in specific organs and then reach specific organelles. The enzyme must get there without being destroyed, and it needs an appropriate delivery system. For example, in lysosomal storage diseases, the cells' normal delivery system must be used to get the enzyme into the lysosome by allowing the enzyme with its carrier to bind to the cell surface receptors as a macromolecule and allowing normal pinocytosis to occur.

Cofactor and Coenzyme Therapy

As discussed in Chapter 9 (see Figure 9.8), many enzymes are holoenzymes, that is, they are composed of an apoenzyme (protein part) plus a cofactor or coenzyme (prosthetic part) that is needed for function. Cofactors are frequently vitamins or metal ions. Many inherited biochemical disorders have both vitamin-responsive and -nonresponsive subtypes. The replacement of a missing or defective cofactor or supplying it in megadoses allows the formation of a functional holoenzyme or allows binding when large amounts of cofactor are available. In this way, they regulate the activity and amounts of apoenzyme. At least 25 vitamin-responsive inherited biochemical disorders are known. Fetal vitamin therapy for certain vitamin-responsive disorders has been accomplished, and the potential exists for the possibility of this approach with the others. Giving vitamins in high doses has been found in some cases to activate other pathways unintentionally with accompanying ill effects, and this must be watched for during therapy.

Recombinant DNA

Briefly, the process of creating recombinant DNA for use in the manufacture of certain proteins, enzymes, and hormones is as follows. So-called foreign DNA from a higher biologic organism or human is cut into specific sections containing the normal-functioning gene of interest by a type of enzyme called restriction endonucleases and is purified. These enzymes also are used to remove a segment from the DNA of a vector or carrier. Vectors most commonly used are bacteriophages (bacterial viruses) or plasmids (a type of bacterial DNA). The foreign DNA and the DNA from the vector are allowed to unite, thus forming a recombinant DNA molecule that is inserted into a host bacterial cell. This bacterium, with its own DNA plus that of the vector with the foreign DNA, multiplies, making identical copies of the foreign DNA inserted and its product—the protein or enzyme—desired. This process is called *cloning* and is being used commercially to produce human insulin, growth hormone, interferon factor VIII, and other substances in large quantities. This has made for the wider use of substances that were formerly limited in production and now are available and has removed the necessity of extraction from pooled blood, thus making safer (free of infectious organisms such as hepatitis or human immunodeficiency virus) product available. Another use of restriction endonucleases is in the creation of gene "probes" for diagnosis as discussed in Chapter 2.

Gene Therapy

Gene therapy is the most direct approach to the treatment of genetic diseases. If it is successful, it eliminates the need for all of the other therapeutic modalities previously described. It has long been known that genetic material has been transferred nonpurposefully from one organism or species to another, as in the case of viruses that invade human tissue and become integrated into the cellular DNA. Gene therapy usually consists of inserting a new gene into somatic or germline cells but may also refer to repair or reprogramming of a gene. The optimal gene therapy would be the replacement of the abnormal gene with a normal copy in the proper location of that gene in every cell with appropriate expression. The new gene must not only be delivered but expressed correctly over time. Among current interests in gene therapy is the understanding of gene regulation and tissue-specific gene expression control that can be manipulated to correct the defect. The concept is illustrated in Figure 5.6. Gene therapy can be used in several ways:

- Replacing a missing function as in the case of absent or deficient gene product that usually occurs in autosomal recessive biochemical disorders
- Enhancing or activating normal functioning
- Providing a new function such as resistance to a disease such as influenza
- Interfering with an undesired or aberrant function such as in the case of an abnormal gene product formed in an autosomal dominant disorder

Gene therapy could be used to treat both genetic diseases and common diseases such as cancer and heart disease, and also as a prevention strategy. The idea of using germ cells for correction of a genetic defect has aroused ethical concerns about whether it is appropriate to alter the human genome for future generations and the effect on those future generations. It is also technically difficult, but it is appealing in that it ideally would correct the genetic defect in all cells and all descendants. Germline gene therapy is not now actively being pursued in humans. Somatic cell gene therapy corrects the defect only in the person treated, not his or her descendants.

The first human gene therapy trial was the insertion of a functional gene into somatic cells (T-lymphocytes) to correct the defect in adenosine deaminase deficiency (ADA), a type of severe combined immunodeficiency disorder, and the return of these cells by infusion to the affected children. This was not permanent, and infusions every one to two months were needed initially, followed by three to six months. Newer approaches involve the insertion of normal ADA genes into bone marrow stem cells. Other examples of conditions in which clinical trials of gene therapy have been done is the introduction of the gene for the low-density lipoprotein (LDL) receptor into the liver cells of patients with familial hypercholesterolemia, and the *CFTR* gene into lung and airway cell in cystic fibrosis patients. Gene therapy trials received a setback when an

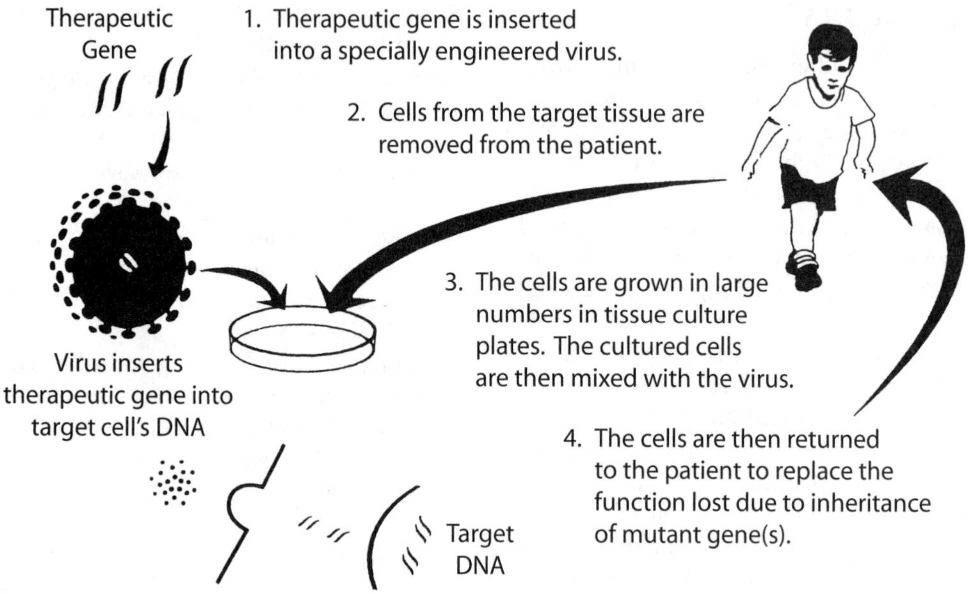

Therapeutic Gene

1. Therapeutic gene is inserted into a specially engineered virus.

2. Cells from the target tissue are removed from the patient.

Virus inserts therapeutic gene into target cell's DNA

3. The cells are grown in large numbers in tissue culture plates. The cultured cells are then mixed with the virus.

4. The cells are then returned to the patient to replace the function lost due to inheritance of mutant gene(s).

Target DNA

FIGURE 5.6   Ex vivo gene therapy. Courtesy of Karina Boehm, NHGRI, NSH.

eighteen-year-old male with ornithine transcarbamylase deficiency who was receiving intravenous infusion of the normal gene via a weakened adenovirus vector developed multiple organ failure and died. After this, the Food and Drug Administration (FDA) and others instituted stricter regulation. In late 2002, the development of leukemia in some children enrolled in a French gene therapy trial using retroviral vectors to insert genes into stem cells for X-linked severe combined immunodeficiency disease led to a temporary halt in 2003 of these types of trials by the FDA.

Somatic cell gene therapy could involve gene insertion not only into the infant, child, or adult but also prenatally. The times for this would be in the zygote before and after fusion of pronuclei (this could be done by the microinjection of DNA into the male pronucleus of the fertilized ovum), in the preimplantation embryo, perhaps in conjunction with embryo transfer, or postimplantation into the embryo or the fetus at an early age of development before damage from the mutant gene has occurred. Newborn gene therapy also appears promising be-

cause of the infant's small size and for other reasons, and ADA has been treated in this way. In some neurologic genetic diseases, damage is detectable by the third month or earlier. In one case, in utero stem cell transplantation of bone marrow from the father to the male fetus was accomplished to prevent the X-linked type of severe combined immunodeficiency disease. Several infusions were necessary using ultrasound-guided intraperitoneal injection, and at 5 months of age, the boy appeared well. The Patent and Trademark Office has allowed patents for gene therapy techniques.

Gene-based therapies have been tested for diseases such as cancer and heart disease. In cancer, one approach has been to alter cells to produce substances that alter the host response to cancer cells. In heart disease, angiogenic factors can be delivered into ischemic heart muscle. In HIV, it has been suggested that introducing drug resistance genes into normal bone marrow cells would allow more aggressive chemotherapy. Genetically engineered islet cells have been transplanted in type 1 diabetes.

Epigenetic Therapies

Epigenetics refers to changes in gene expression not coded for in DNA. Various genetic disorders are due to inappropriate gene silencing or expression. These may occur through such mechanisms as DNA methylation and modifications in chromosomal histones and are discussed in Chapter 2. Thus, it follows that epigenetic therapeutic approaches would be developed. For example, inhibitors of DNA methylation, such as 5-azacytidine, are being examined for their ability to reactivate genes that have been silenced. Applications include certain cancers such as myeloid dysplastic syndrome and certain hemoglobinopathies.

KEY POINTS FOR DISCUSSION

- What are some of the ways in which genetic testing and screening differ?
- Discuss elements to include in programs to prevent genetic disease.
- What are some advantages and disadvantages of nondirective genetic counseling? Should genetic counseling be more directive? Why or why not?
- What are some causes for concern with germline gene therapy?

II

The Integration of Genetics Into Nursing Courses and Curricula

The Application of Genomics to Pharmacology

BiDil, a combination pill of isosorbide dinitrate and hydralazine, was recommended for approval by an advisory committee of the Food and Drug Administration (FDA). What was different about this approval was that it was recommended for a particular ethnic group: Black heart failure patients. This is one of the most recent widespread commercial applications of pharmacogenomics targeted to a specific ethnic group. This and other applications of pharmacogenomics are discussed in this chapter.

CASE EXAMPLE

A 21-year-old male student was brought to the hospital with a fractured leg. He was more worried about anesthesia than about his leg. When taking the family history, it was noted that 10 of his relatives had died after having general anesthesia. You will learn why below.

Differences in how individuals respond to drugs can be due to genetic or nongenetic factors. Different individuals may require different doses of the same drug in order to achieve maximum effectiveness, others may not respond at all to certain drugs, and different adverse reactions may be manifested. This variability is largely genetic, and some families may be at greater risk than the population at large. The well-known and recently discovered polymorphisms in the genes coding for enzymes affecting such parameters as drug metabolism, transport, disposition, excretion, and drug receptors affect large numbers of persons worldwide. The clinical signif-

icance depends on a variety of factors, some of which are not directly genetic, such as age, weight, the condition of organs such as the liver, and the therapeutic index of the drug. Genetic controls can come into play at any stage of the drug-handling process listed in Box 6.1.

Pharmacogenetics is concerned with the consequences of genetic variations in drug handling that affect individual response and tend to refer more to rare individual differences. *Pharmacogenomics* has been coined more recently and refers more broadly to drug effects on the total genome, usually beyond structural variations. It also deals with how drugs act on gene variations and expression and other applications, such as how study of the genome of microorganisms can lead to the development of new antibiotics that can attack genetic vulnerabilities in those microbes. These terms are often used interchangeably.

Genetic variation in drug metabolism and handling can be quantitative or qualitative. For exam-

---

BOX 6.1

Some Stages in Drug Handling Influenced by Genetic Controls

Absorption	Membrane transport
Distribution	Tissue sensitivity
Protein binding	Tissue storage
Metabolism	Elimination
Attachment to membrane receptors	The activation of special responses such as the immune response

ple, mutant genes may produce enzyme variants with high, intermediate, low, or absent activity. The degree and type of variation in an individual's response may not be apparent if there is no important easily detected consequence. Someone who has even a low level of activity for a given enzyme may have enough enzyme product to cope usually unless some unusual stressor such as infection or trauma is encountered. Therefore, this person may be unaware of his/her impairment.

Information about response variation is particularly important in drugs with a narrow therapeutic margin. Many drugs have a wide enough margin of safety so that even with individual-response variation, effectiveness and safety are not compromised. However, practitioners must recognize that persons from diverse racial and ethnic groups may respond differently to medications because of genetic differences. Male and female differences in drug handling and reactions can also be important. Developers of new drugs are increasingly using genetic knowledge to develop approaches to drug treatment.

Receptor mutations are known to cause functional changes that themselves cause disease. An application of this research is in regard to opiate receptor variability and drug dependence. Inherited drug receptor variants leading to resistance to such drugs as vasopressin, estrogen, insulin, and the steroid hormones are known to influence response. Differences in the metabolism of alcohol and of illicit drugs will be identified that will lead to new information about the genetic role in drug dependence and addiction.

Variations can be relatively common in certain populations, in which case the variation may be referred to as a *polymorphism*, or may be relatively rare. Pharmacologically significant variations can be:

- one feature of a person's genetic disorder such as in the porphyrias,
- the only known rare abnormality present, such as in butyrylcholinesterase variation,
- widespread common polymorphisms in enzymes involved in the metabolism and processing of many different drugs such as within the cytochrome P450 system.

In this chapter, both rare pharmacogenetic disorders and common polymorphisms leading to altered response to drugs are discussed, as are pharmacogenomic applications and the ethical problems engendered.

COMMON VARIATIONS AFFECTING DRUG METABOLISM

There are a number of relatively common genetic variations or polymorphisms that affect the way a person handles drugs. These include those in drug metabolizing enzymes such as cytochrome P-450 polymorphisms, acetylator variation, and thiopurine S-methyltransferase polymorphisms. A relatively common human enzyme condition, glucose-6-phosphate dehydrogenase (G6PD) deficiency, is also discussed below. Some other common variations affecting drug metabolism and handling are shown in Table 6.1.

Glucose-6-Phosphate Dehydrogenase Deficiency

Glucose-6-phosphate dehydrogenase (G6PD) deficiency is the most common enzyme abnormality known. It affects millions of people throughout the world, especially those of Mediterranean, African, Middle Eastern, Near Eastern, and Southeast Asian origin. G6PD deficiency was thought to have a protective effect against malaria, leading to its maintenance in the human population. G6PD deficiency results from mutations in a gene located on the X chromosome. Thus, males are hemizygous. Approximately 10–15% of Black males in the United States have G6PD deficiency. In some areas of the Middle East, G6PD deficiency may be as high as 35% of males. Because of this high frequency, more homozygous females are found to be G6PD deficient than any other X-linked recessive disorder. Females who are heterozygous for the mutant gene have two types of red blood cells: those that are normal and those that are deficient. Although the two types of red blood cell populations are usually approximately equal, as a consequence of X inactivation (see Chapter 4), there can be an unequal distribution. If more cells with deficient enzyme are present, such heterozygous females are subject to hemolysis on encountering specific oxidative drugs.

The major consequences if clinically evident can include any of the following manifestations:

- Neonatal jaundice (hyperbilirubinemia)
- Acute hemolysis following exposure to certain oxidative drugs, ingestion of fava beans, or infection

TABLE 6.1   Examples of Other Polymorphisms Affecting Drug Activity and Response

Polymorphism	Comments
ATP-binding cassette subfamily B member 1 (*ABCB1*), also known as *MDR1*	A multidrug transporter, associated with drug resistance in epilepsy therapy. A specific polymorphism (3435 C→T). These results suggest that by genotyping other drugs that are not ABCB1 substrates or drugs that inhibit evade ABCB1, it could be predicted what agents might be more effective in certain people. These areas are a source of intensive pharmaceutical research.
β_2-adrenergic receptor variations	In the treatment of congestive heart failure, responsiveness to therapy with beta blockers such as carvedilol varied.
Bradykinin B(2) receptor gene	Results in the appearance of cough when taking angiotensin-converting enzyme (ACE) inhibitors, commonly used to treat essential hypertension.
Dihydropyrimidine dehydrogenase (*DPYD*)	Is involved in the metabolism of 5-FU, an anticancer drug. About 13 genetic polymorphisms have been identified. Those who have genetically reduced activity show increases in adverse effects with 5-FU such as leukocytopenia, mouth sores, diarrhea, and nausea and vomiting.
KCNE2	Encodes a peptide subunit of the cardiac potassium channel that results in susceptibility for long QT syndrome and drug-induced torsade de pointes after exposure to clarithromycin and also to trimethoprim/sulfamethoxazole.
Thymidylate synthase	Expression in colorectal tumors has been noted to be a predictor of response to 5-fluorouracil therapy in which those with lower expression had a greater response and longer survival.
Vitamin K epoxide reductase variants	Three groups require high, medium, or low dosages of warfarin complex, subunit 1 (*VKORC1*) gene based on 10 gene polymorphisms. African Americans are likely to require large doses, Asian Americans are more likely to require a low dosage.

- Chronic hemolysis leading to chronic hemolytic anemia

G6PD is found in all cells where G6PD is necessary in order to catalyze an important oxidation or reduction reaction in the pentose phosphate pathway and also maintains adequate levels of NADPH (see Glossary) in cells. In most cells, other metabolic pathways can provide the needed end products from the above reaction. The G6PD-deficient red cell, however, usually functions well, but hemolysis can occur when:

- Oxidant- or peroxide-producing drugs are taken up;
- Infection occurs;
- There is exposure to naphthalene in moth balls,
- There is ingestion of the fava (broad) bean (favism).

The severity of the hemolysis varies with the percentage of active enzyme present in the specific G6PD variant. There are more than 400 identified G6PD variants, but not all are clinically significant. Various classifications exist depending on the severity of the enzyme deficiency and the effects seen. Among the variations are:

- G6PD-A, which is most prevalent in Africa, the Americas, and West Indies with 10–60% of normal enzyme activity—class III in the World Health Organization (WHO) classification—and associated with mild or moderate hemolysis
- G6PD-Mediterranean, which is most prevalent in the Mediterranean, North Africa, and the Middle East with 0–10% of the normal enzyme activity usually associated with severe hemolysis—class II in the WHO classification.

Most persons with G6PD deficiency are not detected due only to the presence of opposite clinical manifestations.

Hemolysis following the intake of certain drugs in persons with G6PD deficiency was first identified with the use of the antimalarial drug primaquine. Since the original work, WHO has classified some drugs as those everyone should avoid; those that G6PD-deficient persons of Mediterranean, Middle Eastern and Asian origin should avoid; and those that persons with the African (A–) variant should avoid. In some cases, the decision to use a particular drug depends on how important the need for that drug is and the dosage used. Other factors that influence response to these drugs are other genetic differences, the severity of the G6PD deficiency, the hemoglobin level, factors relating to the red cell, the age of the person, and the presence of other sources of oxidative stress such as infection. Drugs and chemicals listed as associated with adverse effects in persons with G6PD deficiency vary according to author. Selected major drugs to be avoided include acetanilide, dimercaprol, dapsone, flutamide, methylene blue, nalidixic acid, naphthalene, niridazole, nitrites, nitrofurans including furazolidone, nitrofurantoin, nitrofurazone-pamaquine, pentaquine, phenazopyridine, phenylhydrazine, primaquine, sulfacetamide, sulfamethoxazole, sulfanilamide, sulfapyridine, toluidine blue, triazolesulfone, and trinitroluene. In addition quinine water, mothballs, and fava bean should be avoided. Exposure to some of these can present workplace issues, as discussed in Chapter 12.

Hemolysis in the G6PD-deficient person typically begins within 24 to 72 hours of starting the oxidative drug, eating fava beans (a common dietary component in the Mediterranean, Middle and Far East and North Africa), or manifesting an infection, usually a more severe one, such as typhoid fever, rickettsial infections, or viral hepatitis. Favism may be seen seasonally when the fava beans are more readily available. Manifestations include a fall in Hb, Heinz bodies in the red cells, and eventual hemolytic anemia and can include dark urine and back and abdominal pain, along with jaundice. Acute renal failure often follows hepatitis or urinary tract infections in G6PD-deficient persons. Chronic nonspherocytic hemolytic anemia accompanies certain variants and may be made worse by stress, infection, or drug intake. There may be a history of neonatal jaundice, and the person may have gallstones, splenomegaly, decreased stamina, weakness, iron overload, or progressive hepatic damage.

Some researchers believe that all individuals in population groups at risk should be screened for G6PD deficiency before any of the drugs to be avoided are prescribed. Awareness of this deficiency has become important in administering drugs used to treat many patients with human immunodeficiency virus (HIV) infection such as dapsone. In some instances, the need for the drug outweighs the risk of hemolytic anemia. Nursing points are given in Box 6.2.

BOX 6.2

Nursing Points Related to G6PD Deficiency

- Be aware of populations in which G6PD deficiency is known to be more common.
- Review the patient's prior drug exposure history and effects with the individual at the time of treatment.
- Inquire about any drug reactions in blood relatives, and consider whether further testing for G6PD deficiency is merited.
- Once an individual is known to have G6PD deficiency, agents that can precipitate hemolytic anemia should be listed and reviewed.
- Counsel the affected person on what to avoid. Avoidance of the fava bean should be included, as well as discussion of breast-feeding risks if the infant is deficient in G6PD. Mothers who take drugs to be avoided or eat fava beans may transmit these substances in breast milk.
- Advise that family members may be at risk and should be screened for the deficiency in order to identify them.
- Advise the persons to wear some type of medical information and be sure his/her current health care provider is aware of his/her status.

Cytochrome P450 Polymorphisms (CYPs)

The hepatic cytochrome P450 enzyme system comprises a group of related enzymes known as a superfamily. These enzymes are responsible for oxidizing many chemicals and drugs. A separate gene codes for each, and more than 200 have been identified, some of which have multiple allelic forms. They are named according to the following system: CYP followed by a family number, a subfamily letter, and a number for the individual form. While each group has different numbers of variation, clinically they fall into ultra rapid, extensive (considered normal), intermediate, and low functional activity categories. They often vary by ethnic group. In general, poor metabolizers break down drugs processed by this pathway more slowly. This means that blood levels stay higher, and toxicity can be more frequent. Poor metabolizers also need a less frequent dosage so as to get optimum therapeutic effect without side effects or adverse reactions. Persons who are ultrarapid metabolizers, on the other hand, need the same dose more frequently or may not show expected therapeutic effectiveness and be classified as treatment failures. For some variants, genotyping is now available clinically in order to maximize effectiveness and prevent serious adverse reactions. Important variations in cytochrome P450 enzymes are summarized in Table 6.2.

Of particular interest to nurses is the inhibited metabolism of codeine in poor metabolizers of CYP2D6 who therefore receive no analgesic effect from codeine. When a patient is not getting the expected pain relief from codeine, the reason may be genetic, and the nurse needs to find appropriate analgesic relief, not increase the dose of codeine or decide the patient is "faking."

TABLE 6.2   Selected Cytochrome P450 Polymorphisms

Polymorphism	Comments
CYP2C9	Important clinically because of activity with drugs with narrow therapeutic indices such as warfarin and phenytoin. In the case of the anticoagulant warfarin, prescribed for about 1 million persons in the United States alone, persons with the variants CYP2C9*2 and *3 have reduced clearance leading to reduced dose requirements. Failure to recognize can lead to toxicity at standard dosages, including severe bleeding complications. If these persons are given a CYP2C9 inhibitor such as amiodarone (used to treat cardiac arrhthymias) concurrently, drug-drug interaction leads to serious bleeding or neurotoxicity because of diminished enzyme activity.
CYP2C19	Involved in hydroxylation of S-mephenytoin, an anticonvulsant, and metabolism of some proton pump inhibitors, such as omeprazole as well as proguanil; 14–30% of Asians and 2–6% of Whites are poor metabolizers.
CYP2D6	More than 75 genetic variations. Metabolize many antidepressants such as nortriptyline (Pamelor), clomipramine (Anafranil), desipramine (Norpramin); antipsychotics such as haloperidol; beta blockers such as timolol (Blockadren), metoprolol (Lopressor); encainide (Enkaid); flecainide (Tambocor); perhexiline; tamoxifen; oxycodone; phenacetin; and codeine. Poor metabolizers of the beta blockers need only a daily dose, whereas extensive hydroxylators need the same dose two or three times a day for effectiveness. Poor metabolizers show more intense and prolonged beta blockade if the dose is not adjusted, leading to side effects such as bradycardia. Those with ultrarapid metabolism may not show the expected therapeutic effectiveness, and thus demonstrate treatment failure due to low blood concentrations of the drug. Genotyping and phenotyping are available for detection of these mutations
CYP2B6	About 8% of current drugs metabolized by it. Specific genotype (G516T) found in 3% of Whites and 20% of Blacks. This genotype is associated with slow clearance of efavirenz, a nonnucleoside reverse-transcriptase inhibitor used in HIV therapy. Those with it have higher risk of toxicity and discontinuation, especially CNS difficulties. Detecting the high-risk genotypes could lead to dose adjustment.

Acetylator Status and Drug Metabolism

The ability to metabolize and eliminate certain drugs depends on acetylation in the liver by the enzyme N-acetyltransferase with two functional genes, NAT1 and NAT2. Each has multiple alleles. Further descriptors are designated by an asterisk and the allele designation, for example, NAT2*5B. Both drug efficacy and toxicity are linked to the functioning of this enzyme. Individuals can be categorized into the following basic phenotypic groups: slow or poor, rapid, and ultrarapid acetylators.

In North American and European populations, between 50% and 70% are slow acetylators, as are about 90% of some Mediterranean populations such as Egyptians and Moroccans. In eastern Pacific populations such as Chinese, Korean, Japanese, and Thai, about 10–30% are slow acetylators, as are about 4% of Alaskan Natives. The importance of acetylator status was first recognized during therapy for tuberculosis with isoniazid (INH). Drug therapy for which acetylator status is known to have clinical relevance includes INH; dapsone, a sulfone; hydralazine (Apresoline), an antihypertensive; procainamide (Pronestyl), an antiarrhythmic; phenelzine (Nardil), an antidepressant; nitrazepam (Mogadon), a sedative; and sulfasalazine (Azulfidine), a sulfonamide derivative. Caffeine metabolism is also mediated by this system. Slow acetylators maintain higher serum levels of these drugs than do rapid acetylators. In general, slow acetylators are more likely to experience greater therapeutic responses but also a higher incidence of side effects than rapid acetylators when the same medication regime is used for the drugs mentioned above. In regard to NAT2, slow acetylators are also at greater risk for the development of spontaneous systemic lupus erythematosus (SLE) with certain drugs such as hydralazine and procainamide. Fast acetylators who eat meat have been said to have a higher risk for colorectal cancer and slow acetylators have a higher risk for bladder cancer when exposed to arylamines and cigarette smoke, another workplace issue (see Chapter 12).

Thiopurine-S-Methyltransferase (TPMT)

CASE EXAMPLE

Joseph is a 25-year-old who has been diagnosed with inflammatory bowel disease. Consideration is being given to a course of azathioprine therapy. Before this is started, however, his blood TPMT levels were measured and found to be virtually absent. Genotyping determined that Joseph had a homozygous mutation at the TPMT locus. If azothioprine therapy had been started, he would be at high risk for severe adverse effects, especially myelosuppression. This is an example of predictive pharmacogenetics in treatment.

Identified genetic polymorphisms in this system not related to ethnic or racial groups include those heterozygotes with intermediate enzyme levels (11%) and very low or absent levels in about 0.4% of persons homozygous for the deficient allele; the rest (about 89%) have high activities. TPMT is involved in the metabolism of azathioprine, an immunosuppressant, used widely in dermatology and to treat systemic lupus erythematosus and inflammatory bowel disease, as well as part of immunosuppression in liver transplantation. It is also involved in the metabolism of the anticancer drug mercaptopurine (6-MP) used often for acute lymphocytic leukemia (ALL), and thioguanine. When the metabolic pathway is not functioning properly, these drugs are directed to another pathway and form toxic thioguanine nucleotide concentrations that are reciprocally related to leukocyte counts. For azathioprine, those who have very low levels of TPMT are at risk for severe pancytopenia, and those who are rapid inactivators may need higher doses for clinical effectiveness. Thus, absent or very low levels of TPMT may result in pancytopenia, myelosuppression, and profound neutropenia. Those with higher levels of enzyme might be able to tolerate a dose-intensive treatment with 6-MP, for example, in ALL, but could have relapses due to undertreatment with the usual doses. Before beginning therapy with these agents, patients may be tested for TPMT activity or genotyped for allelic variants of the TPMT gene. Those who have high metabolic inactivation can be given a larger dose, and those who have low inactivation of 6-MP may be given a dose that is 10 to 15 times smaller.

LESS COMMON SINGLE GENE DISORDERS

There are a variety of genetic disorders arising from less common defects in single genes that are important in drug response and handling. Malignant hyperthermia and porphyria are described briefly below because they are especially important in terms of impact or prevalence. A selection of others is found in Table 6.3.

Malignant Hyperthermia

Malignant hyperthermia (MH) has been cited as the most common cause of death due to anesthesia. It occurs in about 1:10,000 to 1:15,000 anesthetized pediatric and 1:50,000 anesthetized adult patients. There are pockets of higher incidence of gene mutations in north-central Wisconsin, and some populations in North Carolina, Austria, France, and

TABLE 6.3   Selected Inherited Disorders with Altered Response to Therapeutic Agents

Condition or Disorder	Examples of Agents	Response or Effect
Acatalasia	Hydrogen peroxide	Tissue ulceration
Arene oxide metabolism defect	Phenytoin (Dilantin)	Hepatotoxicity
Butyrylcholinesterase deficiency	Succinylcholine	Apnea
C1 esterase inhibitor deficiency	Oral contraceptives, hormone replacement therapy	Episodes of hereditary angioedema
Crigler-Najjar syndrome	Salicylates, tetrahydrocortisone, menthol	Jaundice, drug toxicity
Down syndrome	Atropine	Increased response
Dubin-Johnson syndrome	Oral contraceptives	Jaundice
Familial dysautonomia	Norepinephrine	Increased pressor response
Gilbert syndrome	Oral contraceptives, alcohol, cholecystographic agents	Increased blood bilirubin, jaundice
Glaucoma (narrow angle)	Atropine, mydriatics	Increased intraocular pressure
Glaucoma (open angle)	Corticosteroids	Increased intraocular pressure
Hydantoin hydroxylation	Hydantoin (Dilantin)	Toxic plasma concentrations defect with severe side effects
Lesch-Nyhan syndrome	Allopurinol, 6-mercaptopurine azathioprine, azaguanine	Drug not metabolized to active form, resistance; formation of xanthine stones (allopurinol)
Methylenetetrahydrofolate reductase deficiency	Nitrous oxide	An infant with a severe form of this defect in folate metabolism died after being anesthetized with nitrous oxide
Mitochondrial 1555A>G	Aminoglycoside antibiotics	Sensorineural hearing loss; mutations in *RNR1*
Osteogenesis imperfecta	General anesthesia	Elevation of body temperature
PKU	Catecholamines	Increased pressor response
Warfarin resistance	Warfarin	Decreased response to warfarin, so 20–25 times usual dose is needed for therapeutic effect; increased requirement for vitamin K

Quebec. There may be MH susceptibility in 1 in 8,500 persons and as great as 1 in 2,000 persons in France. The mortality rate formerly was 60–70%, but improved recognition and management have lowered it to about 10%.

CASE EXAMPLE

The first recognized case was published by Denborough and Lovell (1960) and contained features that are often present. This is a classic case study. A 21-year-old male student with a fractured leg was brought to the hospital, where he turned out to be less concerned about the fracture than he was about having general anesthesia. Since 1922, 10 of his relatives had died as a direct consequence of having general anesthesia. Halothane was used to anesthetize the student, but MH occurred. His recovery, and the subsequent publication of the incident, led to awareness of the previously unrecognized problem.

The symptoms of MH include tachycardia, progressive muscle rigidity especially in the masseters with rhabdomyolysis (muscle breakdown), tachypnea, hypercarbia, cardiac arrhythmias, a rapid rise in body temperature that may reach 42–44°C, and the darkening of blood on the operative field with the later development of metabolic imbalances such as hyperkalemia and respiratory and metabolic acidosis. Cardiac arrest can occur before the rise in temperature. Treatment includes IV dantrolene, hyperventilation with 100% oxygen through an endotracheal tube, and cooling. Myoglobinuria may appear 4 to 8 hours later. After the initial episode, there is a risk of acute recurrence hours later and of disseminated intravascular coagulation.

The underlying defect is a preexisting defect in skeletal muscle affecting the concentration and release of calcium that is manifested after exposure to certain anesthetics. Anesthetics triggering MH include inhalation agents such as halothane, halogenated ethers such ethrane, sevoflurane, desflurane, isoflurane, and enflurane; ether and cyclopropane are also triggers, but they are not used today. MH can also occur after exposure to succinylcholine, a muscle relaxant that may be used before surgery. In some cases of MH, the mutation responsible is in the ryanodine receptor gene (*RYR1*) (a large skeletal muscle calcium release channel gene). More than 100 allelic mutations have been described. The mode of transmission is autosomal dominant, with varying penetrance. This confers susceptibility on exposure to the particular inhalational anesthetic or succinylcholine. Other genetic loci have been implicated as well but much less frequently. MH is also associated with several myopathies such as central core disease, myotonia congenita, Becker and Duchenne muscular dystrophy, and Evans myopathy but the genetic etiology may vary. The model may be that of a major gene with the effect of modifying genes.

Persons who have had an episode of MH should be screened for *RYR1* using mutation analysis, and some recommend that they have the caffeine/halothane muscle contracture test (CHCT) performed. The test requires 500 mg of fresh skeletal muscle tissue to perform, is expensive, and is invasive, and thus is used only in certain circumstances. If the DNA test identifies an *RYR1* mutation, at least first-degree relatives should also be tested. If no mutation is found the relative may wish to have the CHCT test. If the test is negative, the indication is that they are not MH susceptible. At present DNA sequence variation analysis is not ready for general population screening.

The person with MH usually appears well because the myopathy associated with it in the absence of already identified myopathy is subclinical until exposure to a volatile depolarizing anesthetic. Nevertheless, in some, there may be complaints or signs of mild ptosis, strabismus, muscle cramps, muscle weakness, recurrent dislocations, hernia, back problems such as kyphosis or scoliosis, short stature, unusual muscle bulk or other musculoskeletal complaints, or sometimes a cleft palate. A preponderance of heavily muscled young males have been noted to be susceptible to MH. Because the heart is a muscle, it may also be affected. Major stress, high environmental temperatures, strenuous exercise, or trauma may also induce MH in some cases. The combination of succinylcholine and the administration of halogenated inhalation anesthesia is especially provocative, although MH can occur after succinylcholine administration alone. Hyperkalemia, sudden general muscle rigidity, or isolated contraction of the jaw muscles can occur following succinylcholine administration usually after inhalation induction. This type is frequent in children.

BOX 6.3

Nursing Pointers to Decrease MH Morbidity and Mortality

- Before either surgical or obstetric anesthesia is given to any patient, a thorough family and personal history should be taken that includes the following questions: Have you ever had anesthesia? If so, what type? Have you ever had surgery? Was there any difficulty or problem with surgery or anesthesia? Dental surgery should be included, and specific complications such as fever, rigidity, dark urine, or any unexpected reactions should be asked about. The nurse should also ask about any musculoskeletal complaints or known muscular diseases in the family, any history of heat intolerance or fevers of unknown origin, or any unusual drug reaction (some MH patients have been reported to exhibit cramps or fever when taking alcohol, caffeine, or aspirin). The same questions should be asked about all family members, including any sudden or unexplained deaths, particularly while participating in an athletic event. The nurse should review this family history with the person going back two or three generations and include cousins. Any answers indicating sudden death or fever while receiving anesthesia should be further investigated before the individual receives anesthesia. Perhaps the same information should be collected before a student participates in strenuous school sports.

- Anesthesia for the MH-susceptible person can be planned before surgery. Planning may include prophylactic dantrolene administration, although this is somewhat controversial and can cause muscle weakness. Choice of anesthetic is based on avoiding the use of triggering agents. Regional anesthesia is a safe choice for procedures that can be accomplished with its use. Special preparation of the anesthesia machine should be done to remove trace amounts of volatile agents. A safe muscle relaxant such as pancuronium (Pavulon), atracurium (Tracrium), or mivacurium (Mivacron) should be used.

- A high index of suspicion should be maintained for an individual with any or all of the following characteristics, particularly young males with: short stature, cryptorchidism, ptosis, low-set ears, lordosis, kyphosis, pes cavus, strabismus, weak serrati muscles, or antimongolian slant of the palpebral fissures. Cases of MH have followed corrective surgery for strabismus.

- Abnormal electrocardiograms or unexplained cardiomyopathy in young patients may represent a person susceptible to MH and should be investigated.

- Any preoperative or preanesthetic physical examination should include a search for subclinical muscle weakness and the presence of any physical signs previously described, especially related to the muscular system.

- If succinylcholine (Anectine, Quelicin) is administered, the nurse or anesthetist should be alert for any abnormal reaction, such as failure to relax as expected, masseter stiffness, or muscle fasciculations that are greater than usual. Such a response should prompt consideration of postponing the surgical procedure pending further investigation and preparation. About half of children who develop this are later found to be MH susceptible.

- During surgery, the temperature and pulse should be continually monitored. Unexplained tachycardia is often the first sign but may be preceded by a rising end tidal CO_2 as shown by capnography. The development of any symptoms described earlier should mean the immediate institution of emergency procedures, the cessation of anesthesia, and the conclusion of surgery, unless some other reason can account for a rapid rise in body temperature such as excessive draping in a hot operating room, which would be rare today.

- Any rapid rise in body temperature or myoglobinuria, as evidenced by dark red urine occurring in the first 24 hours after surgery,

(continues)

should be considered as possibly caused by MH and should be investigated further.

- Resuscitation equipment and drugs necessary for treating an MH crisis should be standard equipment in all operating rooms.
- Patients known to be susceptible to MH must be cautioned to avoid potent inhalation anesthetics such as those noted. None is considered completely safe. Depolarizing muscle relaxants such as succinylcholine and decamethonium should also be avoided.
- Information regarding MH should be put into written form for the susceptible person. One should be in professional language for his or her personal health care provider, and the other should be in the language that the

patient and family can understand.
- Genetic counseling in MH includes discussing with the patient the necessity for informing relatives of the potential risk for them and urging them to seek further evaluation and to inform their families. The written information mentioned above can be used for that purpose. Referral should be made to a support group such as the Malignant Hyperthermia Association of the United States, http://www.mhaus.org
- Patients who are susceptible to MH should be advised to wear medical alert identification with this information and told how to get one.

Preoperative prophylactic doses of dantrolene (Dantrium) have been believed to protect the susceptible person from an episode of MH, even with inhalation anesthesia. It is preferable to detect the MH-susceptible person before exposure to an inhalation anesthetic or succinylcholine administration so that, if possible, another type of agent can be used. Nurses and nurse anesthetists are in an ideal position to help minimize morbidity and mortality from MH. Nursing points are summarized in Box 6.3.

The Porphyrias

The porphyrias are a group of errors in the heme synthesis pathway leading to excessive porphyrins or their precursors. Most of them are inherited. Each type of porphyria is due to a specific defect in a different enzyme in a step on the heme pathway. Two major classifications are hepatic and erythropoetic or erythroid. The more common hepatic group includes acute intermittent porphyria (AIP), varigate porphyria, hereditary coproporphyria, ALA dehydratase deficiency porphyria (ADP, very rare), and porphyria cutanea tarda. The erythropoietic group includes erythropoietic protoporphyria (EPP) and erythropoietic porphyria (EP). Others classify them as acute (characterized by acute attacks with neurological symptoms) and nonacute

(characterized by photosensitivity), cutaneous or noncutaneous, or by type of inheritance. Most of the porphyrias are inherited in an autosomal dominant manner, which is unusual for disorders of enzyme metabolism. Depending on the type, symptoms can vary. The major types are shown in Table 6.4.

AIP is the most common genetic type, occurring in all races. It is an autosomal dominant disorder caused by deficiency of porphobilinogen deaminase (hydroxymethylbilane synthase). It is genetically heterogeneous with multiple mutations, a few of which are most prevalent. It has an incidence of approximately 1:50,000 to 60,000 worldwide and an incidence in Scandinavia approaching 1:1,500. The prevalence of latent AIP is higher, and many cases never come to attention. AIP is usually latent until puberty or early adulthood, with few cases presenting after menopause. It is often first seen by the nurse during or following an acute attack that results from the exposure to alcohol; certain drugs (including oral contraceptives); or because of infection; fever; reduced caloric intake; or hormonal changes, especially menses and pregnancy; all of which can precipitate attacks. Clinical expression appears more frequent in females, perhaps because of contributing hormonal factors. In AIP, the most common symptoms during acute attacks are severe

TABLE 6.4 Major Types of Porphyria

Porphyria Type	Method of Inheritance	Comments
Acute intermittent porphyria (AIP)	AD	See text.
Erythropoetic porphyria	AR	Sometimes called congenital erythropoetic porphyria. Age of onset varies, but usually cutaneous sensitivity begins in early infancy. Skin blisters on sun-exposed areas with thickened skin and hypertrichosis of face and extremities, hemolysis and hemolytic anemia, splenomegaly, reddish-brown discoloration of teeth. Can be milder adult form. Deficiency of uroporphyrinogen synthase.
Hereditary coproporphyria	AD	Hepatic type due to deficiency in coproporphyrinogen oxidase. Abdominal pain; constipation prominent with acute attacks precipitated by certain drugs. May have cutaneous photosensitivity and psychiatric manifestations.
Porphyria cutanea tarda (PCT)	AD, some cases acquired	The most common type, with an incidence of 1:25,000 in North America; more common in Czechoslovakia. Usually appears in adulthood but can appear earlier. Due to deficiency of uroporphyrinogen decarboxylase. Men seem to be more frequently affected. Cutaneous findings are similar to VP. May show chronic liver disease. May be precipitated by alcohol, estrogens (including oral contraceptives), iron exposure, and polyhalogenated hydrocarbons.
Porphyria variegata (VP)	AD	Particularly frequent in South Africa (an example of the founder effect; see Chapter 3) and in Finland. Manifesting after puberty. Among White South Africans, especially the Dutch Afrikaaners, the prevalence may be as high as 1:300–400, and elsewhere is about 1:50,000–100,000. The defective enzyme is protoporphyrinogen oxidase. Acute attacks precipitated by essentially the same factors as AIP. Lead from moonshine and other sources may precipitate attacks. The clinical picture also includes skin manifestations including severe photosensitivity, skin fragility, milia, erosions, blisters, and bulla with eventual scarring. Hypertrichosis and hyperpigmentation may be seen. Effects are prominent on the face, ears, neck, and back of the hands.

abdominal pain, which may be mistaken for acute surgical abdomen such as appendicitis; nausea; vomiting; constipation; and can include abdominal distention with paralytic ileus; urinary retention; tachycardia; hypertension; neuropathy; predominantly motor that includes muscle weakness (especially of the extremities); sensory disturbances including the loss of pain and touch sensation; mental symptoms including anxiety, insomnia, depression, disorientation, hallucinations, and paranoia. Respiratory paralysis may occur. No skin manifestations are seen. Patients may become violent and are often treated with drugs such as narcotic analgesics that worsen the symptoms. The urine may become the color of port wine during an attack. Some cases of AIP present as respiratory failure. The acute attack can last several days to weeks and can become chronic at a low level. Early-onset chronic renal failure may occur, perhaps because of increased susceptibility to analgesic nephropathy, the effects of the porphyrins, or because of the hypertension.

CASE EXAMPLE

Betty Brown was an 18-year-old college freshman admitted through the emergency department. She had been attending a fraternity party and had been drinking alcoholic beverages. She began having symptoms of nausea and vomiting and complained of abdominal pain. She was in the second day of her menstrual period. Betty had passed dark urine, which initially was attributed to either her menses or trauma. She also was confused and was agitated with visual hallucinations. Tachycardia, pallor, and sweating were present, and she was reported to have had one seizure. Among the considerations for diagnosis initially was acute psychosis. It was not until later the diagnosis of AIP was made. What are some of the teaching considerations for Betty Brown?

After AIP is identified, a primary preventive effort is the avoidance of precipitating drugs, substances, and events. Drugs known to cause attacks in AIP include alcohol, aminoglutethamide, antipyrine, barbiturates, carbamezepine, carbromal, chloramphenicol, chlorpropamide, danazol, dapsone, diphenylhydantoin, ergot preparations, estrogens, glutethamide, griseofulvin, halothane, meprobamate, methyidopa, novobiocin, oral contraceptives, phenylbutazone, phenytoin, progesterone, pyrozolone, sulfonamides, theophylline, tolbutamide, and valproic acid. The nurse should question the prescription of these for a patient with known or suspected porphyria. Family members should be screened for the enzyme deficiency. Smoking, caloric restriction, and malnutrition may also precipitate attacks. Those with a deficiency should be warned to avoid the drugs and agents mentioned above, instructed as to the association between their use and acute attacks, advised to wear a medical identification bracelet indicating that they have porphyria, and instructed to avoid alcohol ingestion, oral contraceptives, and low-calorie diets. If planning surgery, they need to talk with the surgeon and anesthetist regarding porphyria, as both long periods of nothing by mouth (NPO) and certain drugs can be dangerous. In some types of porphyrias, antiseizure medication may be needed. Those with skin manifestations should take care

to avoid the sun and to use opaque sunscreens such as those with titanium dioxide. Topical antibiotics and beta carotene may also be useful. Patients may be seen in pre- or postoperative periods; during severe illness, infection, or fever; or during pregnancy. Support and encouragement are especially important in the care of these patients because the uniqueness of their symptoms may cause health professionals to think that they are faking or result in misdiagnosis.

GENOMIC APPROACHES TO DRUG THERAPY IN COMMON DISEASES

Genomic knowledge has contributed to approaches of the treatment of many diseases including cancer (its complications and metastasis) and heart disease. Some approaches center around gene therapy, while others use knowledge about the pathogenetic mechanisms underlying the disease or about individual susceptibility to certain drugs. Understanding the disease at the molecular level allows that research to be translated into clinical management.

One of the most recent examples illustrating the clinical application of molecular medicine to treatment is that of receptor and nonreceptor tyrosine kinases. Tyrosine kinases are enzymes, and there are a large number of different ones functioning in the body. The tyrosine kinases are highly expressed in many solid tumors. When expressed, they correlate with progression of disease, poor response to therapy, and poor survival rates. Several drugs act to inhibit these tyrosine kinases. The first drug to be clinically used to inhibit tyrosine kinase activity was imatinib (Gleevec/Glivec) in Philadelphia chromosome positive (Ph+) CML (discussed earlier). In these cases, the *BCR-ABL* fusion gene results in activated BCR-ABL tyrosine kinase, which is inhibited by imatinib. Imatinib is being used in newly diagnosed Ph+ adults with CML and in pediatric patients in the chronic phase whose disease has recurred after initial treatment, thus using what is known about the chromosomal translocation and its fusion gene and products.

Another example is in the treatment of non–small cell lung cancer with the drug gefitinib (Iressa). Gefitinib is aimed at the known specific molecular defect: the activation of epidermal growth factor receptor tyrosine kinase by the tumor as it grows. Gefitinib hibits tyrosine kinase. A subset of persons, about 10–15% were found to respond to gefitinib, he others did not. This subgroup was found to have certain mutant tumor variations in the EGFR tyrosine kinase that made these people sensitive to gefinib. Thus, knowledge of genetics allowed therapy to be targeted for these people.

Asthma therapy has also been an area where genetic polymorphisms have been shown to influence response to therapy. For example, one of the treatments for bronchial asthma is inhaled beta agonist therapy. When people who were receiving therapy with salbutamol, those who had the arginine arginine genotype at codon 16 of the beta adrenoceptor (about 15%) instead of glycine glycine or argnine glycine were more susceptible to asthma exacerbations when using salbutamol because of altered response to the drug. Thus, for these people, another drug could be selected.

Another example relates to statin therapy for cholesterol reduction. Statins are prescribed for millions of people. Those who had certain variants or single nucleotide polymorphisms (SNPs) in genes encoding 3-hydroxy-3methylglutaryl-coenzyme A (HMG-CoA) reductase experienced smaller reductions (about 20%) in cholesterol when treated with pravastatin than did those without them. Two tightly linked SNPs were significant and were present in 7% of people in the study. Again, another statin that was more effective could be selected for these individuals.

BiDil was an example given at the beginning of this chapter. BiDil is a combination of isosorbide dinitrate and hydralazine. It is used to treat Black patients with heart failure but is not effective in other ethnic groups. It acts by restoring low nitric oxide concentrations in the blood, and when combined with the usual therapy in a clinical trial of heart failure patients, it was found to reduce the risk of death among Black patients by 43%. One speculation was that the response may be due to ethnic differences in the underlying pathophysiology of heart failure.

Tardive dyskinesia is a condition that may be defined as involuntary abnormal movements, which may be a complication of long-term use of certain antipsychotic medications. These may consist of orofacial tics or other movements and can lead to stigmatization. Two genetic variants appear associated with the development of tardive dyskinesia, DRD3 Ser9Gly and CYP1A2*C734A. DRD3 refers to the dopamine D3 receptor gene. One polymorphism of this gene, Ser9Gly—which denotes the substitute of one amino acid (serine) for another (glycine) at position 9 of the gene—has been signif-

icantly associated with the development of tardive dyskinesia, but this varies in various ethnic populations. By using this information, patients may be able to avoid the development of distressing symptoms. Likewise, abacavir (Ziagen) is a nucleoside analogue reverse transcriptase inhibitor used to treat human immunodeficiency virus infection. It is associated with potentially fatal severe hypersensitivity reactions that occur with use in about 5–8% of patients. The strong association of possession of the HLA-B*5701 allele with susceptibility to abacavir hypersensitivity has led to the suggestion that screening take place before prescribing the drug to lower the possibility of this reaction.

Irinotecan (Camptosar) is an agent used to treat metastatic colorectal cancer by stopping cancer cell growth through inhibition of cell division. Among its adverse effects are neutropenia, with potentially fatal outcomes that may occur in up to one-third of patients treated. An enzyme, UDP glucuronosyltransferase 1A1 (UGT1A1), is involved in catabolizing the active metabolite in irinotecan. More than 30 variant alleles have been identified, including a dinucleotide repeat that influences gene expression. About 10% of the population has the homozygous UGT1A1*28 genotype (also called the 7/7 genotype) and therefore lower functional enzyme activity. These people have a more than nine-fold greater risk of developing grade 4 neutropenia than do those with the normal 6/6 genotype or the heterozygous genotype when receiving the standard dose of irinotecan. Thus, another regimen can be selected for these people until it is known if there is a safe but effective dose they can be given.

ETHICAL, LEGAL, AND SOCIAL ISSUES RELATED TO PHARMACOGENOMICS

As the field of pharmacogenomics has evolved, various ethical concerns have been raised. Some concerns are applicable to other aspects of genetics such as confidentiality and the potential for misuse of genetic information with the potential for stigmatization for various groups. This is because the genotype of an individual specifically pertaining to his/her disease and treatment would be known to the practitioner perhaps just by the drug he/she was receiving.

Further, the potential for selective drug development to benefit specific ethnic groups with a particular frequency of a certain genotype related to disease and treatment might exist at the expense of other ethnic groups or genotypes. This might also occur for those who can afford tailored treatments. As an example, in a clinical trial, if only a small percentage of participants can tolerate a certain drug dosage, then this dosage is likely to become the standard. This means that the larger percentage of persons will not receive larger doses of this drug, which might be more effective and be well tolerated by this larger group. By differentiating compounds based on genotyping, drug therapy can be more effectively targeted. This could create the possibility of insurance companies that might deny coverage to persons who had genotypes requiring more costly treatment for a specific disease. Conversely, those who are in low-risk populations with regard to pharmacogenetic disorders might pay higher premiums because coverage was extended to those in high-risk groups without penalties. Implications also exist in regard to employment and workplace exposures and coverage.

END NOTES

Pharmacogenetics and pharmacogenomics are still young, but their importance is increasingly recognized. Entire journals such as *Pharmacogenomics*, *American Journal of Pharmacogenomics*, *Pharmacogenomics Journal*, and *Current Pharmacogenomics* are devoted to this topic. For the most part, persons taking drugs with broad therapeutic ranges and safety profiles will not usually show significant clinical consequences even if they are poor metabolizers. However, when they are taking drugs with a narrow therapeutic index, such as many antidepressants or isoniazid, the genetic polymorphism becomes clinically important. Eventually the field of pharmacogenomics will allow the determination of a genetic profiles for pharmacological treatment of a specific disease. This will allow drug therapy to be tailored to genetic profiles for maximum effectiveness and also determine the best dosage and allow the withholding of drugs that might be ineffective or result in side effects. Another advantage would be that fewer medications might be needed for a given condition, and therefore patient adherence would be enhanced.

Nurses have observed that different individuals receiving the same dose of the same drug can exhibit different degrees of effective response and can experience variation in the type and degree of side effects for no readily apparent reason. Nurses are in an excellent position to observe interindividual differences in response to drugs that can lead to further research. These will add to the knowledge of the inborn error of drug metabolism and also to the further delineation of genetic diversity of metabolic functions that have both theoretical interest and clinical importance.

An important pharmacogenetic and pharmacogenomic implication in testing new therapeutic agents is for testing the agent in populations of different ethnic backgrounds, as the information obtained regarding metabolism, effectiveness, and side effects cannot be wholly transferred from one population to another. Information regarding polymorphisms and genetic variability is beginning to be incorporated into drug development trials. It is important to remember that the usual effective dose of a drug when given to any individual patient may be effective, ineffective, or even toxic depending on his/her genetic make-up, and the drug itself may be ineffective, as in the 6–10% of those who are unresponsive to codeine. Thus, in regard to drug therapy, one size does not fit all. Recent moves to reduce costs by limiting hospital formularies can have unintended pharmacogenetic consequences. In the future, one can envision designer medications tailored to specific genotypes and labeled as such while others will need to be avoided by certain genotypes. The marketing of DNA chips for both *CYP2C6* and *CYP2C19* to identify poor drug metabolizers is just the beginning of the application of this technology to clinical drug therapy.

KEY POINTS AND QUESTIONS FOR DISCUSSION

- Genetic factors play important roles in response to medications.
- Genetic knowledge is being used to design drugs based on the molecular defect and on designing drugs specific to genotype.
- What are the implications of disclosure of genotypes related to pharmacogenomics?
- It is more likely that female homozygotes for G6PD deficiency will be identified than for other X-linked recessive disorders. What are the reasons for this?

7

Assessing Patients With a Genetic "Eye"
Histories, Pedigrees, and Physical Assessment

The initial recognition of the need for genetic evaluation may arise when an alert practitioner suspects a genetic problem because of family history, physical findings, observation, discussion with the family, or knowledge of a related problem in a known relative. For example, the nurse may notice that the mother of a child being evaluated because of a problem such as cleft palate also has another minor malformation such as clinodactyly (incurving of fifth finger). Such an observation in a family being seen at our cleft palate center led to the uncovering of a four-generation history of an autosomal dominant disorder with mild expression in most members but severe expression in the child. However, at an early point in health care encounters, the taking of an accurate family history can be an important starting point for the detection of genetic contributions to disease or of a genetic condition in a family.

HISTORIES

Family history assessment is a valuable tool that is underused in clinical practice. The importance of family histories to identify conditions in families that may be inherited and require further follow-up, as well as assisting in risk assessment, is enjoying a resurgence. A proper family history can be taken by the nurse and should include at least three generations. Some family history instruments may be found on the website for the National Coalition for Health Professional Education in Genetics (http://www.nchpeg.org) and the American Medical Association (http://www.ama.org).

Exact questions to be asked depend on the reason for the evaluation, the client's responses to questions asked, previous information, and information from observation, laboratory data, or physical assessment. Therefore, it is difficult to prescribe exact questions to be asked when taking the history, except for standard baseline data. Sometimes printed forms that can be filled in by the client or the client's parents are used. Then further questions are designed on the basis of these responses. Other practitioners prefer to collect history information through interview. This can be time-consuming. The incorporation of the history and pedigree into general medical practice could result in the identification of genetic risk factors not otherwise identified.

Family and Health Histories

The importance of family histories to identify conditions in families that may be inherited and require further follow-up as well as assisting in risk assessment is enjoying a resurgence and emphasis in primary as well as specialized practices. The nature of the problem and the answers to questions asked of the family seeking counseling determine the extent of information needed. Some of the questions given below present more detail than may be possible in a general office visit. But they can be important in a thorough genetic investigation. When the condition is in a child, both members of the parental couple should be present if possible in order to get accurate information about both sides of the family. Even if one partner has consulted with the other, the relevant questions may not have been asked. A history should cover at least three generations, including the grandparents, siblings, half-siblings, parents, offspring, aunts, uncles, and cousins. Thus first-, second-, and third-degree relatives should be considered, and more if warranted. Information to be gathered in taking the family history includes:

- The correct legal name of the counselees, including the maiden names of the female members (the same or even very similar names may indicate consanguinity, which the interviewer can then pursue).
- Racial, ethnic, and country-of-origin information (many genetic disorders are more frequent among certain groups).
- Place of birth (certain possible environmental exposures or the suggestion of consanguinity).
- Baseline information, such as address and telephone number.
- Occupation (certain ones suggest the possibility of genotoxic exposures).
- Date of birth, which can be used in determining risk for the development of a disorder. For example, if the brother of an affected person with Huntington disease is the grandfather of the counselee and is 75 years of age and unaffected, the chances of his having the gene are essentially nil, which means that the grandchild will not be at risk.
- Current and past health status should be ascertained and verified when necessary for the problem for each individual in the pedigre. Specific health problems known to have a heritable component should be asked about when ascertaining the status of the family members.
- Age and cause of death of deceased individuals.
- The presence of birth defects, intellectual and developmental disabilities, familial traits, or similarly affected family members.
- Specific inquiries should be made about offspring, miscarriages, stillbirths, and severe infant and childhood illnesses and deaths for each eligible member, even if the inquiries do not appear related to the problem at hand.
- Whether anyone in the family was a twin or multiple, if all the children are the natural children of both parents, and if any prior matings occurred, and if so, any relevant history to the present problem.

Information gathered from the history is used to prepare the pedigree. All information should be confirmed by medical records, laboratory data, photographs, autopsy reports, and other objective methods whenever possible.

Other questions may depend on the replies and on observation. For example, if the index case has osteogenesis imperfecta type III, then when taking the history, the interviewer should inquire specifically about some features of the disorder that might suggest the presence of the condition in a milder form, such as blue sclera, fractures, deafness, discolored teeth, and "loose" joints in other family members. Some questions might be age dependent. One might ask whether at a certain age, any family member showed a specific symptom that relates to the problem at hand. The age of onset of any health problem should also be recorded. Such information is useful in determining whether a person may be at risk for an inherited type of cancer. The health care professional should ask if further questions are based on answers to initial questions. The family history may be useful in devising health prevention. Men with a family history of prostate cancer should have earlier screenings more often than others, for example. Family history is discussed further in this chapter in the "Pedigrees" section.

Reasons for obtaining a negative family history when one child is affected with a genetic disorder within a family can include any of the following:

- The disorder is a new mutation.
- The child was conceived by artificial insemination.
- The child's mother received a donated ovum.
- The child was adopted.
- The family is very small.
- The father is not the biological father.
- There is nonpenetrance in a parent.
- There is minimal expression of the trait in a relative who was missed.
- The trait is rare.
- The person giving the history lacks full knowledge.
- The informant deliberately withholds information.
- The interviewer fails to ask critical questions.
- There is the presence of a chromosome abnormality such as a submicroscopic deletion in the affected person, allowing the expression of a mutant gene present on the other chromosome.
- Gonadal mosaicism is present (see Chapter 4).
- Uniparental disomy is present (see Chapter 4).

Therefore, a negative family history does not rule out a genetic component.

Environmental, Occupational, and Social Histories

Environmental exposures can result from the person's primary occupation, second job, residence location, volunteer activities (e.g., firefighting), recreational activities and hobbies, and, for children, anyplace where they spend time after school or in day care such as a grandparent's home. Information can be gathered in a written form with a follow-up interview or by interview directly, depending on the information collected or the problem at hand. Information should be gathered for both the client and the other persons living in the household, for example, the person doing the laundry may be exposed to fibers on the clothing of the worker. Information to be gathered includes name of the employing company, job title, kind of work done, work schedule, and number of hours worked each week. The interviewer should ask about the kinds of materials that the person is exposed to on the job. It may be more productive to ask about specific materials, such as radiation, chemicals, fumes, dust, fibers, tobacco, gasses, temperature extremes, microorganisms, and vibrations. If the person is not sure, then it may be necessary to get data sheets from the employer about specific substances, depending how critical the information is to the problem at hand. In one case in my experience, a woman with a lung lesion had mesothelioma, a rare form of cancer, in her case involving the lining of the pleural sac associated with asbestos exposure. Her husband was a heating and cooling contractor, and she washed his clothes every day. The asbestos fibers she inhaled from this contact probably acted on a genetic susceptibility to allow this tumor to be expressed. Interestingly, he was free of this condition.

The same type of information should be ascertained for secondary jobs, schools, hobbies, and so on. Sometimes the job itself can alert the interviewer to possibilities of toxic exposure. Clients should also be asked about contact with domestic animals (e.g., cats, dogs, birds) and about the proximity to any farm animals on the job or at home. If it is not clear what the job or hobby entails, then the interviewer can ask exactly what a person with that job title does or ask him/her to describe a typical workday verbally or in writing. Any affirmative answers

about exposure should be followed up to determine the duration of exposure, the frequency, and the last time the person was exposed; whether the person was eating, drinking, or smoking at the time; and the concentration of exposure if possible. Ill effects such as skin reactions should be asked about specifically. A worker who has been noncompliant in the use of protective devices may not wish to tell the interviewer about it, and skill may be needed to elicit the needed information. The person should be asked how long he/she has been at this job and what kind of work he/she did on the last job if pertinent. Someone who is not currently working should be asked what kind of job he/she had last, or what kinds of work he/she has done for the longest period in order to obtain the needed information.

Answers that suggest increased risks should be followed up. For example, a woman who is considering pregnancy and works in a pet boarding kennel can be advised on safe methods of disposal of excreta and handling the animals to minimize her own exposure without jeopardizing her employment. Information to be obtained regarding the place of residence should include its location, the composition of the household, the source of drinking water or food (especially in rural areas), type of community, the proximity of any factories, knowledge of any chemical spills or waste exposure, noticeable air pollution, the type of insulation and heating, insecticide or pesticide exposure, products used to clean the home, and other data as relevant. Social data should be obtained as appropriate. Because exposure to various agents has detrimental effects on reproduction, the client should be specifically asked if he/she or his/her partner have had any problems in this area, including difficulty in conception, changes in libido or menses, spontaneous abortions, stillbirths, infertility, intrauterine growth restrictions, infants with birth defects or intellectual disabilities, and children with developmental disabilities or childhood malignancies. If a problem appears to be job or environmentally related, the client should be asked if anyone at work or in his/her neighborhood has had similar problems (see Chapter 12). Persons should also be asked about any military service and what it entailed.

Medication and Drug Use

It is helpful to ask the client to bring a list of drugs he/she has taken in the relevant time period. If the interview is after the birth of an affected child, then this period should include a few months before pregnancy in both the male and female partner and that during the pregnancy in the female. In some cases, the client can bring in his/her medications and containers. Clients should be asked about prescription drugs, over-the-counter medications, home remedies, botanicals, and "folk" medications. Specific medications can be asked about if they are known to be popular among persons of the client's ethnic group or geographic location. Another method to ascertain drug use is to have a checklist of common types of drugs and ask the client to indicate the ones that he/she has used. If responses are negative, the interviewer can ask about vitamins and mineral supplements, or ask what the client does for headache, stomachache, menstrual cramps, and so on. Many clients may omit items that they do not consider to be drugs or medications. There is also reluctance to discuss street or illicit drug use. Use of social drugs such as caffeine, alcohol, or cigarette smoking must also be explored. For each drug taken, the dose, frequency of use, reason for use, duration, and approximate dates should be obtained. Facilitation of accurate assessment of drug and medication use can be accomplished by teaching and encouraging clients to keep an accurate list of all those taken. The practitioner should also keep a record of prescription and recommended drugs. Cigarette smoking and alcohol and drug use in pregnancy and prevention of ill effects from such use are discussed in Chapter 8. Detailed questions can follow a positive response to a question about alcohol use, such as, "Do you ever drink wine, beer, or mixed drinks?" A nutritional diary that represents what the person has eaten for a week can be used to suggest nutritional concerns. The client and family members should be asked about any past drug or food allergies or reactions. This may elicit a genetic susceptibility or predisposition that can be used to prevent problems in the individual or other relatives, as well as to provide information about the current problem. The client should also be asked whether he/she has ever been told not to take a certain medication or eat a certain food. See Chapter 8 for more information on drugs in pregnancy.

Reproductive, Pregnancy, and Birth History

There is some overlap between the reproductive and family history, as all stillbirths, miscarriages, abortions, infant deaths, or offspring should be noted when discussing the family. Information should be obtained for all pregnancies, but one resulting in an affected child should be considered in depth especially if the diagnosis is unknown. The following information should be included:

- Age at each pregnancy for both parents
- Weight gain
- Exposure to radiation, drugs and medications and alcohol, as well as smoking habits for both parents
- Outcome of each pregnancy, including miscarriages, stillbirths, or infant deaths
- Contraceptive use immediately prior to pregnancy
- Vaginal bleeding or discharge during the pregnancy
- Occurrence of any accidents, illnesses, fevers, rashes, or other health problems during pregnancy
- Work, hobbies, or travel of both parents that might have led to toxic exposure
- Any medical treatments during pregnancy
- Nutrition and food habits, including pica
- Type of delivery
- Presence of blood group incompatibilities (see Chapters 3 and 8)
- Health of all infants previously born, including low birth weight and prematurity
- If all offspring had the same parents
- Medical history of chronic disease, infections, or sexually transmitted disease
- Information about fetal movement, uterine size, and details of labor and delivery (e.g., the amount of amniotic fluid present, length of labor, type of anesthetic and perinatal medications, if any)
- Apgar score, birth weight, and head circumference
- Whether the client has had any difficulty becoming pregnant
- Whether there is any other relevant information that the client feels should be known

Answers to these questions determine the direction of further questions. One of the reasons for asking for this information is to try to determine whether a problem such as intellectual disability could have been caused by environmental factors during the perinatal period. If this seems a likely possibility,

hen this line of questioning must be followed fur-
her. This information should be recorded in detail,
for example, for radiation, the time of pregnancy
during which exposure occurred, the part of the
body x-rayed, the reason for the X-ray, and so on.
Confirmation through records is necessary for accuracy. Detailed prenatal risk assessment forms
have been devised. However, in general, those who
are at greatest risk for a poor pregnancy outcome
related to birth defects and genetic disorders are in
these categories:

- Increased maternal age (35 years and above)
- Increased paternal age (40–45 years and above)
- Decreased maternal or paternal age (especial-
  ly below 15 and 20 years, respectively, which is
  believed in part to be due to nutritional needs
  of the young mother versus the fetus)
- Rapid consecutive pregnancies
- Difficulties with reproduction
- History of alcohol abuse, drug intake, or
  smoking
- Underweight or overweight
- Poor nutrition
- Multiple gestation
- Oligohydramnios or polyhydramnios
- Previous unfavorable pregnancy outcome
- Maternal metabolic or genetic disease
- Maternal chronic disease, especially seizure
  disorders; or infectious or sexually transmitted
  disease in pregnancy
- Maternal-fetal incompatibility
- Previous infant weighing 10 pounds or over or
  with growth restriction as well as those factors
  listed as indications for prenatal diagnosis (see
  Chapter 8)

If the woman is currently pregnant, the date of
the last menstrual period and the expected date of
delivery should be obtained. Large prenatal or pre-
pregnancy clinics may have little time to take detailed histories or conduct in-depth interviews with
every client. Some clinics have attempted to devise a
short questionnaire that acts as a screening device
for potential genetic problems for the pregnancy.
When a client answers affirmatively to any of the
specific questions, the chart is flagged for an in-
depth interview with a geneticist, genetic counselor,
or genetics nurse. The interview may need to be immediate if the need for prenatal diagnosis appears
possible, or it can be scheduled at the next prenatal

visit. Information needing follow-up that can be ascertained on such screening tools are maternal age
of 35 or over; paternal age of 40 or over; specific
ethnic groups with higher risk of known detectable
disorders; previous stillbirth, infant death, or two or
more miscarriages; the birth of a previous child or
member of the family who has a birth defect or genetic disorder; previous prenatal diagnosis; drug or
alcohol use; maternal disease such as diabetes mellitus or maternal phenylketonuria; family history of
retardation or anemia; or any particular problem or
concern that the mother identifies. These question-
naires are usually set up in a simple yes-no format
using simple language. They may need to be in the
native language of the client.

Not infrequently, the taking of a pregnancy history follows the birth of a child with a defect of some
type or a stillbirth. Thus, retrospective information
about the pregnancy is likely to be influenced not
only by the same factors responsible for obtaining a
negative family history, but also by feelings of guilt
(real or imagined) as well as other emotions.

PEDIGREES

A pedigree is essentially a pictorial representation or
diagram of the family history. Clear information
obtained from the family histories can:

- Allow the visualization of relationships of
  affected individuals to the family seeking
  counseling,
- Pinpoint any vital persons who should be examined or tested,
- Elucidate the pattern of inheritance in a specific family,
- Allow for various types of complex pedigree
  analysis and linkage studies if needed and
  applicable,
- Allow other professionals working with the
  family to quickly see what information has
  been collected on which family members, thus
  saving unnecessary repetition and facilitating
  the collection of further data,
- Facilitate the brief notation of other data relevant to effective counseling, such as family
  interactions.

The widespread use of pedigrees requires the
nurse to understand their meaning and to be able to

construct one from a family history. Computer programs specifically for pedigree construction are available. Symbols commonly used in pedigree construction are illustrated in Figure 7.1. There may be some variation in the use of some symbols because there is no formal standard. The family names or

initials should be on the pedigree along with the date, the person who is giving the family history, the name and title of the pedigree recorder, the date of the pedigree, and dates for any subsequent additions. Some guidelines for pedigree construction and interpretation are in Box 7.1.

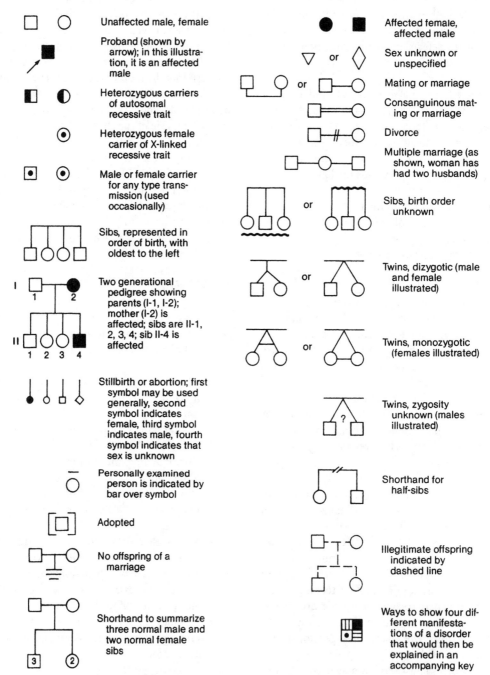

FIGURE 7.1   Commonly used pedigree symbols.

BOX 7.1

Rules for Pedigree Construction

- Pedigree construction usually begins in the middle of the sheet of paper to allow enough room.
- Males are represented by a square and females by a circle (if the person is affected with the disorder in question, the symbol is shaded in).
- An arrow, sometimes with a "P" at the shaft end, represents the proband or propositus, and the pedigree drawing usually begins with this person (if the counselee is different, sometimes a "C" is placed under that person's symbol).
- For a mating or marriage, a horizontal line is drawn between a square and a circle. Sometimes a diagonal line is used for convenience. Traditionally, males in a couple are drawn on the left.
- Offspring are suspended vertically from the mating line and are drawn in order of birth.
- Generations are symbolized by roman numerals.
- The order of birth of siblings within a family is indicated by the use of arabic numbers (the sibship line is sometimes drawn more thickly than the mating line; if birth order is unknown, a wavy line is used).
- The name of each person (maiden names in the case of married women) and date of birth should be included.
- A pedigree should include at least the parents, offspring, siblings, aunts, uncles, grandparents, and first cousins of the person seeking counseling.
- Pedigrees may indicate unmentioned consanguinity or suggest it because of the occurrence of the same name on both sides of the family or because of the same place of birth of an ancestor that is revealed by the history or pedigree.
- When the rough pedigree is redrawn, a mate's family history may be omitted if it adds nothing to the elucidation of the family study, but it should be retained in the file.
- The pedigree should be dated and signed with the name, credentials, and position of the person drawing it.
- Pedigrees can be shortened by grouping large numbers of similar-sexed normal children in one symbol.
- Causes of death or health problems should be noted.
- Adoptions are shown by brackets.
- For assisted reproduction, the donor (D) is drawn to the right of the female partner with a diagonal line to the pregnancy symbol or child. For a surrogate, a straight line is suggested to the pregnancy symbol and a diagonal line follows from the couple.
- For evaluation, both clinical and laboratory data may be listed as an E. E_1, E_2, and so on to denote each individual evaluation defined in the key. A question mark is used if results are not documented or available, and an asterisk is used next to the pedigree symbol to denote a documented evaluation. If the exam is negative, a minus sign is used, a plus sign is used for a positive examination, and if uninformative, a *u* is used.

As part of the examination of the pedigree, one should look for consanguinity, male-to-male transmission, female-to-male transmission, the ratio of male-to-female siblings, whether males and females are affected in equal numbers, the birth order of affected persons, and other characteristics of the patterns of inheritance as discussed in Chapter 4.

Sometimes the mode of inheritance cannot be determined from the history and pedigree because of small family sizes or because there are no instances of certain types of transmission (there may not be the presence of a critical transmission). Sample pedigrees for different modes of inheritance are shown in Figure 7.2.

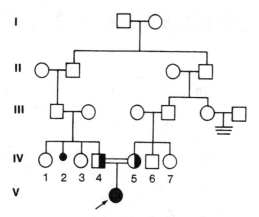

Autosomal-recessive pedigree of T family illustrating consanguinity; the diagnosis indicates that the parents, IV-4 and IV-5, are obligate heterozygotes.

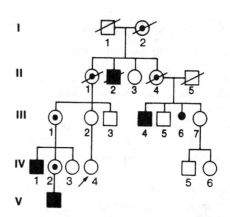

Pedigree illustrating X-linked recessive inheritance; the status of III-2 and IV-4 is not yet known and cannot be determined from the pedigree, although IV-2 must be a carrier because both her brother and son are affected, and retrospectively, this marks III-1 and II-1 as carriers.

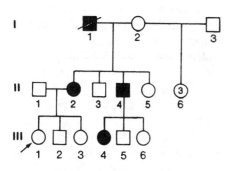

Pedigree illustrating autosomal dominant inheritance in Huntington disease; the age of III-1 must be taken into account when risk is determined.

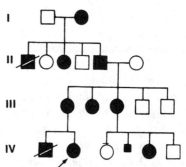

Pedigree illustrating X-linked dominant inheritance; note that all daughters of the affected father are affected, and no sons of the affected father are affected; all affected males have affected mothers.

FIGURE 7.2   Examples of pedigrees in different types of inheritance.

CLINICAL, DEVELOPMENTAL, AND PHYSICAL ASSESSMENT

Information from the history can suggest specific areas for comprehensive physical assessment. Also, certain findings should suggest the possibility of a genetic component and the need for further evaluation. Clinical clues that suggest the need for further evaluation and testing also depend on the age of the person. A newborn girl who has lymphedema should have a chromosome analysis because of the possibility of Turner syndrome (see Chapter 9); however, the lymphedema rapidly disappears, and the next time of suspicion may be when menstruation and the development of secondary sex characteristics are delayed. Likewise, Wilson disease (an autosomal recessive disorder of copper metabolism) should be considered in the child or adolescent who experiences acute liver failure. The appearance of certain features may be considered normal at a certain age and deviant at another

Wrinkled skin in a 65-year-old is unremarkable. In a 1-year-old infant, it might suggest the possibility of progeria (a very rare disorder involving features of early aging). An early age of onset of an adult-type tumor or a common disease such as coronary heart disease should suggest the possibility of a strong genetic influence in this family and should be investigated. The cry of the newborn may reflect nervous system pathology. Certain odors and other typical signs and symptoms are associated with specific biochemical abnormalities especially in the infant or child. These are discussed in Chapter 9.

Between 13% and 39.9% of otherwise normal newborns will have one minor anomaly; less than 1% will have two. Most newborns with three or more may not be normal. The occurrence of two and, especially, three minor malformations in an otherwise normal infant should alert the practitioner to search carefully for one or more major defects and consider chromosome studies (see Chapter 5). Sometimes the major anomalies are not visible (e.g., congenital heart disease) or not yet apparent (e.g., intellectual disability).

Physical examinations of children and adolescents can provide an opportunity for detection of disorders making their appearance around puberty and even provide a forum for preconception counseling for adolescent girls. For girls or women with significant menorrhagia, it is recommended that they be screened for von Willebrand disease (a hereditary bleeding disorder characterized by deficiency of von Willebrand factor needed for optimum platelet adhesiveness), since about one-third of adolescent girls presenting with menorrhagia at menarche were found to have this or for factor V Leiden deficiency (an inherited thrombophilia). It is important to screen before initiation of oral contraceptive therapy since this may mask the diagnosis. Sometimes these examinations take place in a sports physical setting, where screening is rushed and there is pressure to approve a child for sports. It is important, however, to assess the child for such conditions as Marfan syndrome (see Chapter 10) and for other potential causes of genetically based potential impairment.

The objective of this section is to discuss those measures and observations that are of particular importance in genetic disorders rather than physical assessment in general.

Measurements

Measurements used in the detection or confirmation of genetic disorders and congenital anomalies include many that are too complicated or too time-consuming to be practical in the routine examination of the normal infant and child but are useful when an abnormality is suspected. The extent to which the nurse uses such measurements depends on his/her area of practice. For the normal infant and child, height, weight, and head circumference are usual. Other measurements, such as inter-inner canthal distance, inter-outer canthal distance, inter-pupillary distances, upper and lower body segment ratios (U/L), arm span, chest circumference, inter-nipple distance, ear measurements, philtrum measures, palpebral fissure slant, and various craniofacial measures are done only when suspicion so dictates. Craniofacial examination is often evaluated by cephalometrics; three-dimensional craniofacial surface imaging from CT scans, magnetic resonance imaging, and computer-driven techniques.

Usually the practitioner begins with the child's height and weight. The same technique should always be used, as well as the same standardized tables. Measurements should ideally be made at the same time of day. One unusual result should not cause immediate concern, but serial measurements should be kept so that growth velocity can be examined. Growth velocity is greatest in infants, falling until puberty, when a growth spurt occurs. A growth rate of 5 cm per year has been recommended as the lower limit of normal. Children below the third percentile in height who are growing at a rate below 5 cm per year require investigation. When using charts for the comparison of a given child's measurements to standardized tables, it is important to remember that they must be derived from data obtained from the same ethnic group and country and not be based on outdated standards. Parental stature and measurements, the child's birth weight, and maturity should always be considered when evaluating unusual results. Isolated measurements should not be completely relied on but rather the overall rate and pattern considered. Various studies have demonstrated that correlation still persists between birth weight and height and current parameters even in late adolescence and early adulthood. If it appears that height is abnormal, then the ratio of upper body segment to lower body segment, limb lengths, and arm span should be determined to ascertain whether disproportionate growth is present and, if so, of what type. It is important for diagnosis, treatment, and counseling to determine the type of growth disorder. Many chromosome and metabolic disorders have failure to thrive or altered growth as a component. These merit full investigation.

Other growth disorders may be noted. Macrosomia may be seen in the offspring of diabetic mothers. Unusual obesity, associated with hypotonia, and later hypogonadism is a feature of Prader-Willi syndrome (see Chapter 9). Failure to thrive may be organic or nonorganic, and the cause should be determined. The failure of needed substances to be utilized results in failure to thrive in many inherited biochemical disorders. It is important to inquire about feeding practices, gastrointestinal symptoms, and food intolerance. Fatty, foul-smelling stools can indicate cystic fibrosis, whereas bulky, foul stools after weaning from breast milk may indicate acrodermatitis enteropathica. Delayed or precocious puberty can be assessed by means of criteria for pubertal stage attainment. Hypogonadism and delayed puberty are frequent components of many genetic disorders and must be fully investigated.

Head size depends in part on, and reflects the growth of the brain, and therefore it relates to ultimate intelligence. In measuring head circumference, an accurate, nonstretchable tape measure should be used. The child's head must be held still, and the tape is placed over the most prominent part of the occiput, posteriorly, and just above the supraorbital ridges, or eyebrows, anteriorly. The tape is held snugly, and the measurement is read over the forehead. At birth, the average value is about 35 cm with a variation of 1.2 cm above or below in over half of normal full-term infants. There is about a 5 cm increase in the next four months, and an increase of 5 cm more by 1 year of age. Head size should always be evaluated within the context of other factors such as body size, weight, and chest circumference. These should approximate each other in percentile position. For example, an otherwise very small child whose head circumference is above the 50th percentile could have hydrocephalus. Variation in size can be caused by familial characteristics and racial or ethnic group, as well as from other causes. A large head size can result from

hydrocephalus, Tay-Sachs disease (see Chapter 9), a tumor, megaloencephaly, or a large-sized infant. A small head size can result from microcephaly, craniostenosis, developmental disability, or a small-sized infant. Any deviation in size can be reassessed by serial measurements. The earlier in development that developmental disability occurs, the more marked the microcephaly is. Because microcephaly is a relatively common finding after intrauterine infection, this would alert the clinician to look for other common symptoms or signs of congenital infection, such as chorioretinitis (inflammation of the retina), which is seen in congenital toxoplasmosis and cytomegalovirus disease.

Appraisal and Assessment

One should always begin with a general appraisal and observation before conducting a systematic assessment. The photographing of any unusual features provides a permanent record, allows for consultation, and permits later study. Attention should be paid to any concerns of the parents about slow development. Attention should also be paid to the child who is so quiet that his/her parents "hardly know they have a baby." Children with xeroderma pigmentosa (an autosomal recessive disorder with extreme sensitivity to sunlight that leads to malignancies) often cry on sun exposure, an event that occurs before any other signs and symptoms. Parents' recall of developmental milestones, except for walking, is generally thought to be unreliable. Therefore, it may be a good idea for hospitals or offices to give the parents a book in which to record important developmental milestones. Many developmental screening tools and techniques are available for such assessment. During assessment, particular attention should be paid to the head and face area, the skin, and the limbs, because the majority of deviant development has some reflection in these areas. Clinical findings seen in some genetic disorders are organized by region in Table 7.1. This is not an inclusive list.

Indications suggesting specific disorders (e.g., unusual infections in childhood in immune disorders) and those that should suggest the need for further evaluation are given throughout the book and at the end of this chapter. The frequency of syndrome association in blindness, deafness, cleft lip or palate, failure to thrive, and developmental

TABLE 7.1   Selected Minor and Moderate Clinical Findings Suggesting Genetic Disorders

Location and Finding	Examples of Genetic Disorders and Syndromes With These Findings
Head, neck, face	
Macroglossia	Beckwith-Wiedemann syndrome
Lip pits	Van der Woude syndrome
Smooth tongue	Familial dysautonomia
"Tongue thrusting"	Familial dysautonomia
Short philtrum	DiGeorge syndrome; orofaciodigital syndrome
Smooth philtrum	Fetal alcohol syndrome
Long philtrum	Robinow syndrome
Micrognathia	Cornelia de Lange syndrome, Robin syndrome
Broad nose	Fetal hydantoin syndrome
Low nasal bridge	Achondroplasia, Down syndrome, Kniest syndrome
Prominent nose	Rubenstein-Taybi syndrome, trichorhinophalangeal syndrome
Malar hypoplasia	Bloom syndrome
Low-set ears	Potter syndrome
Facial asymmetry	Klippel-Feil syndrome
Frontal bossing	Achondroplasia
Coarse facies	Mucopolysaccharide disorders
Lip pigmentation	Peutz-Jeghers syndrome
Teeth	
Natal teeth	Ellis–van Creveld syndrome, Hallermann-Streiff syndrome
Large teeth	47,XYY
Conical teeth	Ellis–van Creveld syndrome
Hyperdontia (supernumerary)	Gardner syndrome, orofaciodigital syndrome
Reddish or purple teeth	Some porphyrias
Opalescent, brownish teeth	Osteogenesis imperfecta
Hypodontia	Hypohydrotic ectodermal dysplasia
Eyes, ocular region	
Nystagmus	Chédiak-Higashi syndrome, albinism
Cataract (infancy)	Galactosemia
Cherry-red spot (macula)	Tay-Sachs disease (infantile)
Setting sun sign	Hydrocephalus
Blue sclera	Osteogenesis imperfecta, Roberts syndrome
Aniridia	Wilms tumor
Glaucoma	Lowe syndrome
Retinal detachment	Marfan syndrome, Ehlers-Danlos syndrome
Hypertelorism	Aarskog syndrome
Hypotelorism	Trisomy 13
Ptosis	Aarskog syndrome, Smith-Lemli-Opitz syndrome, Steinert myotonic dystrophy
Up-slanted palpebral fissure	Down syndrome, Pfeiffer syndrome
Down-slanted palpebral fissure	Coffin-Lowry syndrome
Short palpebral fissure	Aarskog syndrome, Treacher Collins syndrome
Night blindness	Refsum syndrome
Epicanthal folds	Down syndrome
Kayser-Fleischer ring	Wilson disease
Iris coloboma	Cat-eye syndrome
Arcus corneae (child)	Familial hypercholesterolemia IIa
Synophrys	Cornelia de Lange syndrome

(continues)

TABLE 7.1 (*Continued*)

Location and Finding	Examples of Genetic Disorders and Syndromes With These Findings
Limbs, hands, feet, trunk	
Arachnodactyly	Marfan syndrome, homocystinuria
Polydactyly	Ellis–van Creveld syndrome, trisomy 13
Broad thumb/toe	Rubenstein–Taybi syndrome
Syndactyly	Apert syndrome, Poland syndrome
Joint hyperextensibility	Marfan syndrome, Ehlers-Danlos syndrome
Asymmetric shortening	Conradi-Hunermann syndrome
Clenched hand	Trisomy 13
Clinodactyly	Down syndrome
Brachydactyly	Turner syndrome, Silver syndrome
Crusted lesions on fingertips	Richner-Hanhart syndrome
Broad, shieldlike chest	Turner syndrome
Pectus excavatum	Marfan syndrome, homocystinuria
Skin, hair, nails	
Hirsutism	Cornelia de Lange syndrome, leprechaunism, Hurler syndrome
Widow's peak	Optiz syndrome
Upswept, crewlike hair	Microcephaly
Sparse hair	Ellis–van Creveld syndrome, Menkes syndrome
White streak	Waardenburg syndrome, type 1
White hair	Albinism
Low hairline	Turner syndrome
Stubby, wiry, coarse hair	Menkes syndrome
Xanthomas	Hypercholesterolemia Ia
Café-au-lait spots	Neurofibromatosis
Photosensitivity	Bloom syndrome, the porphyrias, xeroderma pigmentosum
Hyperelastic skin	Ehlers-Danlos syndrome
Loose skin	Cutis laxa, Ehlers-Danlos syndrome
Brownish-yellow skin	Gaucher disease (adult)
Shagreen patch	Tuberous sclerosis
Leaf-shaped white macules	Tuberous sclerosis
"Marble swirls"	Incontinentia pigmenti
Large pores (orange-peel)	Conradi-Hunermann syndrome
Thick skin	Hurler syndrome
Telangiectasia	Ataxia-telangiectasia
Port wine hemangioma	Sturge-Weber syndrome, von Hippel–Lindau disease
Nail hypoplasia	Ellis–van Creveld syndrome
Transverse crease	Down syndrome, Seckel syndrome
Blisters	Epidermolysis bullosa
Growth disorders	
Macrosomia	Beckwith-Wiedemann syndrome
Obesity	Prader-Willi syndrome, Laurence-Moon syndrome
Cry (infant)	
Hoarse, weak	Farber disease
Catlike, mewing	Cri-du-chat syndrome (5p–)
Low-pitched, growling	Cornelia de Lange syndrome

TABLE 7.1   (*Continued*)

Location and Finding	Examples of Genetic Disorders and Syndromes With These Findings
Genitalia	
Hypogonadism	Klinefelter syndrome, Prader-Willi syndrome
Pigmented areas on penis	Bannayan-Riley-Ruvalcaba syndrome
Cryptorchidism	Aarskog syndrome, Rubinstein-Taybi syndrome, Noonan syndrome
Macro-orchidism	Fragile X syndrome
Ambiguous genitalia	Congenital adrenal hyperplasia
Bifid scrotum	Fryns syndrome
Labia majora hypoplasia	Prader-Willi syndrome, 18q- syndrome
Double vagina	18q- syndrome
Micropenis	Klinefelter syndrome, 48,XXXY syndrome
Enlarged clitoris	Fraser syndrome
Other	
Omphalocele	Beckwith-Wiedemann syndrome
Hernia	Hurler syndrome, Beckwith-Wiedemann syndrome
Seizures	Menkes syndrome, Sturge-Weber syndrome
Single umbilical artery	Sirenomelia, VATER association
Photophobia	Acrodermatitis enteropathica, Richner-Hanhart syndrome

Note: Reflexes are not included.

disability precludes discussion here but mandates full evaluation.

Head, Neck, and Face

In an assessment of the head and face, the shape should be observed. Variation can be due to normal factors or pathology. Mild asymmetry may be present in the newborn because of intrauterine factors and birth. In microcephaly, a tapering is noted from the forehead to the vertex. Premature closure of the cranial sutures (craniostenosis) can result in abnormal shape if there is compensatory growth toward sutures that remain open. Palpating a bony ridge suggests premature closure. This is serious either alone or as part of a syndrome. Delayed closure of the fontanels can result from hydrocephalus or from hypothyroidism, whereas premature closure might result from microcephaly, craniostenosis, or hyperthyroidism. A third fontanel located between the anterior and posterior is found in 5–15% of normal infants, but it is found in about 60% of infants with Down syndrome and 85% of those with congenital rubella syndrome. The finding of a large fontanel for age without increased intracranial pressure can be found in many skeletal disorders such as achondroplasia (a disproportionate dwarfism),

Apert syndrome (an autosomal dominant disorder with various craniofacial deformities), osteogenesis imperfecta, various chromosome abnormalities, progeria, and congenital rubella syndrome.

Various facies have been described in syndromes. Not too long ago, the expression "funny-looking kid" was used to describe patients with unidentified dysmorphic features. This is not acceptable terminology. Coarse facies develop in most of the mucopolysaccharide disorders because of the deposition of mucopolysaccharide in the tissue. These are not seen until late infancy or early childhood, when enough accumulation occurs. Observation of the nose and lips should be made. A saddle nose may be a minor variant that is not an anomaly, but wide nasal bridges can be seen with hypertelorism and a low nasal bridge with such disorders as achondroplasia. The philtrum is the vertical groove from the columnella of the nose to the carmine border of the upper lip. It is smooth in patients with fetal alcohol syndrome. Cleft lip and palate may occur as single defects or as part of a syndrome (see Chapter 9). A bifid uvula may be dismissed by the practitioner, but it is important because of its frequent association with submucous cleft palate. The teeth provide another accessible location for examination, as many genetic disorders are reflected here. Hypodontia is found in 2–9% of normal persons (excluding third molars) and also in Witkop syndrome, focal dermal hypoplasia, Rieger syndrome, and Ellis–van Creveld syndrome. Hyperdontia is found in 0.1–3.6% of normal persons and neonatal teeth in less than 1 in 2,000.

Eyes and Ocular Region

Congenital cataract is the most frequent cause of remedial childhood blindness. To prevent the effects of visual deprivation, it is important to perform surgery by the time the infant is 2 months of age. Both unilateral and bilateral cataracts may be manifested by the appearance of a milky, hazy, or white pupil with absence of the red reflex when examined with the ophthalmoscope from about a foot away. Unilateral cataracts may also be noticed because one eye may appear larger than the other, the eye may just "not look right," or a unilateral squint may be present. In bilateral cataracts, parents may report that the infant "does not seem to look at them." By 3 months of age, nystagmus and squinting may be seen. Prompt referral to an ophthalmologist is essential. Cataracts may be inherited, sporadic, part of a syndrome, or a single anomaly. They are often the first abnormality noticed in congenital rubella and some biochemical errors. Different-colored (heterochromic) irises are often seen in Waardenburg syndrome type I, but some families have isochromic pale blue eyes instead. Brushfield spots are speckled areas in the iris that are seen in about 20% of normal children, especially those with very clear eyes, and about 50% of those with Down syndrome. Hypertelorism represents an actual increase in distance between the orbits. Sometimes this distance appears wide because of a low nasal bridge, increased space between the two inner corners of the eye (telecanthus), or short palpebral fissures. The palpebral fissure is from the inner to the outer corner of the eye. It is normally horizontal. Up-slanting palpebral fissures are found in about 4% of normal individuals. Epicanthial folds can be present in about one-third of all newborns, but they are unusual in a normal Caucasian child after age 10 years. These folds are often present in children with Down syndrome. Curly, long, eyelashes and thick eyebrows that meet in the middle (synophrys) are frequently found in

the Brachmann de Lange syndrome. Abnormal eyebrow patterns may be seen in Waardenburg syndrome type I.

Ears

Much variation exists in the external ear. It should be looked at for symmetry, position, type of insertion, and size. "Low-set ears" is a descriptor commonly used. It can be easy for ears to appear to be low set because of other features, such as a short or extended neck, tilted ear, small chin, or high cranial vault, any of which can be present alone or in conjunction with another syndrome. Various researchers have demonstrated that subjective impressions may be due to an optical illusion. Assessment of the position of the ear should ultimately be done by objective measurements. One assessment that is easy to do clinically is to consider that a line (or piece of straight-edged paper) drawn from the lateral corner of the eye normally should intersect the upper point of attachment of the external ear to the head. Another measure to consider is that a line from the midpoint of the eyebrow should approximate the upper edge of the external ear, and a line from the base of the columnella of the nose should approximate the lower insertion of the external ear.

Various degrees of malformation of the ear occur. Besides cosmetic considerations, their importance lies in their association with hidden middle ear anomalies, resulting in deafness, and their association with renal disease (e.g., Potter syndrome). Infants or children (even as young as 1 week old) with even a minor ear malformation should have their hearing tested and renal status evaluated. Early detection of hearing problems may allow either surgical correction or prevention of the development of speech, language, and behavior problems by prompt therapy. Very minor malformations (e.g., preauricular pits or ear tags) may be important in syndrome recognition.

Those infants and children who will be at high risk for hearing impairment and who should be very carefully assessed include the following:

- Family history of hearing loss in early childhood, particularly in parent or sibling
- Maternal illness during pregnancy, especially rubella or cytomegalovirus

- Known prenatal exposure to drugs known to be ototoxic
- Prematurity
- Neonatal icterus (severe)
- Presence of certain congenital anomalies, especially ear malformations, cleft lip, cleft palate, and head or neck malformations
- Anoxia at birth
- Neurologic abnormalities, including neonatal seizures
- Parental reports of failure to respond appropriately to sounds
- Delayed or poor speech
- Chronic ear infections

Parents are most likely to be the first to suspect hearing loss, and their concerns should be followed up. Many states now include screening for congenital hearing loss in their newborn screening programs (see Chapter 12).

Skin, Hair, and Nails

The skin should be inspected for pigmentation, lesions, texture, and hair distribution. Many skin lesions are genetic in origin or are a reflection of other genetic disorders, as the skin is derived from all three embryological layers. A normal variant is the Mongolian spot, which is present in 90% of infants of Black and Asian origin and also occurs frequently in those of Mediterranean origin. The Mongolian spot is a blue or bluish-gray nevus that usually occurs on the back or buttocks. Although it occasionally persists into adulthood, it usually disappears in early childhood. Its importance lies in the fact that it has been mistaken as a sign of child abuse when seen in the emergency room, and it should be realized that this is a benign normal variation. Another benign lesion is the "stork bite," or salmon patch, which is a capillary hemangioma on the eyelids, the forehead, or the back of neck that usually fades within a few months. Port wine stains are intradermal capillary hemangiomas that discolor the skin and range from faint pink to deep purple. They are permanent unless treated appropriately. Certain cosmetic products are available to conceal them. They may be associated with deeper hemangiomas such as those of the nervous system seen in Sturge-Weber syndrome. The finding of depigmented spots that are present at birth in 90% of infants with tuberous sclerosis means that the practitioner should examine the newborn carefully. An ultraviolet light may be necessary to do this in infants with light skin. A butterfly rash that may appear later in childhood is also seen in Bloom disease (an autosomal recessive disorder of chromosome instability leading to malignancy development). Sometimes the dysfunction of other systems is not seen until later in life.

Abnormal hair patterning and development may reflect abnormal brain development or other developmental deviation. Variations such as double whorls may be familial in some cases and not abnormal. A widow's peak may be a normal variant or may suggest hypertelorism and deviant migration of embryonic structures. Hair pigmentation may be altered in a variety of syndromes. Hair is lighter than normal for the particular family in children with phenylketonuria. A patch of white hair may indicate Waardenburg syndrome I and should prompt a hearing test. Facial and body hirsutism may be due to ethnic and racial variation, occurring normally in Native Americans, Latinos, and persons of Mediterranean background. It also may occur in syndromes such as Brachmann de Lange syndrome. Photosensitivity is frequent in such diverse disorders as albinism, porphyria (see Chapter 6), and chromosomal instability syndromes. Abnormalities of hair texture, such as the "steel wool type" hair found in Menkes disease (an X-linked defect in copper metabolism with delay), may represent pathology or be a family variant (e.g., woolly hair, dominantly inherited in certain Caucasian families). The nails also may reflect genetic disorders. Hypoplastic nails may be seen in nail-patella syndrome and the ectodermal dysplasias (a group of related conditions with abnormalities of the hair, teeth, nails, sweat glands, and eyes). They should alert one to look further.

Limbs, Hands, Feet, Skeleton, and Trunk

The hands also may reflect a variety of single malformations or more complex disorders. Polydactyly is one of the more common single malformations, especially in Blacks, but should alert the practitioner to rule out other anomalies.

Clinodactyly (incurvation of the fifth digit) is a variation that is often a component of syndromes that might be missed. Syndactyly denotes webbing of the digits. In some cases, hand positioning may give a clue to other problems or help in diagnosis. Typical of this is the overlapping hand position seen in trisomy 13 and "hitchhiker's thumb" seen in Marfan syndrome. Palmar crease variation, such as the transverse crease, may be found in about 5–10% of normal infants but is more frequent in children with other abnormalities, especially with Down syndrome (see Figure 7.3).

The feet may reflect the same anomalies as the hands. In addition, wide separation of the toes may be easier to notice. "Rocker-bottom" feet are a frequent accompaniment of several chromosome disorders including trisomies 13 and 18. Equinus varus (clubfoot) is a relatively common birth defect. During the first 2 years of life, it is important to be alert for congenital hip dysplasia. In the newborn and infant, the Ortolani and Barlow tests can be used, as can ultrasound for detection. In the older infant and child, extra skin folds can be seen on the side; if the child is supine with the knees flexed, the knees will not be at the same level. When the child walks, limping may be seen, especially when the infant is

tired, and when the child stands on the leg of the affected side only, the pelvis droops on the opposite side. Developmental dysplasia of the hip and its assessment are discussed in Chapter 9. Typical signs and symptoms are not present in cases of bilateral developmental dysplasia of the hip.

When the examiner looks at the trunk, supernumerary nipples and widely spaced nipples should be observed. Internipple measurement standards are available to confirm such suspicions. Examination for sacral dimpling and for a tuft of hair in the lower back area should be done. The latter may represent occult spina bifida, which may not be present in such a mild form in other family members. Particularly in older children and adolescence, observation should be made for scoliosis, which occurs in about 10–13% of early adolescents. Although mild curvature may be of no consequence, that which is progressive needs attention. A history of poor posture, observation of awkward gait, apparent unequal arm lengths, unequal shoulders, one prominent hip, one prominent shoulder blade, and unequal hemlines may provide the clue. It is common for scoliosis to develop in children with prior muscle disease or prior irradiation for malignancy. All school children should be evaluated for scoliosis

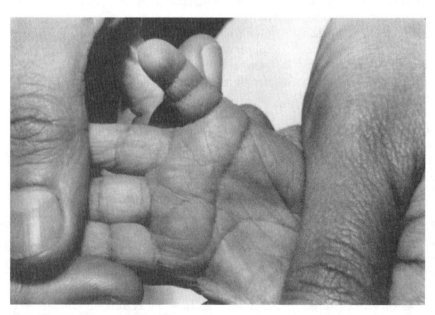

FIGURE 7.3   Transverse palmar crease.

school or a clinic. The skeleton, chest, and trunk should also be examined for conditions such as pectus excavatum (hollow chest) and pectus carinatum ("pigeon" breast) often seen in Marfan syndrome (see Chapter 10) and homocystinuria (see Chapter 2). Observation should be made for lordosis and kyphosis, and upper- and lower-body-segment ratios should be observed.

Neuromuscular

The clinician should test the infant for the usual reflexes. The Moro or startle reflex is exaggerated in the infant with Tay-Sachs disease. In the newborn, poor sucking, reduced activity, and unequal or altered reflexes may provide clues about disorders. The "floppy" infant may demonstrate lack of active movement and unusual posturing. Later, delays in achieving motor milestones are seen. The floppy infant may assume the "frog" position when he/she is lying on the back and also demonstrate head lag. Assessment must be related to gestational maturity, because preterm infants may be normally somewhat hypotonic. In the traction response, the infant's hands are grasped, and he/she is pulled to a sitting position. More than minimal head lag and full arm extension indicates postural hypotonia in the full-term newborn. A protruding ear auricle and ptosis of the eyelid may indicate a neuromuscular disorder. Delay in motor milestones, clumsiness, frequent falling, the inability to climb stairs, and unusual gaits such as waddling and toe walking may be seen in muscle disease. An important aspect of assessment is observation during which the practitioner can assess the child's gait, posture, and play activity. The answers to certain questions determine further direction. Is weakness intermittent? Is it accompanied by atrophy? Muscle cramps during exercise have a different meaning from those that occur at rest. The improvement of fatigue with exercise is different from that in which effort results in fatigue. The enlargement of specific muscle groups, especially in the calves, should be noted in children.

Changes in gait, tremors, seizures, and personality and cognitive degeneration may be features of different genetic disorders and may require investigation, the nature of which depends on the symptom and the age of the client. Seizure activity in the newborn and infant is often associated with inborn errors of metabolism. Seizures can be difficult to detect in neonates and may be manifested as minimal aberrations such as nystagmus, "rowing" or "swimming" motions of the extremities, eyelid flutter, abnormal cry, abnormal positioning of limbs, or apneic periods, as well as overt clonic or tonic movements.

Genitalia

The genitalia are a frequent site of congenital anomalies and are easier to observe in males than females. These anomalies may result from many etiologies including teratogenesis and show great variability in expression. Abnormalities tend to be more frequently observed in males than in females. Sexual development in relation to age may be assessed by use of the Tanner criteria. At birth, an important condition to identify is ambiguous genitalia so that further genetic studies can be done to identify the genetic sex and choose future directions.

SUSPECTING A GENETIC COMPONENT AND REFERRAL TO THE GENETICIST

When a genetic component is suspected because of findings from physical or developmental assessment, family history, or observation, referral to a geneticist should be initiated. Genetic concerns may be sharpened when a couple is contemplating marriage or a family. Development of the nurse's mindset to "think genetically" may result in suspicions of genetic factors that may otherwise be ignored. For example, the early age of onset of a common disease such as coronary heart disease or a common cancer may indicate a heritable component and should be evaluated further. Situations in which genetic evaluation or counseling are indicated include the recent occurrence, discovery, or known presence in the client, his or her mate, or a blood relative of any of the situations shown in Box 7.2. Thus, the nurse should refer such individuals for further genetic evaluation. When in doubt, the clinician can contact the geneticist to discuss concerns. Referral of a person with a suspected genetic problem to a geneticist or genetic clinic is an appropriate and important nursing responsibility.

BOX 7.2

Situations Suggesting a Genetic Component

- Presence of disease in the family known or believed to have a genetic component, including chromosome, single gene, or multifactorial disorders
- Any abnormality affecting more than one member of a family
- Single or multiple congenital abnormalities
- Delayed or abnormal development
- Intellectual disability
- Failure to thrive in infancy or childhood
- Short or extremely tall stature
- Any apparent abnormalities or delays in physical growth
- Unusual body proportions
- Abnormal or delayed development of secondary sex characteristics or sex organs
- Cataracts, leukocoria, or cherry-red spot in retinas of infants or children or blindness
- Deafness
- Familial occurrence of neoplasms
- Occurrence of multiple primary neoplasms or bilateral neoplasms in paired organs
- Occurrence of adult-type tumors in a child
- Early onset of common disorders such as coronary heart disease or cancer
- Appearance of a common disorder in the sex usually less frequently affected, such as a male with breast cancer
- Hypotonia in an infant or child
- Seizures in a newborn or infant
- Skin lesions that may have a genetic component such as café-au-lait spots in neurofibromatosis
- Infertility
- Repeated spontaneous abortions (usually 2 to 3 or more)
- Stillbirths or infant deaths due to unknown or genetic causes
- Consideration of mating or marriage to a blood relative
- Females exposed to radiation, infectious diseases, toxic agents, or certain drugs immediately before or during pregnancy
- Males exposed to radiation, toxic agents, or certain drugs who are contemplating immediate paternity
- Females 35 years of age and older who are considering pregnancy or are already pregnant
- Males 40 years of age and older who are considering paternity
- Members of ethnic groups in which certain genetic disorders are frequent and appropriate testing, screening, or prenatal diagnosis is available
- Unexpected drug or anesthesia reactions
- Any other suspicious sign or symptom suggestive of genetic disease that the nurse believes needs further evaluation

CASE EXAMPLE FOR DISCUSSION

The nurse is examining Brian, 3, and notices six cafe-au-lait spots on his body. She asks Brian's mother, Angela, if anyone else in the family has these. Angela tells the nurse that her husband does and that her husband's brother has some "bumps all over his body." What should the nurse think about and do? Are there other questions the nurse should ask?

KEY POINTS

- A properly taken family history over three generations can help to identify people at genetic risk.
- Pedigrees are essentially pictorial representations of family histories.
- Nurses should look at clients with a "genetic eye" and think genetically when doing assessments.
- Persons with signs and symptoms that suggest the presence of a genetic component should be referred for further evaluation.

8

Maternal-Child Nursing: Obstetrics

Content in maternal-child nursing is heavily influenced by genetic knowledge. Genetic applications begin in the pre-pregnancy period with assessment of risk and application of principles of prevention, and continue into pregnancy with consideration of effects of teratogens on the fetus and prenatal detection and diagnosis with the potential of intrauterine correction. After the child is born, recognition and discussion of genetic disorders (chromosomal, single gene errors of metabolism, congenital malformations) manifested in the pediatric period will be discussed in Chapter 9, as will childhood cancers with genetic components.

PRECONCEPTION OR PRE-PREGNANCY COUNSELING

Preconception or pre-pregnancy counseling may be considered to identify couples at increased risk for a less-than-desirable pregnancy outcome. Good assessment; eliciting family, health, social, occupational and environmental histories; physical examination; and knowledge of genetic risk factors can help to identify such individuals, who are often seen in the primary care setting. Preconception care is a critical component of health care for reproductive age women. Today all women considering pregnancy should have the following areas assessed, evaluated with appropriate education, and referral provided if needed:

- Appropriate diet
- Determination of rubella and varicella titers and vaccinations if necessary

- Appropriate folic acid and multivitamin supplementation.
- Assess and/or determine other risk factors such as diabetes mellitus, maternal phenylketonuria, HIV status, familial genetic disorders and so on.
- Review of medications and drugs they may be using; alcohol, drug, and cigarette use; be advised to avoid hot tubs and take appropriate action
- Determination of ABO and Rh blood types
- A three-generation family history taken
- Discussion of potential risks based on ethnic origin. For example if the couple is of Ashkenazi (Eastern European) Jewish, Cajun, or French-Canadian ancestry or have a family history suggestive of Tay-Sachs disease, carrier testing should be offered before pregnancy.
- Discussi'on of carrier tests available for relatively frequent genetic disorders
- Testing for thromobophilias such as factor V Leiden if indicated
- Stabilization of any diseases such as diabetes mellitus before pregnancy
- Discussion of potential needs for medications in pregnancy such as in the woman with epilepsy who is on medication for seizure control and any necessary adjustments
- Review of measures to prevent infection in pregnancy such as not changing cat litter boxes if possible to prevent toxoplasmosis
- Discussion of any bleeding tendencies in themselves including menorrhagia, especially at menarche, which could prompt evaluation for von Willebrand disease, an inherited bleeding disorder

It is important that women take 0.4 mg of folic acid daily prior to conception, and if they have a previous history of neural tube defects, optimally they should take 4.0 mg of folic acid daily starting at 3 months before conception. Their male partner should also be counseled, for example, to avoid environmental chemicals, cigarette smoking, certain drugs, and radiation. Some may have concerns or be at a risk that prompted them to seek counseling. Identification of such individuals, coupled with appropriate action, can result in a more favorable pregnancy outcome. For example, women with altered maternal metabolism such as those with diabetes mellitus or phenylketonuria (PKU) can benefit from strict control and diet therapy before pregnancy. Someone who had a corrected congenital anomaly, might have anxiety reduced by knowing the actual risk. For women with genetic disorders, such as Ehlers-Danlos disease (a group of connective tissue disorders), the effect of the disorder on the pregnancy that does not include heritability and also the effect of the pregnancy on the disorder should also be considered. Parents may not be aware that relatively minor problems in themselves may in fact mean that they are at increased risk for a more severe outcome in their children, such as in the case of a mother with spina bifida occulta and the possibility of a more full-blown neural tube defect in a subsequent child. In cases of disabilities arising from unknown or nongenetic causes, counseling can still be useful in terms of optimum pregnancy management in a setting best able to cope with any anticipated problems, and also for aspects of identifying the most common hazards likely to be encountered so that they can be prevented, rather than treated, which might involve increased risk to the fetus. An example is the case of the potential for urinary tract infection, the avoidance of factors that might contribute to it, and proactive measures such as adequate fluid intake that could reduce the chance that medication would be necessary.

Persons at risk thus need to consider:

- their chances of conception,
- the effect of a pregnancy on their own health,
- the effect on the developing fetus in the uterus,
- how their risk bears on any pregnancy complications,
- their chances of having a child with a similar disorder if they are themselves affected.

They can then consider reproductive options, therapeutic options, and the possibility of future prenatal diagnosis, if available and desired, before embarking on the pregnancy. Methods of achieving prevention of genetic disorders are also discussed in Chapter 5.

PREGNANCY

Issues relative to genetics are important in pregnancy. Items discussed under preconception counseling should be applied as early as possible in pregnancy, especially if the mother has not benefited from preconception counseling. They will not be repeated here. This section discusses in more detail effects of teratogens on the fetus and prenatal screening, detection and diagnosis, and assisted reproductive technology.

An important element is screening for both ABO and Rh(D) incompatibility so that maternal fetal incompatibility such as erthyroblastosis fetalis can be prevented. During the first prenatal visit, it is important for the woman to have Rh(D) blood typing and antibody testing as well as that for ABO. All unsensitized Rh(D)-negative women should have Rh(D) immunoglobulin after repeated antibody testing at 24 to 28 weeks gestation. This should also be done after amniocentesis or abortion and perhaps other procedures such as chorionic villus sampling unless the biologic father is Rh(D) negative. If the infant is Rh(D) positive, Rh(D) immunoglobulin should be repeated within 72 hours after delivery. (More information is in Chapter 3.)

Through personal and family history, women will be identified who should have carrier screening early in pregnancy for genetic disorders that are more frequent in certain ethnic groups. This is important so that a full range of options, such as prenatal diagnosis, will be available to a couple in which the fetus is at risk for a specific genetic disorder. In addition, recent recommendations are that carrier screening for cystic fibrosis should be offered to all pregnant women. Some of the voluntary carrier screening that should be offered to women and couples in specific ethnic groups either preconception or in early pregnancy are shown in Table 8.1 It is important to understand that a negative screening test for either partner does not guarantee that the child will not be affected because screening can-

ABLE 8.1   Prenatal Carrier Screening for Genetic Disorders by Ethnic Background

Ethnic Group Background	Genetic Disorder Amenable to Carrier Screening	Carrier Frequency in Pregnancy	Description in This group
African-American	Sickle cell disease	1 in 12	May include sickle cell anemia and other forms of hemoglobinopathies such as sickle cell disease and S-thalassemia; see the text
	Beta-thalassemia		See below
Ashkenazi Jewish	Tay-Sachs disease	1 in 30	See the text
	Bloom syndrome	1 in 100	Poor growth, susceptibility to cancer and infection, facial telangiectasias, death usual in early adulthood
	Canavan disease	1 in 40	Similar to Tay-Sachs disease; death usual in early childhood
	Fanconi anemia Type C	1 in 89	Short stature, developmental delay, severe anemia, increased risk for anemia, intellectual disabilities, other congenital malformations; often die by early adolescence
	Familial dysautonomia	1 in 32	Various sensory and autonomic disorders including gastrointestinal dysfunction, altered sensitivity to pain and temperature, vomiting crises, autonomic crises, labile blood pressure, absent tearing, feeding difficulties
	Gaucher disease type 1	1 in 12–15	Varies in severity from mild to severe, enlarged liver and spleen, bone pain, anemia, chronic fatigue, easy bruising, nosebleeds
	Mucolipidosis IV	1 in 127	Neurodegenerative lysosomal storage disease with psychomotor and growth delay, retinal degeneration; most affected persons do not advance past the level of a two-year old, but life span is near normal
	Niemann-Pick disease type A	1 in 90	Lysosomal storage disease with enlarged liver and spleen, poor growth, and a neurodegenerative decline with death usual by age 5 years.
Cajun	Tay-Sachs disease		See the text
French-Canadian	Tay-Sachs disease		See the text
Mediterranean (Greek, Italian, some Arab groups)	Beta-thalassemia		See the text. Severe anemia causing poor growth, bone deformities; requires frequent transfusions
	Sickle cell disease		See the text
Southeast Asian	Alpha-thalassemia	1 in 20	Severe anemia, which can result in death of fetus or infant; see the text
	Beta-thalassemia		See above and the text

Note: This list is not all inclusive. Cystic fibrosis testing should be offered to individuals from all ethnic groups. All the above are autosomal recessive disorders not test for every possible gene mutation but only the most frequent ones in the population. For detailed information or complicated situations, the couple should be referred for genetic counseling. More about genetic variation in population groups is given in Chapter 3.

THE VULNERABLE FETUS AND TERATOGENESIS

The fetus is vulnerable to many influences, some of which may emerge many years postnatally. The practitioner treating a pregnant woman has two patients: the mother and the fetus. The term *teratogen* is often used to describe agents that cause structural or functional damage to the unborn child. The term *fetus* as used in this chapter also includes the embryo. In a given exposure during pregnancy, a teratogen can have any of the consequences shown in Box 8.1.

Complex and multifaceted maternal and fetal factors influence the consequences to the fetus of drugs, radiation, and chemical and infectious agents

---

BOX 8.1

Possible Consequences of a Teratogen

No apparent effect	Prenatal or perinatal fetal death
Congenital anomalies	Altered fetal growth (e.g., growth retardation)
Carcinogenesis	Postnatal functional and behavioral deficits and aberrations

---

(Figure 8.1). These are shown in Table 8.2. Drug and chemicals can cause fetotoxic effects not onl by direct fetal interaction, but also through interfe ence with maternal systems (e.g., circulatory, en docrine, excretory, appetite regulating). Some c the problems involved in determining whether specific substance is injurious to the fetus are show in Table 8.3.

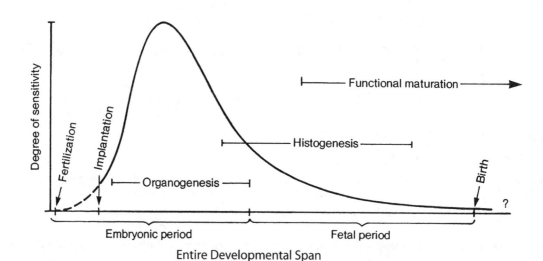

FIGURE 8.1   Periods of fetal growth and development and susceptibility to deviation. The highest sensitivity, at least to structural deviation, occurs during the period of organogenesis, from about days 18 to 20 until about days 55 to 60. The absolute peak of sensitivity may be reached before day 30 postconception. As organogenesis is completed, susceptibility to anatomical defects diminishes greatly, but probably minor structural deviation is possible until histogenesis is completed late in the fetal period. Deviations during the fetal period are more likely to involve growth or functional aspects because these are the predominant developmental features at this time. Wilson JG: Environment and Birth Defects. New York: Academic Press. 1974. Figure used with permission.

Drugs and Chemical Agents in Pregnancy

In spite of the bitter lesson of thalidomide, pregnant women continue to take a substantial number and variety of self- or physician-prescribed drugs. Several questions must be asked before recommending a drug for a pregnant woman, as shown in Box 8.2.

These questions are not always easy to answer. To begin, the statement that a drug "has not been shown to be a human teratogen" does not mean that it is safe; it may never have been tested in the pregnant human female. Establishing drug safety is difficult because of the previously discussed problems and factors influencing fetal effects (Table 8.3). In addition, drug testing for safety may not use a species that is sensitive to the effects of the drug when doing animal and laboratory studies. Thalidomide had appeared harmless in the species in which it was tested. Drugs tested in humans before mass marketing may be in specific population groups, from which generalizations should not be made, or have few or no pregnant women in the sample because of ethical concerns for safety. If the effect is one in which the increased incidence of defects is small and nonspecific, then the number of subjects in preliminary tests before marketing may not be sufficient to demonstrate the effect. Cost and time are also limiting factors on the extent of testing that is carried out, as there are pressures to get new drugs on the market quickly.

BOX 8.2

Questions to Consider Before Recommending a Drug in Pregnancy

- Is pharmacologic intervention necessary for this condition?
- Are other effective alternative therapies available?
- Is the risk increased if no treatment is given?
- Is this specific drug the agent of choice for both the condition and the pregnancy?
- Does the risk of the disorder or its consequences outweigh the risk of the drug?
- Does the value of the drug to the mother for treatment of the disorder weigh favorably against any possible detrimental effects to the fetus?

After distribution, the association of a drug with detrimental fetal effects can be made by case reports, surveillance, and epidemiologic studies. The teratogenicity of thalidomide was discovered because of the sudden increased incidence of a previously rare type of limb defect (phocomelia) that coincided with the widespread use of thalidomide by pregnant women. The numerous case reports

---

TABLE 8.2   Factors Influencing the Effects of Teratogens

- Agents often act differently in different species, and on individuals within the species (e.g. differences in genetic constitution, variability in metabolic pathways). This applies to both the mother and fetus.
- The age of the fetus at the time of exposure. Generally when the fetus exposed to agents affecting the period from fertilization to implantation, the result is either death or regeneration. During the period of organogenesis, the result is usually gross structural alterations. After organogenesis in the fetal period the result is usually related to alterations in cell size and number, although the central nervous system, and external genitalia remain vulnerable through most of pregnancy.
- Access to and disposition within the fetus.
- Chemical, biologic, and physical properties of the agent (for microorganisms—type, virulence, and number).
- Interactions with other agents and factors (e.g., environmental, nutritional, other drugs).
- Level and duration of dosage or exposure.
- Maternal biochemical pathways and mechanisms for handling drugs and chemicals are altered by pregnancy.
- The degree of interference with maternal systems and the extent of modulation that occurs.
- The genetic constitution of both mother and fetus; dizygotic twins have been born with one having anomalies typical of a drug effect and the other being normal.

TABLE 8.3   Some Problems in Determining Whether a Specific Substance Causes Fetal Injury

- Different effects may be seen depending on the time of gestation at which the fetus is exposed, and the exact date of pregnancy is not always known.
- The number of pregnant women getting a certain drug or disease at the same time of gestation are few, and a slight increase in an anomaly may not be statistically significant. Even then, differences in their environment, the reason for giving the drug, ethnic differences, and other factors make associations and generalizations difficult
- The difficulty in detecting minor anomalies or delayed deficits.
- One fetotoxic agent can have several different effects; drugs rarely produce only one type of defect.
- Many fetotoxic agents can show the same effect.
- Long-term problems cannot be detected easily (e.g., the administration of diethylstilbestrol in pregnant women and the appearance of clear cell adenocarcinoma of the vagina in their daughters).
- In humans, all of the interacting and modulating factors such as genotype of both mother and fetus, environmental chemicals, and nutrition may differ and cannot be controlled.
- Bias in recall. Mothers who give birth to infants with defects are more likely to recall adverse events such as illness and medications in their pregnancies than women who have normal infants.
- Effects may be subtle (e.g., behavioral alteration).
- Agents do not need to harm the mother in order to damage the fetus.
- Difficulties in extrapolating data from animal studies.
- More than one drug may interact, as may the drug and the disease process.

appearing at the same time in the literature led to the establishment of the association and its withdrawal from the market at that time. Thalidomide is available again, this time as an investigational drug particularly for erythema nodosum and aphthous ulcers. Retrospective studies can be done after the birth of a malformed child when a woman is asked to recall details of her illnesses and medications used during her pregnancy but is subject to recall bias. Epidemiologic surveillance and reporting of congenital anomalies, especially the frequency of certain sentinel defects, is carried out by the Centers for Disease Control and Prevention at several sites across the United States in order to detect any changes in patterns or incidence that might reflect an environmental influence.

Prescription drugs are labeled as to their pregnancy category. The Food and Drug Administration (FDA) has established five categories:

A—Controlled studies show no risk. Adequate well-controlled studies in pregnant women have failed to demonstrate risk to the fetus.

B—No evidence of risk in humans. Either animal findings show risk, but human findings do not; or if no adequate human studies have been done, animal findings are negative.

C—Risk cannot be ruled out. Human studies are lacking, and animal studies are either positive for fetal risk or lacking as well. However, potential benefits may justify the potential risk.

D—Positive evidence of risk. Investigational or postmarketing data show risk to the fetus. Nevertheless, potential benefits may outweigh the potential risk.

X—Contraindicated in pregnancy. Studies in animals or humans or investigational or postmarketing reports have shown fetal risk that clearly outweighs any possible benefit to the patient.

Even those listed in Category A should not be used unless "clearly needed." About two-thirds of drugs listed in the *Physician's Desk Reference* are in Category C. Schwarz, Maselli, Norton, and Gonzales (2005) reported use of a class D or X medication in 1 of 13 women of childbearing age in ambulatory practices. Certain fetotoxic drugs are discussed below, and others are presented in Table 8.4. Absence from the table does not imply safety, and some adverse fetal ef-

TABLE 8.4   Selected Drugs Known or Suspected to Be Harmful or Teratogenic to the Fetus

Drug	Reported Effects
Alcohol	See the text
Antibiotics	
Aminoglycosides	Amikacin, gentamycin, kanamycin, tobramycin (see streptomycin).
Chloramphenicol	Effects in neonate from administration in second and third trimester include gray baby syndrome, hypothermia, failure to feed, collapse, and death.
Streptomycin	Ototoxic to fetal ear, eighth cranial nerve damage; other aminoglycosides may also cause this.
Tetracycline	Yellow/brown discoloration of tooth enamel, enamel hypoplasia, inhibits bone growth.
Anticancer drugs	
Alkylating agents	Chlorambucil has been associated with renal agenesis. Busulfan has been associated with growth retardation, cleft palate, microphthalmia, and increased incidence of multiple malformations; all apparently cause a risk of increased spontaneous abortion.
Aminopterin	Cranial dystosis, hydrocephalus, hypertelorism, micrognathia, limb and hand defects, multiple congenital malformations.
Antimetabolites	Cyclophosphamide has been associated with increased incidence of multiple malformations, especially skeletal defects and cleft palate.
Methotrexate	Increased incidence of miscellaneous congenital malformations, especially of the central nervous system and limbs.
Anticoagulants	
Warfarin (Coumadin)	Fetal warfarin syndrome, facial abnormalities, nasal hypoplasia, respiratory difficulties, hypoplastic nails, microcephaly, hemorrhage, ophthalmic abnormalities, bone stippling, developmental delay.
Anticonvulsants	Also see text.
Phenytoin	Fetal hydantoin syndrome, growth retardation, mental deficiency, dysmorphic feature, short nasal bridge, mild hypertelorism, cleft lip and palate, cardiac defects, transplacental carcinogenesis (neuroblastoma).
Trimethadione (Tridione)	Apparent syndrome of developmental delay, V-shaped eyebrows, and paramethadione low-set ears, high or cleft palate, irregular teeth, cardiac defects, (Paradione) growth retardation, speech difficulties, increased risk of spontaneous abortion.
Valproic acid	Spina bifida.
Antimalarial	
Chloroquine	Slight risk of chorioretinitis; may cause ototoxicity.
Quinine	Deafness, limb anomalies, visceral defects, visual problems, other multiple congenital anomalies.
Antithyroid	
Iodides and thiouracils	Depression of fetal thyroid hypothyroidism, goiter.
Carbimazole	Scalp defects, dysmorphic facial features, other possible anomalies.

(continues)

TABLE 8.4   (*Continued*)

Drug	Reported Effects
Hormones	
Adrenocorticoids	Intrauterine growth restriction; neonates may show adrenal suppression and possible increased susceptibility to infection; there are conflicting reports of increased incidence of cleft lip and palate.
Androgens	Masculinization of female fetus.
Clomiphene	Questionable increase in incidence of NTDs.
Diethylstilbestrol	Developmental of vaginal adenocarcinoma, usually in adolescence or young adulthood, reproductive tract structural alterations; in exposed males, testicular abnormalities, sperm, and semen abnormalities have been reported.
Oral contraceptives	Association of increased incidence of cardiac and limb defects, (progestogen/estrogen) VACTERL syndrome; conflicting research reports, may not be teratogenic.
Psychotropics	
Chlordiazepoxide (Librium)	Possible overall increased incidence of congenital malformations.
Diazepam (Valium)	Hypotonia, hypothermia, withdrawal symptoms at birth (?), increase in incidence of cleft lip and palate.
Haloperidol, trifluoperazine, prochlorperazine	Suspected of causing slight increase in incidence of limb defects in exposed fetuses; weigh against need for mother.
Lithium	Increase in stillbirths, neonatal deaths; edema, hypothyroidism, goiter, hypotonia, cardiovascular anomalies such as Ebstein anomaly. Use another drug during pregnancy if possible.
Meprobamate	Possible increase in cardiac defects or major malformations.
Others	
Aminoglutethamide (Cytadren)	Pseudohermaphroditism, increased incidence of fetal deaths, increased incidence of malformations.
Angiotensin-converting-enzyme inhibitors	Hypoplasia of skull, some skeletal anomalies, oligohydramnios, IUGR, patent ductus ateriosus (degree of risk uncertain).
Metronidazole (Flagyl)	Midline facial defects, cleft lip and palate (?), chromosome aberrations with long-term use (?); carcinogenic and mutagenic in nonhuman systems, debated in humans.
Misoprostol (a prostaglandin E_1)	Moebius sequence.
Nonsteroidal inflammatory drugs	
Indomethacin (others may also have these effects)	Premature closure of ductus arteriosus, oligohydramnios.
Penicillamine	Connective tissue defects (e.g., cutis laxa).
Retinoids	See the text.
Salicylates	The use of aspirin has been associated with "postmaturity syndrome" and with a slight possible increase of hemorrhage, especially in premature infants, and possibly some anomalies (debated).
Sulfonylureas	Chlorpropamide and tolbutamide may be associated with increased congenital anomalies and increased fetal mortality (debated).
Thalidomide	Phocomelia and other limb defects, eye and ear malformations and abnormalities.

Note: All exposed fetuses will not show these effects. Absence from this table does not imply safety. Heavy metals and anesthetic gases and hyperthermia are discussed in Chapter 12. See the text for discussion.

ects are not teratogenic. It is not possible to present an inclusive list here, and reports on the safety (or onsafety) of drugs in pregnancy often conflict. Nevertheless, these drugs are best avoided when a less harmful, more efficacious one can be substituted. Selected drugs are discussed in more detail below.

Diethylstilbestrol (DES)

DES is a synthetic estrogen that was introduced in the 1940s and used extensively in pregnant women in the 1950s and 1960s to treat habitual abortion, bleeding, premature delivery, and toxemia. Many women (as many as 7% of all pregnant) took DES before the hazards to the fetus were identified. In 1971, the association between an epidemic in young women of clear cell adenocarcinoma (CCA) of the vagina and cervix and the use of DES during pregnancy in their mothers was made. The magnitude of the DES exposure problem is not completely known because many women did not know the precise medication they took or knew only the trade name and did not recognize that they had been exposed despite wide publicity in the lay press. It is estimated that there may have been about 4 million male (DES sons) and female (DES daughters) exposed offspring. The association between DES use by the mother and CCA in their daughters years later has been well documented. Less widely recognized consequences in women include nonneoplastic alterations of the reproductive system, especially in the vagina, uterus (often T-shaped), or cervix, which may be seen in 25–35% of exposed women, and an increased incidence of spontaneous abortion, ectopic pregnancies, and prematurity. In exposed males (DES sons), sperm and semen abnormalities, testicular abnormalities, including benign cysts in the epididymis, and small and undescended testes have been reported as more prevalent than in controls, but no excess risk of cancer has been reported after long-term study. Some investigators report altered social behavior, but others disagree. DES daughters should not be given estrogen and should be advised to have continuing care. DES sons should see a urologist and be taught the technique and importance of self-examination of the testes. DES is a proven teratogen.

Anticonvulsants

The use of anticonvulsants for maternal seizures such as epilepsy during pregnancy needs to be care- fully considered, balancing the risk of malformations with the risk to the fetus of uncontrolled seizures. Phenobarbital and phenytoin (Dilantin) are given together about three-quarters of the time, so the individual effects of each drug have been hard to separate. Phenytoin and other hydantoins are associated with a risk of orofacial clefts, especially cleft lip and palate, and congenital heart disease of 5 to 10 times and 2 to 3 times that of the general population, respectively. In addition, a fetal hydantoin syndrome consisting of any or all of the following has been reported: growth retardation, mental retardation, dysmorphic facial features such as short nasal bridge, bowed upper lip, mild ocular hypertelorism, and hypoplastic fingers and nails. These consequences must be weighed against the ill effects of prolonged, uncontrolled seizures. Risks have been variously estimated and appear to be about 10% for the full syndrome, and up to an additional 30% for part of the syndrome. If possible, it seems best to use monotherapy or a single agent at the lowest possible effective dose that might be divided, particularly in the first trimester, taking into consideration the stage of pregnancy most affected by the particular agent coupled with monitoring of blood levels and untoward effects. Nurses should be aware that in infants whose mothers took phenytoin during pregnancy, about 48 to 72 hours after birth the infant may show vitamin K deficiency. Such infants should be observed for this hemorrhagic complication so that Vitamin K can be given to the mother during labor for prevention.

Anticancer Drugs

In general, these drugs are both teratogenic and mutagenic. They can cause spontaneous abortion, fetal death, congenital anomalies, and systemic toxicity in the fetus (e.g., hematopoietic depression). The severe effects of these drugs must be weighed against the risk that delay in treatment may jeopardize the health and life of the mother. If possible, therapy should be delayed until the second trimester, and combination therapy should be avoided, with the least toxic agent used. Both males and females taking anticancer drugs should avoid pregnancy or procreation for at least one year after therapy is discontinued. Males may wish to take advantage of sperm banking before beginning therapy, and women may wish to consider harvesting and saving ova.

Other Drugs

As new drugs come on the market, occasionally there is concern about their teratogenic potential. In addition to the drugs already discussed, the Vitamin A derivatives such as isotretinoin (Accutane) used in acne treatment are a cause for concern. These drugs are associated with certain anomalies and an increase in spontaneous abortion. Pregnancy should be avoided within six months of use. They are of concern because of use in teenage girls who might share their medication with friends without awareness of the danger should they inadvertently become pregnant. An association has been found between the use of elective serotonin-reuptake inhibitors in pregnancy after the 20th week to treat depression and persistent pulmonary hypertension of the newborn, which can lead to death or serious consequences such as neurologic abnormalities, hearing loss, and cognitive delay. The use of paroxetine in the first trimester has been associated with an increased risk of birth defects, especially cardiac defects.

Nursing Pointers

- Be proactive. Do preconception counseling.
- Teach females of reproductive age seen in various settings that medical and social drug exposure of certain types can affect the fetus, especially early before the woman realizes she is pregnant.
- Encourage the client to tell her pharmacist, physician, nurse, and other health practitioners involved in her care that she is pregnant.
- Identify those most likely to be users of medications and drugs (including alcohol, caffeine, and cigarettes), and inform those who are considering pregnancy or who are already pregnant of the hazards.
- Teach women that over-the-counter products, including extra vitamins, herbals, and iron, are considered drugs.
- Integrate the above information into school health programs.
- Educate men that taking certain drugs just prior to conception may affect the sperm and be injurious to the fetus; advise waiting 90 days after the last dose before conceiving.
- Educate women as to the dangers of self-medication in pregnancy.

- Provide teaching related to nondrug management of common conditions such as relaxation techniques for tension instead of medication.
- Involve the client in decision making if drug therapy is being considered as an informed partner in her own care.
- Instruct the client to keep an accurate list of all medications ingested during pregnancy, with the date, dose, length of time taken, and the reason.
- Maintain a record of all prescription or recommended drugs with the same information. This should be in a handy form for easy reference as part of the patient profile.
- If drug therapy is necessary, the lowest effective therapeutic dose of the least toxic agent should be used.
- The risks and benefits should always be considered, and doses should be individualized.
- Question any drug that appears contraindicated in pregnancy, as the practitioner prescribing it may not know that the patient is pregnant.

Alcohol in Pregnancy

The harmful effects of alcohol in pregnancy were noted long ago. Aristotle observed that drunken women often had feeble-minded children, and the Old Testament (Judges 13:7) states: "Behold, thou shalt conceive, and bear a son; and now drink no wine or strong drink." In late 1980 the Surgeon General advised pregnant women not to drink alcoholic beverages and to be aware of alcohol content in other foods. A warning addressed to pregnant women is on alcohol containers and in stores selling alcohol that contains language such as, "According to the Surgeon General, women should not drink alcoholic beverages during pregnancy because of the risk of birth defects."

Influences on Effects of Alcohol in Pregnancy

Factors such as genetic susceptibility, genetically determined differences in the metabolism of alcohol, the time of fetal exposure, maternal nutritional status, and the dose of alcohol all play a role in the extent of fetal consequences. Consequences include decreased birth rate, growth retardation, increase in spontaneous abortion rates, and stillbirths, a well as congenital anomalies and functional deficits. Fetal alcohol syndrome (FAS) represents the extreme upper end of the spectrum of effects that occur as a result of maternal consumption of alcohol in pregnancy, whereas lowered birth weight and minimal functional deficits represent the lower. The effects of maternal alcohol abuse in pregnancy are often difficult to separate from the use of other drugs, cigarette smoking, and malnutrition.

Fetal Alcohol Spectrum Disorders (FASD)

Fetal alcohol spectrum disorders (FASD) is the recent term that encompasses alcohol-related effects, alcohol-related neurodevelopmental disorder (ARND), alcohol-related birth defects (ARBD), and the most clinically evident category, fetal alcohol syndrome (FAS), which is considered with and without confirmed maternal alcohol exposure. FASD is not considered a diagnostic term but is defined as an umbrella term for the other alcohol-related conditions. Alcohol consumption can affect reproduction and offspring in the following phases:

- Before conception—lowered fertility
- Prenatal—risk of spontaneous abortion and prematurity
- Perinatal and birth—stillbirth, low birth weight, growth restriction, FAS, alcohol-related effects, ARBD, other anomalies
- Newborn and infant—hyperactivity, fretfulness, failure to thrive, poor sucking and feeding, sleep disturbances, and behavioral and learning deficits, which may be part of FAS or ARND
- Childhood—hearing loss, vision impairment, ARND, behavioral and learning deficits, hyperactivity, sleep disturbances, and other
- Adolescence—behavioral and learning deficits, maladaptive behaviors, ARND

A variety of dysmorphic features and congenital anomalies have been associated with FAS. A dysmorphology scoring system has been devised, and cognitive and behavioral patterns have been identified to assist with diagnosis. Among the most frequent features found are microcephaly, growth deficiency, short palpebral fissures, smooth philtrum, and thin upper lip border. Cognitive and behavioral findings include emotional lability, motor dysfunction, poor attention span, deficient social interactions, commu-

nication and speech problems, disorganization, and hyperactivity. Long-term studies of adolescents and adults with FAS found deficits in socialization, communication skills, attention deficits, and hyperactivity, and about half were mentally retarded. The facies were not as distinct, but microcephaly and shortness persisted. A detailed description of FASD can be found in Hoyme et al. (2005).

The incidence of FAS is estimated at 1 to 3 per 1,000 live births overall but may be as high as 10 to 15 per 1,000 in some high-risk populations. Alcohol-related effects may be more frequently seen. These may be low estimates because diagnosis may not be made until later in life when functional deficits are more noticeable. FAS is many times higher among those of low socioeconomic status (SES) and is higher in some ethnic populations, but these data may be confounded because of SES. Various researchers have examined the outcomes from women who used alcohol in pregnancy. The results of studies vary because of different definitions of mild, moderate, and severe alcohol use; different alcohol content in different alcoholic beverages; and varying patterns of alcohol consumption, ranging from a regular daily amount, to periodic binges, to a combination of both. Nevertheless, it is estimated that the risk for any major or minor congenital anomaly in an alcohol-abusing pregnancy ranges from 38–71%, with an overall adverse pregnancy outcome average of 50%. Data as to the magnitude of risk for the pregnant woman who ingests a minimal amount of alcohol either consistently or sporadically are less clear-cut. Some researchers suggest that alcohol does not need to be totally avoided during pregnancy and that it may be more realistic for women to restrict their intake to one standard measure (1 oz equivalent of absolute alcohol) per day. They fear that unnecessary guilt may arise in mothers of children with birth defects who drank mildly during pregnancy. However, others disagree, and presently, no minimum safe level for alcohol consumption in pregnancy has been established. Pregnant women should avoid drinking alcohol and be aware of the alcohol content in food and drugs.

Although there is a relationship between the dose of alcohol consumed, the time of pregnancy, and the severity of defects in the fetus, studies in animals and humans have determined that benefits are accrued if maternal consumption of alcohol ceases, even if this occurs after the first trimester.

Thus, it is important to identify individuals who are still using alcohol by the first prenatal visit, if not at a contraceptive or general gynecologic visit. In general, women want to have healthy babies, and this provides motivation even in the severe alcoholic. It has also been found that there is a decrease in the desire for alcohol during pregnancy. Both of these factors may help to support efforts by the concerned nurse geared at eliminating alcohol use in pregnancy.

Nursing Pointers

- Be aware of FASD when assessing newborns and infants. In children who have some features, consider the question, "What is the probability that this problem is secondary to alcohol exposure in utero?"
- A woman with chronic alcohol consumption is likely to be at increased risk in the perinatal period for abruptio placenta, precipitous delivery, tetanic contractions, or infection. Anticipate these problems.
- The infant of an alcohol-abusing mother may be at risk for altered glucose metabolism, withdrawal symptoms, or show FAS at birth. Therefore, be alert for respiratory problems, seizures, and tremors. The need for resuscitation is not uncommon.
- If FAS or alcohol-related effects are detected in newborns, look carefully for other defects.
- Nurses working with women of reproductive age should familiarize themselves with common signs and symptoms of alcoholism: neglect, family disruption, partners who abuse alcohol, agitation, tremors, and laboratory signs (e.g., macrocytic anemia, liver function abnormalities).
- The growth-restricted infant resulting from FAS or alcohol-related effects can be masked by the appearance of an apparent cause such as placental insufficiency; therefore, all small-for-date infants should be closely followed for several years.
- Be aware that the infant with alcohol-related effects may have poor sucking, and therefore failure to thrive may be compounded by the difficulty the mother has in feeding the infant.
- Support and help for the mother should begin in the immediate postpartum period and be reassessed and reinforced on return to the clinic or health practitioner.
- In the postpartum period, mothers with alcohol problems may be unable to form adequate bonding with their infant. Therefore, observe for these problems and promote bonding. There may be a prolonged recovery period, and alcohol abuse in the hospital should be watched for. Home follow-up should be arranged before the mother leaves the hospital.
- Education in parenting with demonstrations may be useful at various stages.
- Nurses do not necessarily need to become alcohol experts, but they do need to know where to obtain information and where to refer clients for help.
- Affected children and families should be referred for such support as early intervention programs, counseling, family therapy, and appropriate language, speech, and learning services
- Ongoing contact with a family who has had alcohol problems during pregnancy is necessary. Children who later manifest fretful behavior, hyperactivity, and abnormal sleep may be more prone to child abuse in an already unstable situation.
- School nurses may need to continue follow-up of the children, some of whom have learning deficits that become manifest in the school years. These children often superficially appear to have a large vocabulary and thus may not be detected early.
- Practitioners should take care not to cause women who drink to relieve tension or depression to switch to drugs as an alternative. Drugs may be more harmful than the alcohol.
- Encourage women identified as alcohol abusers to discontinue or decrease their intake before conception.
- Include the rest of the family when making assessments and referrals.

Cocaine and Use of Other Social and Street Substances

The use of cocaine and crack cocaine has become epidemic; estimates are that 1% of the U.S. population has tried cocaine. Many women who use cocaine also use other street drugs such as marijuana or metamphetamines or alcohol and may also suffer from poor nutrition, stress, infections and other confounding conditions, making effects on the fetus difficult to isolate to one agent and difficult to evaluate. Multiple drug use may also be synergistic. Street drug use is probably more dangerous to the homeless woman without prenatal care than to the middle-class woman. In general, cocaine use can result in intrauterine growth restriction (IUGR), low birth weight, increased fetal loss, prematurity, obstetrical complications, microcephaly, urogenital and other congenital malformations, and neurological and behavioral effects such as irritability, excitability, poor state regulation, and poor sleep. Later, poor feeding and poor visual and auditory tracking may occur. Cognitive and attentional process deficts as well as language delay and behavioral problems seem to persist. The results of studies are difficult to evaluate for the reasons listed above.

Cigarette Smoking

Between 19% and 30% of pregnant women continue to smoke. Maternal cigarette smoking in pregnancy is related to detrimental effects. These include an increased spontaneous abortion rate, an increased perinatal mortality rate, an increased incidence of maternal complications such as placenta abruptio and placenta previa, decreased birth weight and size in later childhood, an increased incidence of preterm delivery, and lower Apgar scores at 1 and 5 minutes after birth. The last is a source of particular concern because low Apgar scores have been associated in other studies with developmental and neurologic disabilities in later life.

Ionizing Radiation

Radiation occurs naturally in the background such as cosmic radiation, and people on flights have some exposure depending on altitude and length of time. This is usually significant only for pregnant frequent flyers such as pilots and flight attendants. A frequent reason for seeking genetic counseling is radiation exposure during pregnancy. The consequences of the effects of low-dose radiation to the fetus are still somewhat unsettled. There is probably no threshold level that can be considered absolutely safe for radiation exposure. The type of radiation emitted, its affinity for certain tissues, and the actual dose absorbed by the fetus are factors to consider. The most sensitive stage for spontaneous abortion due to radiation is just before or after the time of the first menstrual period after becoming pregnant when neither pregnancy nor the loss may be real-

ized. However, radiation may be detrimental to the fetus in any stage of pregnancy, including fetal death, malformation, tissue effects, or cancer, especially leukemia. In the past, pelvimetry was used in pregnancy to detect fetopelvic disproportion, but it now is not useful in making decisions to perform cesarean sections.

The major hazard associated with in utero radiation exposure is an increased risk of childhood cancer for the fetus, no matter which trimester in which it occurred. Estimates vary, but the chance for leukemia to develop after in utero exposure of 1 to 2 centiGray (cGy) [1 cGy = 1 rad] is increased by a factor of 1.5 to 3 over the natural incidence. Doll and Wakeford (1997) estimate the excess risk for childhood cancer after irradiation of 10 mGy or more is approximately 6% per Gy. Larger doses of radiation (e.g., 50 cGy) have been known to result in microcephaly, intellectual disability, microphthalmia, genital and skeletal malformations, retinal changes, and cataracts. Another unit of measure used is the sievert (Sv) or millasievert (mSv) (100 rem = 1 Sv). As discussed in Chapter 12, the largest radiation accident occurred at the Chernobyl nuclear power plant in the Ukraine on April 26, 1986. Some children exposed in utero were said to exhibit intellectual disability and behavioral effects.

It is obviously preferable to prevent inadvertent or unnecessary radiation exposure of the pregnant woman. Some measures that nurses should be aware of to do this are as follows:

Nursing Pointers

- In women of reproductive age, limit radiation exposure to that which is clearly indicated, necessary, and for which information or treatment cannot be obtained any other way.
- Women of reproductive age who receive radiation to the lower abdomen or pelvis should be advised to use contraception and delay conception for several months after exposure.
- All clients should be encouraged to ask exactly why an X-ray film is being ordered and how necessary it is.
- Clients should keep records of the X-ray films that they have had so unnecessary duplication does not occur.
- Women should be encouraged to let a health professional know if there is a possibility of pregnancy before receiving radiation.

- Health professionals should always ask female patients in a nonjudgmental way if there is a possibility of pregnancy before the woman receives any radiation. It is particularly important to be nonjudgmental and appropriate in manner when asking this of an adolescent.
- Be aware that pregnancy can mimic some gastrointestinal and genitourinary disorders.
- Pregnant nurses and other female employees should not work with patients receiving radioisotopes.
- The minimum number of radiographs in the smallest field, with the lowest duration and intensity of exposure, should always be used.
- Before X-ray or radioisotope therapy is given to a female patient, determine the date of the last menstrual period, determine if pregnancy is possible, and if it is, communicate this information to the physician ordering the therapy and ask that necessity and risk be discussed with the woman, with the possibility of delay being considered.
- A pregnancy test may be done if there is considerable doubt.
- The gonads should always be effectively shielded. Clients should be encouraged to request this because a recent study showed that in about one-third of exposures, no shielding was used.
- If possible, delay the procedure until onset of next menstruation or within the 10 days following the first day of the last menstrual period, unless data are important because of immediate illness of the woman.

Infectious Agents and Intrauterine Infections

The first recognized association between an infectious disease in the mother and congenital abnormalities in the newborn was made for syphilis in 1850. A definitive cause-and-effect relationship between a virus and specific congenital malformations was first established by Gregg after a rubella epidemic in Australia in 1941 led to a significant excess of congenital cataracts and heart disease in infants whose mothers had contracted rubella in the first trimester. Fetal consequences of maternal infection may include:

- embryonic or fetal death (If in the first few weeks, the embryo may resorb; otherwise spontaneous abortion or stillbirth will occur);
- premature or term delivery of a normal infant;
- premature or term delivery of an infant with IUGR/low birth weight, congenital infection, congenital anomalies, or persistent postnatal infection.

Congenitally infected infants may show clinical or subclinical infection with or without immediate or long-term consequences. Fetal death may be due to either direct fetal invasion by the microorganism or to severe maternal damage (e.g., fever, toxins). The degree of damage to the fetus is not related to the severity of the maternal infection. Many infections with severe fetal consequences can occur in mothers with few or no signs of illness.

Some problems that nurses should be aware of in identifying the stage of fetal development or relating abnormalities to maternal infection include doubt as to the date of the last menstrual period; infection may have been subclinical or very mild; lack of maternal awareness of the importance of the infectious disease and failure to note the dates her illness encompassed; and lack of objective evidence of infection (e.g., laboratory tests due to expense, limited availability, nonrecognition of illness, or difficult techniques).

The most important intrauterine infections in the United States traditionally were syphilis, toxoplasmosis, rubella, cytomegalovirus, and herpes simplex, known by the acronym STORCH. Since others such as human immunodeficiency virus (HIV) infection have become important, the acronym is not used as widely. Infection with some organisms is so rare in pregnancy that their effects are almost impossible to distinguish from chance events. One of the chief roles for nursing lies in prevention of infection in pregnancy. The most important diseases resulting in congenital anomalies in the fetus are individually discussed below. Rubella, toxoplasmosis, cytomegalovirus infection and syphilis, are discussed in detail. Other information is found in Table 8.5.

Rubella

An epidemic of rubella resulted in the birth of more than 20,000 infants with congenital rubella syndrome in the United States in 1964. The develop-

TABLE 8.5   Harmful Effects of Selected Infectious Agents During Pregnancy

Agent/Disease	Increased Reproductive Loss	Effects Congenital Malformations	Prematurity or Growth Retardation
Viral			
Coxsackie B	+	?*	0
Cytomegalovirus	+	+	+
Chicken pox (varicella-zoster)	0	+	+
Herpes simplex 1 and 2	+	+	+
Mumps	+	?	0
Parvovirus B19	+	?	+
Polio	+	0	+
Rubella	+	+	+
Rubeola (measles)	+	?	+
Venezuelan equine encephalitis	+	+	0
Bacterial			
Syphilis (*Treponema pallidum*)	+	+	?
Tuberculosis	+	0?	+
Listeriosis (*Listeria monocytogenes*)	+	0	+?
Group B streptococcus infection	+	0	?
Chlamydia trachomatis	+	0	+
Neisseria gonorrhoeae	0	0	+
Q fever	+	0	0
Parasitic			
Malaria (*Plasmodium* spp)	+	0	+
Toxoplasmosis (*T. gondii*)	+	+	+
Chagas' disease (*Trypanosoma cruzi*)	+	0	?
Fungal			
Valley fever (*Coccidioides immitis*)	+	0	+

+ = established, 0 = no present evidence, ? = possible, not established.
*suspected of causing fetal cardiac anomalies.

ment of a vaccine in 1966, concerted vaccination efforts, recognition of the effects of maternal infection, and increased social acceptance of therapeutic abortion resulted in a marked decrease in cases of congenital rubella syndrome, with 22 cases reported in the United States in 1975. Since that time, the number of cases has risen due to decreased levels of vaccinated persons in the community, and outbreaks may occur among religious communities refusing vaccination. An estimated 10–15% of women of childbearing age lack rubella antibody and are at risk for developing rubella during pregnancy. Since 50% of individuals with rubella may not develop a rash and because the disease can be mild in adults, about one third of pregnant women who contract rubella either do not recognize or do not report their illness.

The risk of fetal eye and cardiac malformations is greatest when infection occurs in the first 8 weeks of pregnancy, and the risk of deafness is greatest between 5 and 15 weeks of pregnancy. Data are insufficient for the consequences of infection acquired after the fourth to fifth month, but delayed development and hearing deficits have been described when infection occurred as late as the 31st week of pregnancy.

The frequency of specific clinical features of the rubella syndrome varies. Approximately one-third of defects are missed in the neonatal period and become noticeable later in childhood. The classic features described in the early literature, such as cardiac malformations (especially patent ductus arteriosus and pulmonary stenosis), eye abnormalities (especially cataracts, retinopathy, microphthalmia, and glaucoma), and permanent hearing loss (bilateral and unilateral), are still seen. To them, the following features of the expanded syndrome can be added: growth restriction, one manifestation of which is low birth weight for gestation; microcephaly; bone lesions and radiologic changes in long bones, often described as "celery stalk"; thrombocytopenia, petechiae, and purpura, which give the newborn a "blueberry muffin" appearance; jaundice; hepatosplenomegaly; pneumonitis; and encephalitis. Among the abnormalities often not detected in infancy are genitourinary anomalies, adrenal insufficiency, behavioral manifestations of minimal brain dysfunction, intellectual disability, autism, various thyroid disorders including hypothyroidism, and growth hormone deficiency. Hearing loss may not be evident until later childhood, after secondary learning and speech disabilities have accrued These findings plus progressive panencephalitis seen in the second decade and diabetes mellitus, which develops in 10–20% of affected infants, may be caused by the persistence of virus in tissues. Approximately 30% of infants with congenital rubella syndrome die in the first four months. Because the risk of fetal damage is substantial, therapeutic termination of pregnancy should be discussed with any pregnant woman known to have contracted rubella during pregnancy, one with known exposure, or one to whom rubella vaccine was inadvertently administered during pregnancy.

Nursing Pointers

- Because there is no treatment for congenital rubella, all efforts must be directed at prevention. Women who are considering pregnancy should have serologic evaluation to determine whether rubella antibody is present.
- Susceptible women of childbearing age should be vaccinated only in the documented absence of pregnancy; instructions should include the necessity to use contraception and avoid pregnancy for at least three menstrual cycles after vaccination.
- Vaccination should be followed by serologic determination that appropriate antibody response has occurred.
- Vaccination as a routine part of childhood immunization programs should be supported and encouraged.
- Identified pregnant women who are susceptible to rubella should be vaccinated immediately postpartum and postabortion.
- Rubella titers and vaccination if indicated should be done for all female staff on obstetrics and newborn units or clinics, and in day care centers, schools, prisons, and facilities for the intellectually disabled.
- Seek confirmation of suspected exposure to rubella (i.e., examination of contact).
- Because infected infants shed virus through the nasopharynx and urine, they should be kept away from women in their childbearing years, isolated in the hospital, and kept apart from susceptible women in clinics and offices.

Toxoplasmosis

Toxoplasmosis is caused by the protozoan *Toxoplasma gondii*. Adults may acquire the organism from the ingestion of raw or undercooked meat or by contamination of soil, litter, and food by the feces of infected cats. Acquired infection is usually found in children or young adults and can be detected by serum antibody screening. Overall 20–30% of women of reproductive age in the United States have such serum antibodies, but this varies with geographic location, socioeconomic level, and cultural practices. The following are estimated rates of transmission to the fetus according to when the mother acquires toxoplasmosis: the first trimester 15%; second trimester 25%; and third trimester 50–65%, with an overall risk of about 40%. Accurate transmission rates are difficult to determine because 70% of newborns later found to have congenital toxoplasmosis are asymptomatic at birth The risk for severe manifestations is highest in the first trimester.

Congenital toxoplasmosis is almost always caused by acute primary infection in pregnancy (estimated at 0.2–1.0%), which can be asymptomatic or consist of any of the following: mild fever, enlarged lymph glands, headache, or muscle aches —all of which may be easily dismissed or unappreciated. Thus, only those who became infected during pregnancy would be at risk for fetal compli

cations or stillbirths. Antenatal testing would usually have to be done twice to determine this—once
to detect negative individuals and again to see if sero-
conversion occurred. Drugs used in treatment are
considered toxic with possible teratogenic effects, so
therapeutic abortion is an option that should be
discussed with patients who clearly have had sero-
conversion.

Congenital toxoplasmosis shows varying manifestations that may include chorioretinitis, cerebral
calcification, hydrocephalus, microcephaly, convulsions, anemia, seizures, hepatosplenomegaly,
anemia, rash, and intellectual disability. Late-
manifesting sequelae include intellectual impairment, developmental delay, hearing loss, nystagmus,
strabismus, and late-developing chorioretinitis resulting in blindness. Screening has been proposed
for women before or during pregnancy and also for
newborns. Prenatal diagnosis of fetal toxoplasmosis
can be accomplished. Treatment has been attempted during pregnancy, and there is indication that it
may be of benefit to the fetus without harm. The
treatment of infants with congenital toxoplasmosis
for a year with pyrimethamine and sulfadizine giv-
en with leukovorin shows promise for achieving essentially normal neurologic, cognitive, and auditory
outcomes (McLeod, Boyer, Karrison, Kasza, Swisher, roizen, et al., 2006). Other points that nurses
should include in health teaching are to advise
pregnant women to do the following:

- Eat only well-cooked meat (heated to 66°C),
  or freeze all meat if they want to cook it less
  than well done.
- Avoid close contact with cats.
- If they have a cat in their home, someone else
  should change the cat's litter daily and dispose
  of feces in a sanitary manner. The cat should
  be fed only cooked, dry, or canned food; it
  should be kept away from wild rodents.
- Practice good handwashing before eating or
  handling food and after gardening or handling
  uncooked meat or touching pets.
- Do not eat raw eggs.
- Wash all raw fruits and vegetables carefully.
- Control flies and roaches, and limit their
  access to food.
- Use special precautions if their work involves
  animals in a lab or as a veterinarian.
- Cover children's sandboxes.

Cytomegalovirus

Cytomegalovirus (CMV) belongs to the same family as the herpes virus. Approximately 0.2–2.2%,
with an average of 1%, of live-born infants have
congenital CMV, but this varies considerably in different populations. It is said to be the current most
frequent cause of intrauterine infection in the United States, estimated to occur in about 44,000 U.S.
infants per year. Intrauterine infection occurs usually because of primary maternal infection, but it
can also result from reactivation of latent infection.
The rate of transmission to the fetus after primary
maternal infection in pregnancy can vary but is
about 40–50%. Those at highest risk for primary
CMV in pregnancy are young primiparas of the
lower socioeconomic groups.

Classic cytomegalic inclusion disease is seen in
only about 10% of infected newborns and can include
the following: microcephaly, hepatosplenomegaly,
jaundice, petechial rash, cerebral calcifications, motor
disabilities, chorioretinitis, microphthalmia, hydrocephalus, and hernia. A small percentage has milder
disease. Primary teeth may show characteristic enamel defects such as discoloration, opacity and rapid
wearing. However, the majority of infants are asymptomatic at birth, and many later show long-term sequelae such as sensorineural hearing loss, minimal
brain dysfunction, intellectual disability, dental defects, motor defects, or poor school performance.
Chorioretinitis may not be detected at birth but may
be seen later. The magnitude of long-term insidious
effects has only begun to be appreciated. Early detection helps children to achieve their maximum potential through early remedial efforts.

Nursing Pointers

- Because even asymptomatic infected newborns
  shed virus through urine and saliva for up to
  three years after birth, thus disseminating infection, they should be kept from direct contact with pregnant women, including the staff,
  when in the hospital, home, office, or clinic.
- Infants with suspected or proven disease should
  be closely followed up for detection of delayed
  effects (including perceptual deficits and dental defects) and for appropriate medical, educational, and family support.
- Serologic testing should be done on the first
  prenatal visit in order to detect seroconverters,
  especially in high-risk groups.

- CMV should be suspected in women with mononucleosis-type symptoms, and diagnosis should be pursued.
- Documented maternal infection, especially in the first trimester, is a reason to discuss pregnancy termination with the client.
- Antibody determinations should be done in female employees. Those without antibodies who are planning pregnancy should not be assigned to obstetric or newborn units or seek employment in day care centers, schools, or congregate living facilities.
- If a blood transfusion is needed for a pregnant woman, use citrated blood that is more than three days old, if possible, because CMV can be transmitted in fresh whole blood.
- Emphasis should be placed on good hand washing for women throughout pregnancy, and especially after contact with potential infective sources.
- Care in handling blood and urine specimens is essential.
- Enforcement of good hand-washing techniques in hospitals, day care centers, and clinics is essential. Hospital personnel appear at increased risk for CMV, and full infection control measures may be warranted with known infected cases.

Syphilis

Syphilis is caused by the spirochete *Treponema pallidum*. It is still a significant sexually-transmitted disease in the United States with about 20,000 new cases a year and over 300 cases of congenital syphilis per year. Infants with reactive tests or whose mother had untreated or inadequately treated syphilis are classified as not infected, confirmed case, or probable case. The major route of infection is through sexual contact, but it can also be transmitted through contaminated injection equipment, especially among drug users, or through direct nonsexual contact with infectious lesions. The infected pregnant woman can transmit syphilis to the fetus at any stage of her pregnancy and in any stage of the disease. Transmission occurs in 70-100% of cases; if the fetus is not treated, 25% die in utero.

Congenital syphilis can be manifested as *early* (before 2 years of age) or *late* (after 2 years of age), but overlap occurs. In early syphilis, the most common symptoms are rhinitis or "snuffles," hepatosplenomegaly, generalized lymph node enlargement, jaundice, rash, and bone involvement including osteomyelitis. Often attention is first sought for affected infants because of rhinitis, persistent diaper rash, or failure to thrive. If not diagnosed or not treated completely, the manifestations of late congenital syphilis may be seen, including teeth changes (Hutchinson's teeth, Moon's or mulberry molars), eye lesions (keratitis, photophobia, uveitis, corneal scarring), deafness, bone changes (saddle nose, hard palate perforations, saber shins, impaired maxillary growth), neurologic involvement (paresis, convulsive disorders), and intellectual disability.

Nurses should be aware that all pregnant women should be tested for syphilis at their first prenatal visit because of the success in minimizing fetal damage when treated with penicillin. If a pregnant woman has a positive result, the underlying cause should be determined so that treatment can be instituted if necessary. Women at the greatest risk for developing syphilis should be retested later in pregnancy. Some factors identified as associated with increased risk are women who are unmarried, very young mothers, drug use in the woman or her partner, sexual promiscuity, contact with known syphilitics or those with sexually transmitted diseases (STDs), history of past STDs including HIV, tattooed women, members of disadvantaged urban minority groups, and women who have unexplained lesions or rashes. Syphilis is disproportionately prevalent in the southeastern United States. A high index of suspicion is needed to consider syphilis in pregnant woman. Factors associated with risk at the time of delivery are premature delivery with no explanation, unexplained large placenta, hydrops fetalis, unexplained stillbirth, or no prenatal care. Further investigation and a blood test should be carried out in order to minimize severe fetal effects. The Centers for Disease Control and Prevention (CDC) recommends blood tests for pregnant women at both 20 and 28 weeks.

Other Infections

As new or newly recognized infectious diseases emerge, there is a need to address the effects of the causative microbial agent on pregnancy outcomes. For example, little information is available on monkeypox, a zoonotic disease caused by an orthopoxvirus. In one case, a woman infected at 24 weeks gestation delivered an infant with a monkeypox-like rash who subsequently died at 6 weeks of age. In regard to pregnant women infected by severe acute respiratory syndrome (SARS) associated coronavirus, their infants did not show congenital malformations but two of the five in one study had growth retardation, and two of five had severe gastrointestinal complications, including necrotizing enterocolitis (Shek et al., 2003). Both the hepatitis B and hepatitis E viruses have a high rate of transmission to the fetus which may result in severe fetal hepatitis. In regard to West Nile virus infection caused by a flavivirus, the CDC has issued interim guidelines and is collecting data on the effects of maternal infection in pregnancy. It has been recommended by the Practice Committee of the Society for Assisted Reproductive Technology that those with suspected or confirmed West Nile virus infection be deferred from gamete donation (2006). The same is true of certain other infections, and the Society can be contacted for further information.

Maternal Environment

The maternal environment and metabolism affects the developing fetus in many ways. Effects derive from interaction of maternal and fetal genotypes, as well as their interaction with internal and external environmental effects. The influence of maternal nutrition and risks of pregnancy and childbirth to adult women with genetic disorders such as Marfan syndrome (see Chapter 10) are beyond the scope of this book. Major genetically determined alterations, such as diabetes mellitus and maternal PKU, are discussed below.

Diabetes Mellitus

The incidence of major congenital anomalies in the offspring of diabetic women is three to four times that of controls. Maternal metabolic influences appear to be the primary determining factor. Although all major anomalies are increased, those of the cardiovascular system (especially a hypertrophic type of cardiomyopathy), kidneys, and skeletal system are most prominent, with caudal dysplasia or sacral agenesis present in 1%. Infants frequently have macrosomia; they are large for their gestational age but are physiologically immature, have increased total body fat, and have enlarged viscera. Nurses should anticipate that the infant of a diabetic mother frequently exhibits lethargy, hypotonia, polycythemia (hematocrits above 65%) leading to other complications, a poor sucking reflex, and metabolic imbalances such as hypocalcemia (present in up to 50%), hypomagnesemia (present in up to 38%), hyperbilirubinemia, and hypoglycemia and plan accordingly. Careful observation is necessary because the neuromuscular system is often very excitable. Respiratory distress, often from hyaline membrane disease, is five to six times that found in normal newborns. Long-term effects include obesity (by 8 years of age, 50% of the weight of offspring were over the 90th percentile), cognitive impairment, and developmental delays. All these effects are more frequent with suboptimal control. Perinatal and maternal mortality are higher in diabetic women. Increase in glycosolated hemoglobin is seen in poorly controlled diabetics and correlates with increased hyperglycemia. Diabetic women who want children should probably be helped to plan these at a younger age before diabetic-related pathology worsens. Prenatal diagnosis that includes ultrasound, amniocentesis, and alpha-fetoprotein level determination should be used to monitor the pregnant woman. Before conception, folic acid in recommended doses to help to prevent neural tube defects is recommended. The time of delivery may be geared to the determination of fetal lung maturity.

It is currently believed that poor diabetic control (hyperglycemia) and ketoacidosis are responsible for the above findings. In order to minimize these effects, it is necessary to rigorously control metabolic balance and blood sugar from preconception through delivery, carefully monitor other potential risks such as hypertension, follow thyroid function closely, and use folic acid supplements daily. Success is best if an expert in the management of diabetic pregnancy is consulted. Because this control may be more stringent than that needed for everyday management of the nonpregnant diabetic, the mother's full cooperation and understanding is vital. Basic education as to the benefits of such control beginning prior to planned conception should be integrated in teaching programs for diabetic women of reproductive age.

Nurses should also be aware of some risk factors associated with potential gestational diabetes:

- Family history of diabetes
- Previous infant with birth weight over 4 kg–4.5 kg (8.8 lb–9.9 lb)
- Neonatal hypoglycemia or anomaly
- Previous or current polyhydramnios
- Unexplained perinatal death or recurrent spontaneous abortions
- Previous episode of latent diabetes
- Obesity (20 lb above ideal weight)
- History of toxemia, pyelonephritis, recurrent urinary infections, glycosuria, or abnormal glucose tolerance test

It is estimated that 20–30% of women who develop gestational diabetes become overt diabetics within five years, so such women should be followed with this in mind. Since about 4% of all women develop gestational diabetes, screening should be conducted during pregnancy.

Maternal Phenylketonuria and Hyperphenylalaninemia

The successful early dietary treatment of children with PKU or hyperphenylalaninemia (PHP) has prevented early, severe mental retardation and resulted in nonretarded adult women with PKU or PHP who then had their own children. In the late 1950s and early 1960s, it became apparent that a substantial number of non-PKU, non-hyperphenylalaninemic (non-PHp) offspring of these women were retarded. Fetal damage appears because of the prenatal exposure to the high concentration of either phenylalanine or its metabolites in the mother. Such women also have an increased frequency of spontaneous abortion. The major untoward fetal effects include intellectual disability, microcephaly, congenital heart disease, esophageal atresia, neurologic problems (convulsions and spasticity), and growth restriction. Although diet restrictions are now thought to be lifelong, diet therapy for PKU typically ceased in childhood and so many women were on a normal diet (see Chapters 5 and 12). The reinstitution of a low phenylalanine (phe) diet throughout pregnancy is believed to prevent or minimize the fetal effects. Maternal weight and nutrient intake need to be monitored. Diet recommendations are those that maintain

blood phenylalanine concentrations between 2 and 6 mg/dL. Levels that are too low can impair fetal growth. Reports of the success of these efforts have been both positive and negative, and adherence may be one factor. It is believed that such therapy should begin before conception and be in effect at conception for optimal benefit. Thus, females with PKU or PHP should be followed over a long period, and information about maternal PKU should be included in their health teaching. Recalling girls at 12 years of age for information about maternal PKU and reproductive counseling may be effective. To do this, all PKU persons would need to be entered into a registry at diagnosis, presenting logistical and ethical problems. Adolescents with PKU or PHP may need to accept a greater level of responsibility if they choose to become sexually active.

The nurse should see that data regarding the outcome of maternal PKU or PHP are discussed with women known to be at risk, so that they may explore the options available. The nurse should then assist her in obtaining optimum dietary counseling with monitoring from a nutritionist experienced with maternal PKU and also help her to obtain products and recipes. It is recommended that serum levels of phe be monitored twice a week and that fetal development be monitored with ultrasound. I once counseled a multigenerational family with PKU. The mother with PKU, who had one infant with both maternal effects and PKU because the father was a PKU carrier, was seeking counseling before a second pregnancy.

Other Maternal Metabolic and Genetic Disorders

Improved detection and treatment in infancy and childhood has led to women with other biochemical disorders reaching adulthood and becoming pregnant. This is also true of women with disorders such as congenital heart disease, which can affect the fetus in an indirect biochemical sense, for example, through anoxia. Women with myotonic dystrophy (an autosomal dominant disorder with cataracts and muscle weakness) have increased rates of spontaneous abortions, stillbirths, and perinatal deaths, and polyhydramnios in such women may be correlated with an affected fetus. Women with acute intermittent porphyria (see Chapter 6) have exacerbations of disease in pregnancy and increased rates of prematurity and spontaneous abortion. It has been suggested that women such as those with maternal PKU use in-vitro fertilization and implantation of the pre-embryo in a surrogate mother for gestational carriage to term. Other problems experienced in pregnancy may not be directly connected to the biochemical milieu, but will not be discussed here. For example, women with Marfan syndrome (see Chapter 10) may experience stress on the already compromised cardiovascular system, and women with Ehlers-Danlos syndrome may have a higher incidence of hernias and delivery complications. Women with sickle cell anemia may deliver small-for-gestational-age infants and need to be watched for complications, and those with spina bifida can be at risk for premature labor.

Hyperthermia

Hyperthermia has been shown to be teratogenic in animals and may cause an increased risk of neural tube defects. Major sources of hyperthermia for pregnant women include fever, baths, saunas, and hot tubs. Data on fevers are confounded by effects of the microorganism such as a virus. For example, possible teratogenic effects of influenza and the common cold may be related to the accompanying fever. However, it is wise to prevent the effects of high fever in pregnancy by using a "safe" antifever drug. Some advocate additional folic acid supplementation as well.

Other Environmental Exposures in Pregnancy

Evidence of environmental contamination by toxic chemicals often comes to the light because of the observation of what appears to be a high frequency or clustering of birth defects, spontaneous abortions, or miscarriages, and may be observed by citizens or professionals. One of the first widespread examples was discovered in 1956 in the Minamata Bay area of Japan. Industrial waste from a fertilizer company containing methylmercury was discharged into the bay that was used for fishing. Many pregnant women either aborted or gave birth to infants with a congenital neurologic disorder resembling cerebral palsy, although the women often showed no ill effects themselves. Follow-up studies have shown that many who were exposed in utero later showed other developmental deficits and mental deficiency. In Iraq, imported grain from Mexico that was treated

with methylmercury as a fungicide was used for bread, instead of planting, by large numbers of individuals. The warning about toxicity was in Spanish and was not understood. Many of the infants subsequently born to women eating bread made with the grain also showed a cerebral palsy–like illness that included blindness and brain damage. In the United States, a family in New Mexico that ingested pork that had been fed grain contaminated by organic mercury used as a fungicide also became ill, and the pregnant mother gave birth to an infant with features of the disorder. In all these cases, some persons were more susceptible to the mercury; not all those who ate contaminated products evidenced toxicity. High levels of mercury (above 1 parts per million) are present in certain fish such as swordfish, tilefish, shark, whale meat, and mackerel in the United States. Pregnant women should minimize the amount of these fish that they eat.

Toxic exposure to lead has occurred by means of environmental and workplace pollution and hobbies, as discussed in Chapter 12. A comparison of pregnancy outcomes was done in two Missouri cities: Rolla, in the lead mining belt, and Columbia, which is not. In Rolla there was a statistically higher rate of prematurity and molar pregnancies. It is believed that the fetus may be sensitive to lead but not manifest such sensitivity until early childhood in the form of impaired intelligence; subtle neurobehavioral changes; growth delay, including decreased height and weight; speech, language, or attention deficits, behavior abnormalities; and developmental deficits. Microcytic anemia may be seen. It can be difficult to sort out prenatal effects from environmental exposure in infancy and childhood. Low birth weight may be associated with lead exposure. Various genetic factors may influence the vulnerability of the brain to lead as well as lead absorption. "Acceptable" lead levels in children have been decreased over time, and it is thought that the current "acceptable" level may be too high.

In areas where the drinking water is high in lead, nurses can advise women planning pregnancy to have their water checked and use an alternate source, such as bottled water, for drinking if necessary. Additionally, household substances such as paint, dust in contaminated areas, or contamination through employment such as construction work can pose a risk to the worker and the family. It is important to advocate safe environmental lead levels and to provide the necessary education and resources such as public health departments to make homes and communities safe from lead contamination. Good preconceptional counseling and prenatal care can help the mother reduce lead exposure in pregnancy and after.

PRENATAL DETECTION AND DIAGNOSIS

Methods of prenatal detection and diagnosis are both invasive and noninvasive. Detection techniques usually involve screening applied broadly to the pregnant population, while diagnostic techniques are targeted because of one or more specific reasons for increased risk. These methods include the techniques shown in Box 8.3.

Ideally, preconception counseling can precede pregnancy, and therefore prenatal diagnosis, so that potential preventive steps such as rubella titer determination and vaccination before conception can be taken if necessary, and folic acid, other vitamin supplementation, and other preventive measures can be accomplished to reduce some risks.

Although prenatal diagnosis has long been a standard of care for women 35 years and older, women younger than 35 years now deliver 75–80% of all infants born with Down syndrome. These younger women would not ordinarily be candidates

for prenatal diagnosis. Current obstetrical practic in the United States usually includes the first and/or second-trimester prenatal screening an detection techniques of maternal serum analyt screening with ultrasound. Ultrasonography ma be used for routine screening in both the first an second trimesters as well as for diagnosis at mor sophisticated levels. Ultrasound is also now used fo measurement of nuchal translucency (sometime called NT screening test, the translucent or clea space in back of the fetal neck on ultrasound) i conjunction with screening of a small sample o blood for maternal serum free beta human chori onic gonadotropin (hCG), and maternal-serun pregnancy-associated plasma protein (PAPP-A) t detect Down syndrome as early as possible in th pregnancy. Higher levels of hCG and lower levels o PAPP-A are associated with Down syndrome. Th time for using this combination is 11 to 13 week gestation. At this time, some practitioners also loo' for the presence or absence of the nasal bone, an these data, along with maternal age, gestational age and any chromosome abnormalities in any previ ous pregnancies, are entered into a computer pro gram. This combination of markers is used to give specific risk mainly for Down syndrome, trisom 13, and trisomy 18. Other chromosome abnormal ities found with increased NT measurements o more than 3 mm include other chromosome ab normalities such as Turner syndrome and triploidy and some other birth defects such as certain ab dominal wall defects and cardiac septal defects a well as some other genetic syndromes such as vari ous skeletal dysplasias and Noonan syndrome. Sus picious findings should prompt further testing an counseling.

It must be remembered that this is a screening not a diagnostic test. When all of these markers are used, the accuracy of the risk assessment for Dowi syndrome can be as high as 97% and is about 80% using NT alone. Those determined to be at in creased risk may wish a diagnostic test such a chorionic villus sampling, which can be done early or amniocentesis, done slightly later. Sometime women who are at increased risk because of mater nal age over 35 years who have a lower risk after thi screening will decide not to have more invasive pre natal diagnostic testing, although they may wish t have targeted ultrasound and maternal serum test ing for neural tube defects. First-trimester screening

---

BOX 8.3

Most Common Methods of Prenatal Detection and Diagnosis

- Maternal serum screening (detection)
- Ultrasonography (detection and diagnosis)
- Amniocentesis (diagnosis)
- Chorionic villus sampling (diagnosis)
- Embryofetoscopy (diagnosis)
- Fetal blood and tissue sampling (diagnosis)
- Preimplantation diagnosis (diagnosis)
- The analysis of fetal cells and cell-free fetal DNA in maternal circulation (investigational)

has become a standard of care in Europe and is on its way to such acceptance in the United States.

At 15 to 22 weeks (16 to 18 optimal) in the second trimester, the use of maternal serum screening for alpha-fetoprotein (MSAFP) and for other markers for detection of certain defects, particularly open neural tube defects (NTDs), where AFP is elevated, and certain chromosome disorders, depending on the markers used, has become commonplace in pregnancy. It is important to stress, however, that this is a screening test, not a diagnostic test. Therefore, the finding of any abnormal results requires prompt diagnostic investigation. About 90% of infants with NTDs are born to mothers with no prior history or known high risk; therefore, they would not be predetermined to be at high risk and would not be referred for amniocentesis or targeted ultrasound. The severe burden of NTDs made this screening highly desirable. In maternal serum, typically these tests are called the multiple marker tests or screen, and include determination of AFP; hCG, either total or free β; and unconjugated estriol (μE_3). These are used in screening maternal serum for fetal aneuploidy, usually with at least one other indicator depending on trimester such as pregnancy-associated plasma protein-A (PAPP-A), inhibin-A, often in conjunction with ultrasound determined fetal nuchal translucency measurements, and sometimes determination of the presence or absence of the nasal bone.

AFP is a glycoprotein, similar to albumin, that is first synthesized in the fetal yolk sac and later in the fetal liver. It can be detected in the amniotic fluid and the maternal serum. The source of AFP in amniotic fluid and maternal blood originates from the fetal cerebrospinal fluid, gastric fluid, meconium, bile, and urine. The outcome of AFP's variety of origins in the fetus means that elevation of AFP occurs not only with open NTDs, but also with other fetal anomalies, making AFP a nonspecific test. For example, in gastrointestinal anomalies such as esophageal atresia, normal clearance of AFP through fetal swallowing cannot occur. In renal disorders, such as congenital nephrosis, excess fetal serum AFP is excreted and thus is elevated in the amniotic fluid.

AFP is used as a specific test when both parents are known carriers of congenital nephrosis, especially of the type frequent in persons of Finnish extraction. In renal agenesis, AFP is very low or absent. In closed NTDs, the layer of skin or tissue

present prevents AFP from leaking out through the fetal cerebrospinal fluid, and so AFP levels are not elevated. Thus, AFP cannot be used to detect the approximate 20% of spina bifidas and 94% of encephaloceles that are closed, while 90–100% of anencephaly is detected. The following major genetic conditions have been identified by elevated MSAFP levels during pregnancy:

- Open neural tube defects—spina bifida, anencephaly, and encephalocele
- Ventral wall defects—omphalocele (midline defect with herniation of abdominal organs into a membrane covered sac), gastroschisis (extrusion of abdominal organs anteriorly with no covering membrane)
- Congenital nephrosis (Finnish type)
- Cystic hygroma (sometimes in association with Turner syndrome)
- Other fetal defects such as Turner syndrome, teratomas, hydrocele, certain congenital skin conditions, and esophageal and duodenal atresia

AFP in maternal blood rises during pregnancy until the 30th gestational week and then falls. The concentration of amniotic fluid AFP (AFAFP) is highest at the end of the first trimester. AFP levels are reported in multiples of the median (MoM). Some degree of overlap occurs in AFP levels between normal pregnancies and pregnancies with NTDs (see Figure 8.2). If the cutoff level is set low enough to include almost all NTD pregnancies, then a large proportion of non-NTD pregnancies will be included, giving a high proportion of false-positive results. If the cutoff level is set so high that few unaffected pregnancies would be included, then a large proportion of NTD pregnancies will be missed, giving a high proportion of false-negative results. The usual cutoff is 2.0 to 2.5 MoM. These must be interpreted in relation to other factors.

A number of variables influence how laboratory results are calculated. Some are patient characteristics such as maternal weight, race, gestational age, maternal diabetes mellitus, and population norms. Various formulas and tables have been developed to determine the probability of a given woman with particular findings and characteristics for having a fetus with a NTD that are also population adjusted for the population frequency of NTDs, and

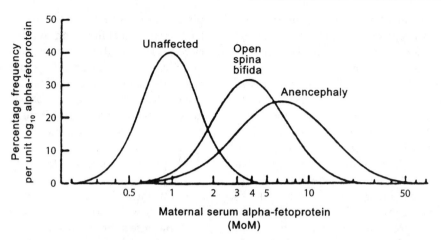

FIGURE 8.2   Frequency distribution of alpha-fetoprotein values at 16 to 18 weeks gestation. From the United Kingdom Collaborative Study on Alpha-Fetoprotein in Relation to Neural Tube Defects (1977). *Lancet, 1,* 1323. Reproduced with permission from Elsevier.

combination with the results from testing other analytes increases diagnostic accuracy.

While the chief reasons for elevated AFP levels other than diseases being screened for are errors in calculation of gestational age, low maternal weight, and membership in the Black race, there can be other reasons for high MSAFP levels. Some of these relate to pregnancy outcome, whereas others are population or biological in nature regarding interpretation when the MSAFP results are being evaluated. These include:

- Multiple pregnancy
- Prior amniocentesis or fetoscopy
- Fetal death
- Severe Rh incompatibility
- Threatened abortion
- Placental distress
- Levels in past pregnancies
- Bloody contamination

When MSAFP levels are elevated, the reason is sought. Typically an ultrasound examination is performed that includes confirming gestational age and fetal viability, and ruling out multiple gestation if possible. If the gestational age used for the MSAFP interpretation was wrong, then a recalculation is done. If gestational age is correct, then targeted ultrasound is done to look for the malformations known to result in high MSAFP levels.

Some clinicians will repeat the MSAFP, while others believe that targeted ultrasound or amniocentesis is warranted immediately.

Waiting for serum analyte screening results engenders anxiety. Parents should be informed promptly of both normal and abnormal results. They should not be told to assume normality if they do not hear from the clinic or center. Those having abnormal results require sensitive and appropriate counseling and referral for appropriate prenatal diagnosis.

ACOG has recommended multiple marker (MM) screening as standard care for women under 35 years of age. Clinicians should be sure that clients receive clear, nonbiased information about the meaning of the results of the MM screen, and that those with abnormal levels are promptly referred for ultrasonography and amniocentesis. Table 8.6 summarizes serum screening results for NTDs and chromosomal abnormalities.

Identifying Candidates for Prenatal Diagnosis

Practicing nurses should be able to recognize which individuals may be candidates for prenatal diagnosis, which is different from prenatal screening and detection suggested for the entire pregnant population with no known risk elevations. This information should be included with the rest of the care

TABLE 8.6   Association of Selected Maternal Serum Analytes and Selected Abnormality

Analyte	Abnormality		
	NTDs	Trisomy 21	Trisomy 18
Maternal serum AFP**	↑	↓	↓
hCG	Normal	↑	↓
uE3	Normal	↓	↓
PAPP-A	NA	↓*	↓
Inhibin A**	NA	↑	NA

* = 1st trimester. ** = 2nd trimester.

being provided. This assessment includes both maternal and paternal information. It may be appropriate to identify candidates for prenatal diagnosis before the individual is pregnant and include that information in preconceptional counseling when it occurs. This assessment may be accomplished by interview, questionnaire, and history. Amniocentesis and chorionic villus sampling (CVS) are the most common invasive diagnostic methods now used. Genetic indications for prenatal diagnosis are listed in Table 8.7. Various prenatal diagnostic procedures are listed in Table 8.8.

These indications identify individuals who will be at increased risk and thus form the basis for assessing which pregnant women are likely candidates for

TABLE 8.7   Some Current Genetic Indications for Prenatal Diagnosis

Indication	Possible Standard Prenatal Diagnostic Technique
Pregnancy at risk for chromosome aberration	
Maternal age of 35 years and above	Amniocentesis, CVS
Previous child with chromosome abnormality or instability disorder	Amniocentesis, CVS
Chromosomal abnormality in parent (mosaicism, translocation carrier, other aneuploidy)	Amniocentesis, CVS
Previous stillbirth or perinatal death (cause unknown)	Amniocentesis, CVS
History of infertility in either parent	Amniocentesis, CVS
Habitual abortion history	Amniocentesis, CVS
Previous child with malformations (no chromosomes analyzed)	Amniocentesis, CVS, Ultrasound
Intracytoplasmic sperm injection	Amniocentesis, CVS
Abnormal serum levels of multiple markers	Amniocentesis, CVS, Ultrasound
Pregnancy at risk for NTD	
High maternal serum level of AFP	Amniocentesis, Ultrasound
Previous child with NTD	Amniocentesis, Ultrasound
NTD in either parent or close relative	Amniocentesis, Ultrasound
Pregnancy at risk for X-linked inherited disorders	
Mother a known carrier	Amniocentesis, CVS
Close maternal male relative affected	Amniocentesis, CVS
Pregnancy at risk for detectable inherited biochemical disorder	
Parents known carriers or affected	Amniocentesis, CVS
Previous child born with known detectable biochemical disorder	Amniocentesis, CVS
Close family member with a known inherited biochemical disorder	Amniocentesis, CVS
Other	
High degree of parental anxiety	Amniocentesis, CVS, Ultrasound
Significant exposure to radiation, infection, chemicals, or drugs	Amniocentesis, Ultrasound, CVS
Diabetes mellitus in mother	Ultrasound, Amniocentesis
Previous child with structural abnormality	Ultrasound, Amniocentesis, CVS
Family history of structural abnormality	Ultrasound, Amniocentesis, CVS

Note: NTD = neural tube defects; AFP = alpha-fetoprotein; CVS = chronic villus sampling. Ultrasound refers to targeted or extended ultrasound.

TABLE 8.8   Selected Prenatal Diagnostic Procedures

Name	Comments
Amniocentesis	A sample of amniotic fluid is withdrawn from amniotic sac after ultrasound guidance. Ideally done between 15th and 18th gestational week. See text.
Chorionic villus sampling	A sample of chorion villi is obtained abdominally or cervically to test for chromosomal abnormalities and other genetic conditions at 10 to 12 weeks gestation. Fetal loss of 1% over baseline.
Early amniocentesis	Done at 12 to 14 weeks gestation. Have found increase in pregnancy loss and congenital foot deformities. No apparent advantage over CVS or amniocentesis.
Fetal blood sampling	Also known as percutaneous umbilical blood sampling (PUBS). Usually umbilical cord blood is sampled through an ultrasound-guided needle inserted in maternal abdomen. Used for diagnosis of genetic disorders that cannot be diagnosed any other way and rh disease; ascertain fetal blood chemistry such as acid-base balance. Fetal loss rates range from 2% to about 9%.
Fetal cells and fetal cell-free DNA circulating in maternal blood	Known that fetal cells and fetal DNA sequences are present in maternal circulation but in very small numbers. Once enriched and amplified, various technologies may be used to determine fetal sex and certain chromosomal abnormalities.
Preimplantation diagnosis	Genetic analysis is carried out on embryos in the 4- to 8-cell stage, and unaffected embryos can be transferred to the uterus. Often done after assisted reproductive technique such as in vitro fertilization.
Ultrasound	Alone used to detect fetal structural abnormalities between 18th and 20th week ideally. Sound waves are converted to images. Also used in conjunction with other procedures and tests such as for early detection of certain chromosome disorders using nuchal translucency and nasal bone, along with analysis of certain serum analytes.

prenatal diagnosis. The most common reason for recommending prenatal diagnosis is advanced maternal age (usually defined at age 35 years), a reflection of a trend for many women to have children later in their lives, after they have embarked on a career. However, some believe that prenatal diagnosis for chromosomal problems should be offered for maternal age of 31 years if there is a twin gestation.

Individuals who belong to an ethnic group with an identified high frequency of a specific detectable inherited disorder should be asked whether they have had their carrier status determined. If they have not, a first approach (depending on the stage of the pregnancy) may be to ascertain the carrier status of the father because, for some disorders, pregnancy makes accurate maternal determinations inaccurate. If he is a carrier or if the pregnancy is already advanced to a time period when carrier determination could not be carried out before the optimal time for amniocentesis was past, then amniocentesis may be appropriate and should be discussed. Pregnancies at risk for an X-linked recessively inherited disorder for which no specific assay or molecular diagnosis is available are especially problematical. The usual procedure is to determine the fetal sex. One option for this in addition to the more common techniques is preimplantation genetic diagnosis discussed below. If the fetus is a male and the mother is a known carrier, there is a 50% risk for it to be affected. If a decision is made to terminate such a pregnancy, the risk of aborting a normal male fetus is 50%. Obviously, such a situation calls for support for parental decisions from all professional staff involved with the patient and also for the provision of supportive counseling, which may need to be ongoing. It is not the place of anyone involved with the clients to express their own views, especially if they differ from those of the clients. An extreme degree of parental anxiety, regardless of actual risk, is considered by many to be an acceptable psychological indication for prenatal diagnosis. Such an indication demands more intensive counseling and explanation of what can be determined before the procedure is undertaken. Both young and advanced paternal age can increase the risk of chromosome aberrations and other birth defects in the fetus. Advanced paternal age increases the risk of some dominant gene mutations (as discussed in Chapter 4) that are potentially detectable by ultrasound.

It is the role of the professional practitioner and a standard of care to thoroughly inform clients who may be at increased risk of the availability of prenatal screening and diagnosis and to inform all pregnant women of the option of screening alone or as part of a multiple marker test as described earlier as well as for level I ultrasound. Many require that informed consent be signed whether the procedure is desired or not desired. If such diagnosis or expertise is not available in the area, it is the professional's responsibility to refer the client to a center that does provide the needed expertise or service, and assist in making arrangements for the service.

Client Information Before Prenatal Diagnosis

Before clients can make a decision of whether to have prenatal diagnosis, they should understand basic information. Even what obstetrical practitioners may consider routine screening (such as an initial ultrasound or maternal serum screening) for their population may not seem so to the clients. The nurse should be able to explain, clarify, and interpret the information at a level that the client can understand, that is culturally sensitive and appropriate and free from any coercion, and to evaluate that understanding. This should be accomplished as early as possible in the pregnancy, so that the client can think about the options and discuss them again. Written reinforcement that the client can take with her is an excellent way to supplement information. Information provided should include that shown in Box 8.4.

An integral part of the nurse's goal for the client at this time should be to establish and build a supportive relationship for counseling during the rest of the pregnancy, especially after prenatal diagnosis, if this is the option that has been chosen, as well as for pregnancy termination if that option has been selected or after delivery.

Amniocentesis

Amniocentesis preceded by ultrasound is still the most extensively used method of prenatal diagnosis. Rapid advances in the field make a list of specific disorders that are diagnosable obsolete before it goes to press. In order to provide up-to-date information for the concerned parents-to-be who are at risk for a known specific disorder, referral should be made to a geneticist who keeps abreast of the current developments in that disorder and knows the location of major research centers or directly to a major center. All chromosome disorders are potentially diagnosable, but as some may arise sporadically in women who are younger than 35 years of age and are not at risk for another disorder, not all will be detected prenatally unless all pregnant women were to have fetal chromosome analysis. Also high-resolution karyotyping to visualize submicroscopic chromosome changes is not done routinely unless there is a prior reason for doing it. The risk of chromosome abnormalities at different maternal ages is discussed in Chapter 4. The determination of AFP levels and other parameters for NTDs is usually routine at the time of amniocentesis even though maternal serum may have already been tested for AFP and other markers. Many inherited biochemical disorders can be diagnosed by specific biochemical assays or DNA assays, and the latter are used to detect hemoglobinopathies (e.g., sickle cell disease and the thalassemias). Thus, prenatal testing may be at the level of the mutant gene (DNA), chromosome, gene product (biochemical), or phenotype (morphology).

Amniocentesis refers to the withdrawal of a sample of amniotic fluid from the amniotic sac. It is usually done at the 15th to 18th week of gestation, when the uterus has reached the pelvic brim, the amniotic fluid volume is adequate (150–250 ml), and enough fetal cells are present to be able to carry out analysis (see Figure 8.3). Fetal cells in the amniotic fluid come from the skin and mucous membranes of the respiratory, digestive, genital, and urinary tracts as well as the umbilical cord and amnion. This also allows analysis to be completed in time for the parents to exercise the option of termination of the pregnancy if they so choose. The actual procedure is usu-

BOX 8.4

Client Information to Include Before Prenatal Diagnosis

- The reason prenatal diagnosis is considered appropriate for this woman or couple
- What will be analyzed (e.g., chromosome and alpha-fetoprotein analysis are usually routinely done regardless of the primary reason for seeking amniocentesis; thus, unexpected results could occur).
- What information will be obtained (e.g., the couple should know that a search for chromosome abnormalities is broader than only for Down syndrome even if the latter is the reason that the couple is interested in prenatal diagnosis).
- The risk of having an affected child in this pregnancy before prenatal diagnosis.
- What the procedure being considered entails, including description, cost, length of time, where it is to be done, and aftercare.
- What the risks of the procedure are—the magnitude and the kind.
- What can and cannot be detected—this should include the information that while some disorders can be virtually excluded (e.g., chromosome disorders if an amniocentesis is being done), a completely normal infant cannot be ensured, both because of a slight risk of error and because no procedure can detect every possible defect.

- The length of time between the procedure and when the results are obtained.
- How the results will be communicated to them.
- That prenatal diagnosis can be done even if the couple does not wish to consider abortion as a viable alternative; if the results are negative, it may relieve anxiety; and if they are positive, they may either change their minds, seek fetal therapy, plan for the delivery of the infant in an expert care center, and have time to think about alternative plans for care of the infant.
- In those now relatively uncommon cases where an X-linked recessively inherited disorder is in question and cannot be assayed for specifically, they should understand that a specific test will not be done. The fetal sex will be determined, and that decision making will proceed on that basis.
- Unintended possible psychological consequences if a problem is detected.
- Potential unintended consequences such as pressure from insurance companies not to carry an affected child to term, or termination or diminution of benefits or coverage for the pregnancy, for the child, and aftercare.

ally done on an outpatient basis, paying careful attention to asepsis. Most practitioners recommend a dose of Rh immunoglobulin to all unsensitized Rh negative women to prevent Rh isoimmunization. With increased frequency of use, amniocentesis has become a safer procedure than it initially was. An accepted risk figure for fetal loss due to amniocentesis that is above the figure for losses in the same period of pregnancy has been given as 0.25–0.5%. An increased incidence of fetal loss and of other complications was associated with an increased number of needle insertions to obtain a sample, uncertain placentation or anterior placentation, and the use of needles with gauges of 19 or larger.

Overall complications from amniocentesis are relatively infrequent. There have been questions raised as to whether infants of mothers having amniocentesis are more likely to develop respiratory problems and emphysema development that may be caused by chronic leakage of amniotic fluid, interfering with normal lung development, and this continues to be a concern, although it is estimated to occur in a very small percentage. Maternal complications can include vaginal bleeding, amniotic

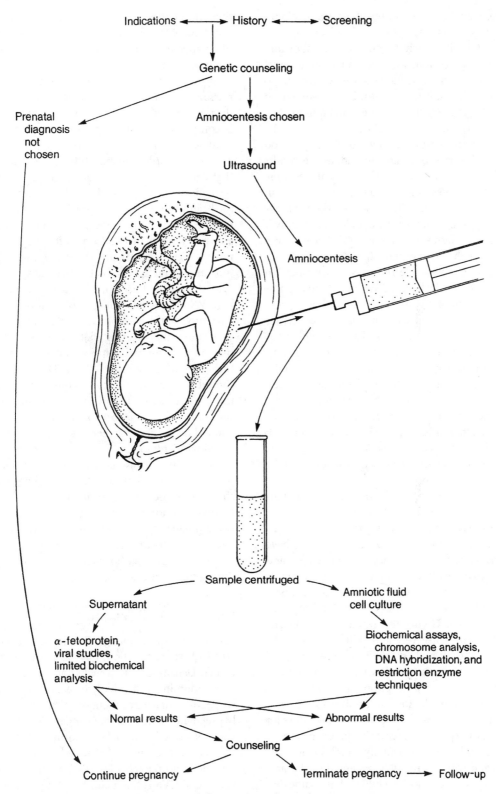

FIGURE 8.3   Amniocentesis: Options and disposition of samples.

fluid leakage, infection, Rh sensitization, precipitation of labor, and perforation of the bladder or placenta. Fetal risks include spontaneous abortion, needle puncture injuries, and injury because of withdrawal of amniotic fluid such as amniotic band syndrome. It is not uncommon for the woman to have cramping, vaginal spotting, and amniotic fluid leakage as transient after-effects.

After amniocentesis is done, the waiting period between the procedure and obtaining the results can be 2 to 3 weeks, although rapid chromosome culture techniques can be used to provide results in about a week or earlier. This may be a time of anxiety and apprehension for the couple, particularly if they have undertaken amniocentesis because of a previous birth with a genetic disorder. Indeed, amniocentesis has been referred to as a crisis situation in terms of the psychosocial stress and anxiety imposed on the normal stresses surrounding a pregnancy. Unresolved past problems, unconscious feelings of guilt and failure, and stresses within the family are exacerbated during this period, especially in families that have experienced the birth of a child with a genetic disorder. Some mothers feel that a conditional relationship was imposed between the mother and fetus. Awareness of these aspects, the establishment of a good relationship with the family, and a clear, mutual understanding of the information prenatal diagnosis provides will be helpful during this period.

If abnormal findings result from the prenatal diagnosis, the couple has a limited time period in which to make a decision in regard to the continuation or termination of the pregnancy if they have not already done so. They may need discussion and specialized counseling that may include conferences with experts in treating the disorder and with parents of children with the disorder, in addition to other supports. Giving the results to the family must be done sensitively and skillfully, and both members of the couple should be told in person by the practitioner in a private setting when there is time to discuss issues and options. Liberalized abortion laws have made amniocentesis a meaningful procedure in terms of removing the Russian roulette atmosphere of attempting pregnancy when in a high-risk group. For many couples who have had a child with an inherited genetic disorder and have a high risk for another child with the same disorder, the availability of prenatal diagnosis offers

them the chance to have an unaffected child. Without it, 50–90% of couples who have a 25–50% risk of an affected child would not have attempted another pregnancy.

In a pluralistic society, it is important for the nurse and other professional practitioners to support the right of individual clients to make a decision that is compatible with their personal philosophy and lifestyle and to provide support for that decision. The World Health Organization (WHO) has stated that decisions following prenatal diagnosis should be made by the couple and that the responsibility of the health care worker is to provide the information in a manner that can be understood. Although abortion for genetic indications after prenatal diagnosis is regarded by many who disapprove of abortion in general as legitimate, there can be a great deal of stress that accompanies that decision making. While prenatal diagnosis is more routine currently, both maternal and paternal feelings of depression after hearing that the fetus is affected may occur. Family disruption can also occur after the birth of an affected child. Thus, the nurse should be aware that ongoing counseling and contact are necessary after pregnancy termination and should make every effort to ensure access to such counseling for both partners. Studies of stress associated with amniocentesis indicate stress is greatest when waiting for results and, if the results are abnormal, when making a decision. Feelings may be similar to those waiting for the results of diagnosis following abnormal screening tests discussed later. If the pregnancy is terminated, then stress is great after the procedure, as well as just before it. Plans for nursing intervention should include support during these periods.

Chorionic Villi Sampling

Chorionic villus sampling (CVS) is typically done at 10 to 12 weeks gestation, but has been performed earlier. Usually CVS is done by the transcervical or transabdominal route. Early detection allows wider scope for in utero treatment or, if chosen, safer early pregnancy termination. Cytogenetic, enzymatic, and DNA studies can all be performed on chorionic villi, and the amount of material obtained makes this method preferable for DNA analysis. A disadvantage of CVS is that neither AFP testing nor any other assay needing amniotic fluid can be done n CVS specimens. Thus, women who have CVS should be referred for MSAFP screening at 15 to 20 weeks. Another disadvantage is the higher rate of cytogenetic ambiguous results than are seen in amniocentesis samples called confined placental mosaicism (CPM) or chromosomal anomalies confined to the placenta (CACP), and not present in the fetus. Few effects immediately follow CVS except for vaginal bleeding. The major serious fetal sequelae from CVS is for transverse limb deficiencies or reduction effects. There appears to be a small but real risk of transverse limb deficiency that overall is 0.03–0.14% after CVS. The risk for spontaneous fetal loss from CVS is approximately 1.64–2.5%. This is lower using the transabdominal route. As with most of the other prenatal diagnostic procedures, CVS should be done in the context of an experienced center, practitioner, and program for best results. Usually chromosome results from direct preparations are available as early as 24 to 36 hours, with cultures for confirmation in about 1 to 2 weeks.

Ultrasonography

Ultrasonography alone is the major method for detecting fetal malformations. Ultrasound consists of vibrations that are inaudible to the human ear. This high-frequency sound produces a mechanical pressure wave, causing vibration consisting of the contraction and expansion of the body tissues and fluids through which it passes. The waves are transmitted into the body through a transducer, and echoes at boundaries between adjacent tissues are reflected. These are converted into electrical signals and are amplified and processed so that they can be visually displayed on an oscilloscope and videotaped or photographed. Fluid-filled or surrounded structures are visualized especially well. The use of oil or gel on the abdominal wall is necessary to diminish the loss of waves. Ultrasound can be used in different ways or modes. In pregnancy, the frequencies used usually avoid known tissue effects from ultrasound that in some instances are the basis for its use, such as heat and tissue destruction. Ultrasound is noninvasive and non-ionizing. Patient preparation is minimal.

Screening ultrasound in early pregnancy at 10 to 13 weeks is usually to accurately date the pregnancy by measures such as crown-rump, but because of better resolution than previously, part of the scan includes examining the fetal anatomy and measuring fetal nuchal translucency (abnormal thickness at the posterior aspect of the neck of a fetus less than 13 weeks, after which it is called nuchal thickening, nuchal fold, or cystic hygroma). The absence of the fetal nasal bone may also be assessed since it is associated with Down syndrome. Alone, a nonvisualized nasal bone during the second trimester of pregnancy was said to identify 40–45% of Down syndrome pregnancies.

The prenatal uses of ultrasound may be either primary or adjunct. The placenta and internal and external fetal structures can be visualized. Ultrasound is used in conjunction with (1) amniocentesis, chorionic villus sampling, fetoscopy, and fetal blood and tissue sampling as a guide to increase safety and diagnostic accuracy and (2) abnormal AFP and/or multiple serum analyte test levels to rule out false positives and false negatives due to inaccurate gestational age assessment, fetal death, or multiple pregnancy or to define the abnormality present. Alone ultrasound can be used for a number of reasons:

- Detecting certain fetal abnormalities in pregnancies identified as high risk. This now can include such features as increased nuchal translucency or cystic hygroma, abnormal fetal bone length or absent fetal nasal bone, and certain other indicators that might be associated with fetuses with trisomy 21 and other aneuploidies.
- Monitoring fetal growth and allowing fetal measurements such as crown-rump length and biparietal fetal head diameter to be made.
- Determining the number of fetuses.
- Determining fetal presentation.
- Assessing gestational age.
- Ascertaining fetal hypoxemia.
- Ascertaining if the fetal environment is normal, including amniotic fluid volume, assessment of the umbilical cord, blood flow, and evaluation of the placenta for anomalies or maturity.
- Detecting ectopic pregnancy.
- Assessing structural and functional integrity.
- Evaluating immediate fetal risk for optimum management and treatment.
- Assessing fetal viability.
- Detecting hydatidiform mole.

In addition, the extended or detailed examination and targeted imaging for fetal anomalies (TIFFA) are terms used for examination to detect fetal anomalies. Those who should be referred for targeted, detailed ultrasonography have these characteristics:

- Previous child or family history of detectable structural malformation or anomaly (including congenital heart defects)
- Those who are at other known high risk for detectable fetal anomaly such as:
  - maternal condition predisposing to fetal anomaly;
  - drug/alcohol exposure in pregnancy;
  - maternal infection in pregnancy.
- Abnormal pregnancy progression
- Abnormal maternal serum AFP or multiple serum analyte screening results
- Abnormal AFP results on amniocentesis
- Intrauterine growth restriction
- Suspicious findings on routine ultrasound

The availability of high-resolution ultrasound machines incorporating both curvilinear and multifocal transducers allows for obtaining good views of the fetus and making a diagnostic interpretation in the hands of the skilled ultrasonographer. These can be translated into clinical outcomes. For example, if esophageal atresia is diagnosed, the esophageal pouch can be aspirated at birth and oral feedings avoided until repair is accomplished, thus preventing aspiration and pneumonia and decreasing morbidity. Moving structures such as the beating fetal heart (using Doppler), the placenta, and fetal movement can be observed, and four-chamber views of the heart allow for referral for fetal echocardiography and other procedures if needed. Sonographic screening effectiveness for detection of cardiac lesions varies with the type of defect. Advances in ultrasound imaging in three and four dimensions (real-time three-dimensional imaging) are beginning to be used in prenatal diagnosis.

Basic ultrasound is a screening procedure that is done on pregnant women who have no clinical indication (low risk) for ultrasound. Increasingly in the United States, ultrasound may be first offered during the first trimester at about 10–13 weeks, followed by an option of more detailed ultrasound screening early in the second trimester for women who have no known risk factor. Some structural abnormalities may be identified during the first trimester and combined with maternal serum screening for Down syndrome and other chromosomal anomaly detection.

Ethical, Social, and Legal Issues Associated With Prenatal Diagnosis

Some of the issues surrounding prenatal diagnosis really relate to the option of pregnancy termination after the results are available, because a second trimester abortion is viewed by some as both an ethical and a medical problem. One may, on the other hand, view prenatal diagnosis as protective of life because it allows many couples with a high genetic risk to undertake pregnancies that they would not have dared to otherwise risk; if the pregnancy is unplanned, it allows them to carry to term an unaffected fetus that might otherwise have been aborted. The option of selective abortion allows meaningful reproductive alternatives to be presented to a couple at risk for a fetus with a known defect. The entire question of abortion is complex and fraught with emotion, which cannot be addressed here adequately, but will only be looked at in a limited way as it relates to prenatal diagnosis.

A professional nurse may have to recognize and separate his/her personal beliefs from those of the clients in order to provide quality care. It is important that clients get accurate, clear, unbiased, comprehensible information, and then have assistance in carrying out whatever decision they make. Because 95% of amniocenteses have resulted in the detection of a normal fetus, the procedure may be very reassuring to couples at risk. In addition, some parents who before the procedure thought that they would not consider pregnancy termination may in fact change their minds if they discover that they are carrying a fetus with a poor prognosis or inevitable death. They may also arrange delivery at a site with specialized care. In some cultures, it may be preferable to accept what is given and have a child with a birth defect rather than no child.

Other issues include the right of the person to refuse to participate or to have a prenatal diagnostic procedure, disclosure, confidentiality, access to information, the right to privacy, ownership of the samples taken, and ambiguous finding (see Chapter 13). Others include aspects of autonomy and choice sex selection, and "trivial" reasons for prenatal diagnosis, and the related issues of enhancement, individual versus societal rights, obligations of the health care provider, and testing for diseases with uncertain outcomes or manifestations in adulthood. Other issues relate to access and how socioeconomic factors might influence the availability of prenatal diagnosis, especially for women who may not be defined as high-risk, thus creating conditions of health disparity.

Patients seeking to determine fetal sex as the primary reason for prenatal diagnosis fall into two categories: those at risk for an X-linked inherited disorder for which no specific assay is available and those who wish to exercise sex selection. In the first situation, there is little problem if the fetus is a female. If the fetus is a male and the mother is a carrier, then the chance the fetus will be affected is 50%. If pregnancy termination is selected without further testing, 50% of the time a normal fetus will be aborted. This is a difficult situation for the family. Genetic counseling before prenatal diagnosis will clarify some of the issues. Parents may be less inclined to seek abortion if the condition is a treatable one. If it is one that is ultimately fatal (e.g., Duchenne muscular dystrophy), then the couple may find it totally unacceptable for them to give birth to this child. Molecular diagnosis is now offering new testing options for these conditions. The use of preimplantation genetic diagnosis offers additional choices.

The second group poses a different type of problem. Generally prenatal diagnosis for social sex selection and the implied pregnancy termination if the "wrong" sex is being carried is considered a trivial reason for procedures that carry a small risk of fetal loss and injury above that which would normally be present.

Another situation is that in which the pregnancy is at risk for a relatively minor defect, such as cleft lip and palate. One must ask whether or not the practitioner can judge what a minor defect is to the couple concerned. Coping with necessary surgery and rehabilitation may be beyond the capacity of that particular couple's resources—financial, emotional, and physical. It may produce additional stresses to the rest of the family or to the marital relationship, of which the practitioner cannot be aware. A positive action that can be taken is to provide immediate (because the time element is so critical), expert counseling for the couple in order to try to elicit the true concerns and problems and help them arrive at a decision that is realistic for the couple, not the practitioner. A broader question is: Who decides normality? Should abortion be condoned or condemned for a defect such as an extra digit on the extremities?

Unexpected or ambiguous findings can result from prenatal diagnosis and can present dilemmas. The practitioner may or may not feel obligated to completely disclose such findings if there was an agreement before testing that limited what would be disclosed. For example, if a woman at risk for Down syndrome in the fetus was found to be carrying a fetus with a small chromosome inversion about which little is known, the practitioner may only wish to tell her that the fetus does not have Down syndrome, and not mention the inversion. However, this paternalistic approach is probably not legally or morally viable. Current knowledge and trends favor openness and honesty in informing the parents of such situations, combined with expert supportive counseling. The limitations of current knowledge should be made clear. Ambiguous findings may also arise after ultrasound screening that identify what is called fetal "soft" markers found on ultrasound such as choroid plexus cysts in the fetal brain or mild renal dilatation, which not too long ago was believed to be associated with Down syndrome but is now known to be present in 1–2% of normal fetuses.

Other issues regarding prenatal diagnosis have more recently been discussed. For example, suppose a test for a behavior such as homosexuality were to be available. Would a couple be able to select testing, and what would be the ethical issues involved if they were to select pregnancy termination? An interesting dramatization of this dilemma is *Twilight of the Golds*, a television movie and play. What are the issues for diseases that emerge in adulthood? What are the issues, concerns and rights of parents to select pregnancy termination or life for a fetus for a disease such as Huntington disease or Alzheimer disease that will most likely not be symptomatic until that fetus is an adult? What about the risk for inherited, or susceptibility to, cancer? What is the meaning of the finding of a gene mutation such as *BRCA1* if found in the fetus? What will guide decisions when cancer development is not certain? These issues may not involve only disease states but issues of living such as life insurance, health benefit coverage and stigmatization. An issue that has occurred in preimplantation genetic diagnosis is that of late-onset genetic disorders such as Huntington disease in which parents wish to ensure that their offspring is disease free but do not wish to know their own carrier status, and ask that a disease-free embryo be selected. Another application has been using preimplantation genetic diagnosis for selection of an embryo based on HLA type to serve as a stem cell donor for a sibling in need of such treatment. Other issues also include the possibility of the finding of a future cure for a late-onset disease that is not now available. In the future, will selection of embryos after preimplantation genetic diagnosis be only for disease, or will preferred traits eventually be sought, for example, taller stature or pleasing facial features if those could be determined, and should this be allowed?

A somewhat related situation is that in which prenatal diagnosis reveals that the mother is carrying a fetus with a disorder that will be extremely costly to society to treat and to educate and which she decides to carry to term. How will society regard such families in the future? Will society continue to assume financial responsibility? Should the values of the individual or of society prevail? If a woman has the right to choose to terminate a pregnancy, shouldn't she also have the right to choose not to terminate it? Can society morally deny services to a disabled child because of his or her parent's decision? All of these are complex fundamental issues that have to do with the rights of the individual and the good of society, freedom and equality, and the quality of and the right to life. Certainly simplistic, rigid methods cannot be used to solve them; a thoughtful, individualized approach should be taken. Professionals can help to emphasize the importance of the preservation of choice and to safeguard these choices in their practice.

ASSISTED REPRODUCTIVE TECHNIQUES

It was in July 1978, that the first "test tube" baby, Louise Joy Brown, was born in the United Kingdom using in vitro fertilization; in 1992, the first birth using intracytoplasmic sperm injection occurred. It is now estimated that assisted reproductive procedures are used in 1 in 150 births in the United States. The use of assisted reproductive technology (ART) including in vitro fertilization and embryo transfer, intracytoplasmic sperm injection (ICSI), and other approaches, including the cryopreservation of both reproductive cells and embryos, has vastly benefited infertile couples but has created a variety of questions and ethical issues. Many experimental techniques are being used in order to find the most effective and safest approaches that minimize multiple pregnancies and unwanted side effects. In spite of these successes, questions have been raised that focus on the health and development outcomes of children born after ART and of ethical issues that have emerged from this technology. Among the problems in examining health and development of children born using ART are that the procedure is generally done in a population in which at least one parent is infertile, and the effects of parental age, parity, the cause of the infertility, whether hormonal or other therapy is used to maintain pregnancy, the maturity of sperm used, and delayed fertilization of the oocyte are all factors that may influence results. In ICSI, most natural selection mechanisms are bypassed. ICSI has become commonly used in as many as 80% of all ART procedures. In regard to ICSI, in which a single spermatozoon is injected into the oocyte cytoplasm, lower birth weights have been observed. There is also an increase in multiple pregnancies, which in and of themselves can lead to complications. ICSI has been associated with a higher number of major birth defects than naturally conceived children, especially in regard to chromosomal defects, including those of the sex chromosomes. Those conceived using IVF had a greater number of cardiovascular and urogenital defects, particularly hypospadias.

A variety of social, legal, and ethical issues are engendered by ART. These have to do with the creation of multiple embryos for ART and their potential selection for characteristics of sex not related to a genetic disorder; the possibility of the use of unused embryos who are under 14 days postconception and those between 14 and 18 days for research purposes; induction of twins; the use of eggs, sperm, or embryos for research when the donor has not given explicit consent; induction of twins through division of embryos; creation of embryos for research purposes; constructing embryonic cell lines from unused embryos; and selective reduction of multifetal pregnancies after ART. In some of these, issues of informed consent and the right to keep and store cells and tissues for later research and other purposes are of concern. Issues have also been created by mistakes during IVF that in one case involved implantation of the "wrong embryo," and in another, a White woman's eggs were fertilized by mixed sperm due to a poorly sterilized pipette. She gave birth to one Black and one White twin, so her partner was not the father of both her children. Such instances have looked at what determines what is a parent and what determines parental rights and duties. Another issue has been the potential for ART children to seek their donor parent in much the same way people who are adopted have done, and issues of disclosure and confidentiality for gamete donors.

SCREENING GAMETE DONORS

Sperm donation for artificial insemination or in vitro fertilization is a genetic reproductive option when both parents are known carriers of a deleterious autosomal recessive gene or the male is affected or at risk for carrying an autosomal dominant or X-linked mutant gene. Yet there is still misunderstanding and inappropriate use of the procedure. A major issue lies in the screening of donors. A recent study showed inconsistencies between what screening actions should be taken and those that are actually taken. There is a question of how far such screening should go. The couple should always understand that a normal infant cannot be guaranteed, although with the advent of various prenatal diagnostic techniques such as preimplantation genetic diagnosis, selection of embryos is possible but "normality" in all arenas can never be assured. For example, Gebhardt (2002) described a case of a man who had been a sperm donor for 18 children who later was found to have an adult-onset type of auto-somal dominant neurologic disease. This type of situation is one reason to limit the number of inseminations per donor. Every effort should be taken to exclude those ova and sperm donors at greater risk than the general population. Some possible indications for exclusion include:

- Presence of a single gene disorder, chromosome abnormality, or serious multifactorial disorder in the donor or close blood relative,
- Rh or ABO blood group that might cause incompatability between mother and fetus,
- A male donor who is 40 years of age or older,
- A female donor over 34 years of age,
- Exposure to drugs, radiation, certain infectious diseases, or chemical mutagens,
- Unexplained stillbirths, multiple miscarriages, or fetal deaths in their own children or close blood relative.

KEY POINTS

- The preconception period and pregnancy are important points in time for preventing genetic disorders
- Appropriate folic acid supplementation beginning pre-conception if possible, and other preventive measures should be accomplished before pregnancy to minimize chances for untoward genetically-related fetal outcomes
- Prenatal screening and diagnosis have become relatively safe and have entered standard obstetric practice
- Nurses should recognize couples who are candidates for prenatal screening and diagnosis
- All candidates for prenatal screening and diagnosis should have certain information as discussed in this chapter

9

Maternal-Child Nursing: Pediatrics

Genetic disorders are frequently recognized at or around birth or identified in the infant or child. At birth, visible congenital malformations that are isolated defects or part of a syndrome may be evident. Disorders of metabolism may become manifested after feeding begins. Newborn screening is an important way to detect some metabolic disorders such as phenylketonuria (PKU) or congenital hypothyroidism so that treatment can be initiated. Because of early discharge procedures, samples drawn for such testing may or may not be done within the hospital setting, and communication of results largely occurs once the mother and baby are back in their communities. For this reason, newborn screening is discussed in Chapter 12. Assessment is discussed in Chapter 7. This chapter discusses the most common chromosome disorders, important single gene disorders recognized in infancy and childhood, and common birth defects such as neural tube defects. Issues of genetic testing in children, often related to inherited forms of common diseases such as cancer, are discussed in Chapter 5.

Regardless of the type of genetic disorder diagnosed in a child, certain reactions are often seen. A number of factors influence these reactions, such as religious beliefs and partner relationships and whether the disorder is visible, such as Down syndrome, or hidden, such as congenital heart disease. Most parents mourn the loss of their "perfect" child and lose dreams and expectations. There are short- and long-term effects not only for the parents and the affected child but also for siblings and grandparents as well as other relatives. The way in which the family is told of the disorder, the supports provided and referrals made, as well as familial strengths and problems, influence short- and long-term coping. A full discussion is beyond the scope of this text, but elements of coping and adjustment are similar to chronic diseases in general. Eventually it is important for families to have genetic counseling and be aware of options relating to treatment, prenatal diagnosis, reproductive options, anticipatory guidance, short- and long-term plans, ways to cope with associated symptoms and conditions such as short stature in achondroplasia (discussed below), who and how to tell about the disorder, insurance issues, resources, and school or work issues. (See Lashley, 2005, for a detailed discussion.)

BIRTH DEFECTS

The terms *birth defects* and *congenital anomalies* are essentially synonymous. The visual appearance does not tell etiology. For example, a cleft palate may be an isolated anomaly or part of a syndrome; it may be caused by a chromosome aberration, a single gene disorder, an environmental insult, a combination of genetic and environmental factors, or unknown causes. Prenatal development is extremely complex, involving cell proliferation, differentiation, migration, programmed cell death, fusion between adjacent tissues, proper chemical communication between tissues, and induction. The correct sequence and timing is crucial. Birth defects may be caused by any of the factors in Box 9.1.

ing in the literature. Definitions of the ones most likely to be encountered by the nurse and examples of each are shown in Box 9.2. Other terms that describe various anomalies, such as *agenesis*, *aplasia*, *dysplasia*, *hyperplasia*, and *hamartomas*, are defined in the glossary at the end of this book.

BOX 9.1

Causes of Birth Defects

- Chromosome disorders (e.g., trisomy 13)
- Single gene defects (e.g., Meckel syndrome)
- A combination of genetic and environmental factors (multifactorial)(e.g., anencephaly)
- External physical constraints of the fetus in utero (e.g., torticollis)
- Infectious agents (e.g., rubella), drugs, or chemicals (e.g., thalidomide)
- Radiation exposure in utero (e.g., microcephaly)
- Maternal metabolic factors (e.g., diabetes mellitus)
- Other environmental causes (e.g., methylmercury exposure)
- Unknown causes

Various estimates have been made for the frequency of birth defects in the general population. Differences arise depending on the type of population surveyed, criteria used to record an anomaly, and the age at which estimates are made. For example, neural tube defects have a high frequency in Ireland, and internal urinary tract anomalies are not usually detected at birth. The frequency of major congenital anomalies (defined as those that require surgery or interfere with normal livelihood) identified by 1 year of age is estimated to range from 4–7% and is about 3% at birth. The frequency of minor anomalies (e.g., a supernumerary nipple) is estimated at 10–12%. A higher incidence of congenital anomalies is found in twins. The United States maintains active surveillance for selected birth defects through the Centers for Disease Control and Prevention. This section concentrates on birth defects that are believed to be of multifactorial causation.

Terminology

The nomenclature associated with birth defects varies. Terms like *malformations*, *anomalads*, and *complexes* have not been used with consistent mean-

BOX 9.2

Nomenclature Associated With Birth Defects

- Association—Nonrandom occurrence together with a pattern of multiple anomalies, but that are not yet known to be a syndrome or sequence (e.g., VATER association—*v*ertebral defects, *a*nal atresia, *t*racheo-esophageal fistula with esophageal atresia, *r*adial dysplasia, and *r*enal defects).
- Disruption—The initial developmental process is normal, but a defective organ or part of an organ or tissue results from interference (usually external) with the process (e.g., limb defects resulting from thalidomide; amniotic band syndrome).
- Deformation—An abnormal form, shape, or position of a previously normal body part caused by mechanical forces (usually molding) on normal tissue (e.g., intrauterine restraint resulting in clubfoot).
- Malformation—A morphologic defect of an organ or part of an organ with poor tissue formation that results from an intrinsic abnormal developmental process (e.g., cleft lip).
- Syndrome—A recognized pattern of multiple anomalies presumed to have the same etiology (e.g., Down syndrome).
- Sequence—A pattern of multiple anomalies derived from a single prior anomaly; this replaces anomalad or complex (e.g., Robin sequence—micrognathia, large tongue, cleft palate).

Multifactorial Causation and Inheritance

The common congenital anomalies often have a familial basis, but they usually do not fit a Mendelian inheritance pattern or show an association with a chromosomal abnormality. Although exact causes remain unknown for the most part, it is believed that many of the common congenital malformations and isolated birth defects are inherited in a multifactorial manner, involving the interaction of several genes and the environment. Some congenital anomalies show sex bias in their expression. Females seem to show tissue anomalies, while males often have more organ-specific findings (see Table 9.1). The reasons for these are under investigation. In some cases, newer techniques have demonstrated nonmultifactorial causes for congenital anomalies

TABLE 9.1   The Occurrence and Sex Distribution of Selected Congenital Anomalies

Congenital Anomaly	Incidence	Sex More Frequently Affected
Anencephaly	1:1,000	Female
Spina bifida	1:1,000	Female
Cleft lip with or without cleft palate	1:1,000—Caucasian 1.7:1,000—Japanese 0.7:1,000—Blacks	Male
Cleft palate alone	1:2,000–1:2,500	Female
Congenital heart defect	6–8:1,000	Equal
Developmental dysplasia of the hip	1:100–1:1,000	Female
Pyloric stenosis	5:1,000—males 1:1,000—females	Male
Clubfoot	1:1,000	Male
Hirschsprung disease	1:5,000	Male
Hypospadias	6:1,000—Caucasian males 2:1,000—Black males	Males only

Note: Frequency in the United States unless stated otherwise.

such as submicroscopic chromosomal deletions and duplications. An example is DiGeorge or velocardiofacial syndrome (VCFS), where microdeletions of chromosome 22q11 are associated with ventricular septal and conotruncal heart defects in association with an absent thymus, facial abnormalities, hypoparathyroidism, immune deficiencies, and others. Thus, even if a person had chromosomal or other testing that was negative years ago, it may be useful to repeat such testing in order to provide updated genetic counseling information. Multifactorial inheritance is explained in Chapter 4.

Congenital Heart Disease

The overall frequency of congenital heart disease (CHD) in the North American population is about 75 per 1,000 if trivial lesions are included and 19 per 1,000 live births if moderate and severe forms are included. Unlike most other congenital malformations, the sexes are about equally affected for the overall category of CHD. The etiology varies, with about 5–10% being of chromosome or single gene mutation origin and 1–2% being of environmental origin. CHD may be due to:

- teratogenic agents (e.g., lithium, alcohol, dilantin, retinoic acid, valproic acid);
- infection (congenital rubella);
- maternal environment disturbances such as maternal PKU;
- chromosomal origin (e.g., Turner syndrome, trisomy 21);
- single gene disorder (e.g., Holt-Oram syndrome, an autosomal dominant disorder resulting from mutation of the *TBX5* gene that encodes a transcription factor and consists of upper limb skeletal defects and cardiac anomalies);
- mitochondrial inheritance;
- multifactorial inheritance mechanisms;
- uncommon inheritance mechanisms, such as imprinting, germline mosaicism, or uniparental disomy.

An important consideration for nurses, especially those involved in routine physical examinations of infants, and children, is that persons with CHD frequently have one or more extracardiac defects, ranging from 25–45%. Thus, all children known to have CHD should be carefully evaluated in order to detect such other anomalies. Some anomalies, such as cleft palate, are readily apparent, but others, such as those of the urinary tract, are more difficult to detect. The most frequent extracardiac defects associated with CHD are those of the genitourinary tract, gastrointestinal tract, and musculoskeletal system. Nonimmune fetal hydrops (generalized edema and ascites in the fetus) is estimated to have a cardiac cause in as many as 25% of the cases. The most frequent congenital heart defects found in association with other anomalies are patent ductus arteriosus, atrial septal defects, atrioventricularis communis, tetralogy of Fallot, coarctation of the aorta, ventricular septal defects, and malposition defects. Some tend to be associated with specific syndromes (e.g., coarctation of the aorta and Turner syndrome). About 10% of all CHDs are part of a syndrome. It is important to recognize these syndromes in order to provide accurate genetic counseling and management. Recurrence risk figures vary for the type of defect as well as for other factors previously discussed. If the CHD is multifactorial, an overall risk to a future sibling of an affected individual is 2–4%. This increases to 6–12% if a second sibling is affected.

Because of effective early interventions, many persons with CHD survive into adulthood. There are clinicians who specialize in adult CHD, and it has been noted that some carry over from "precious" babies to "precious" adults, and may seek medical care accompanied by their parents even into their 30s.

Developmental Dysplasia of the Hip (DDH)

DDH was formerly known as congenital dislocation of the hip (CDH). The interaction of genetic and environmental factors in DDH is striking. It is now thought of by most as a deformation rather than a true congenital malformation, with an incidence of about 1% of all live births, depending on the criteria used and the age of assessment. A full range of severity, from a lax dislocatable hip to a dislocated hip that cannot be reduced, is possible. DDH is five to eight times more common in females, 60% are firstborn children, and 30–50% are delivered in breech presentation. Environmental factors present after birth may contribute to DDH development.

Cultures such as the Lapps and some Navajo Indian tribes in which infants are wrapped to a cradle board or swaddled, with legs in forced extension, show an incidence of DDH that is 10 times greater than normal. A lower-than-usual incidence is seen in societies that keep infants in a "protective" position, in which the hips are partially abducted, as in the Hong Kong Chinese, who carry infants on their back. Intrinsic factors leading to DDH have also been identified. These include the nature of the hip joint (e.g., a shallow-angled acetabulum is more susceptible to dislocation) or lax connective tissue from either heritable causes or hormones (e.g., inborn errors of estrogen or collagen metabolism, maternal estrogens, or hormones that may be given before delivery).

The nurse should carefully assess neonates and infants for clinical features of DDH by examining for shortening of the thigh with bunching up of tissue and skin fold accentuation, limitation of abduction, or other signs. The Ortolani or Barlow test may also be done. However, DDH may not be detected at birth, and surveillance should be maintained. See Box 9.3. Ultrasound screening of the neonatal hip has become more common and has a specificity and sensitivity of over 90%. DDH is relatively easy to treat early, but if it is discovered after 1 year of age, it requires more complex management, and complete correction may not be possible. Nurses should be especially alert in examining infants who are female, firstborn, and delivered in a breech position. Health teaching should include information about optimum positioning.

> ## BOX 9.3
>
> ### Common Presenting Signs and Symptoms of DDH
>
> - Limping
> - Walking on tip-toe
> - Unequal leg length
> - Difficulty in crawling
> - Delayed walking
> - Noticeable short leg
> - Asymmetric thigh creases
> - Uneven shoe wear

Neural Tube Defects

One of the biggest public health success stories in prevention of genetic disorders has been the ability to prevent many neural tube defects (NTDs) by the periconceptual administration of folic acid, as discussed later. In addition, a large proportion of NTDs can be detected prenatally by ultrasound and measurement of alpha-fetoprotein (AFP) in maternal serum and amniotic fluid.

The embryonic structure that gives rise to the central nervous system is the neural tube. Errors in its development encompass a group of malformations that include those in Box 9.4. Neural tube defects may be open or closed. In open NTDs, neural tissue is either exposed or covered with a thin transparent membrane. In closed NTDs, neural tissue is covered with skin or a thick, opaque membrane. Closed lesions may not be detected by alpha fetoprotein determinations. Hydrocephalus may accompany spina bifida. Anencephaly and spina bifida are related etiologically and are generally discussed together. After having an infant with either anencephaly or spina bifida, the recurrence risk is for either one, not just for the anomaly that was present in the affected infant. An infant with a meningomyelocele is shown in Figure 9.1.

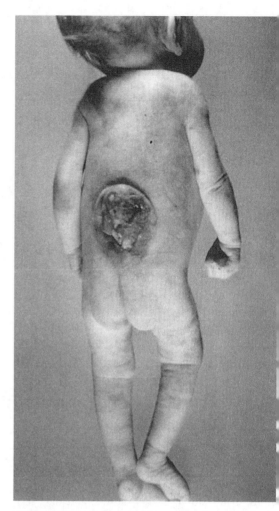

FIGURE 9.1   Infant with a meningomyelocele. Courtesy of Dr. John Murphy, Southern Illinois University School of Medicine, Springfield, Illinois.

BOX 9.4

Major Neural Tube Defects

- Anencephaly—the vault of the skull is absent, with a rudimentary brain
- Spina bifida, which includes:
  - Spina bifida occulta—one vertebra is not fused, and a tuft of hair may be present over the skin of the area.
  - Meningocele—meninges protrude or are herniated from the spinal canal, but the cord is in its usual position.
  - Myelomeningocele—the meninges and the spinal cord protrude from the defective vertebrae.
- Encephalocele—meninges and brain protrude through a gap in the skull, so part of the brain is outside the skull. This is less common than the others.

Many epidemiological studies have been carried out, and many factors related to the occurrence of NTDs have been identified. It is now believed that at least four separate closures of the neural tube occur early in embryonic life. Each seems to be sensitive to different environmental agents, and each has a different result when it fails to close. For example, "zipper" 1 is susceptible to folic acid deficiency, while "zipper" 4 is susceptible to hyperthermia. The multiple closure theory helps to explain the varying epidemiological observations about NTDs. A consistent observation has been that NTDs are more frequent in poorer socioeconomic groups and after conditions that result in poor diets, especially folic acid deficiency, but also possibly deficiency in ascorbic acid, zinc, and others. Some studies have found a higher risk of NTDs in obese women that is independent of folic acid intake.

The highest incidence is found among the Irish and in the United Kingdom, where the incidence is 4:1,000 to 5:1,000. It is also high among Sikhs and in parts of Egypt, Pakistan, and India; the incidence is lowest in Blacks, Ashkenazic Jews, and most Asians. Females predominate, especially in anencephaly. In the United States overall, the incidence is 2:1,000 with a higher rate in the eastern and southern United States, decreasing in the West. Hyperthermia, from either maternal illness with fever or environmental, such as that with sauna or hot tub use, during early pregnancy has been shown to be capable of causing NTD, especially anencephaly. Surgical repair may include the placement of a shunt, and the extent of surgery depends on the severity of the defect. Long-term rehabilitation, often requiring bowel and bladder training, may be necessary. In some centers, fetal surgery is being performed to close myelomeningoceles to decrease shunting and improve motor function.

The appearance of an infant with anencephaly is so shocking that often parents equate the severity of the infant's appearance with the risk of recurrence. In fact, it falls into the same general range of the other multifactorial disorders. Recurrence risks must always be adjusted to the population incidence, ethnic background, the number of affected relatives, epidemiological factors when known, and so on, but in general, the risk of recurrence in the United States for a Caucasian couple after having one affected infant and no other affected relatives is believed to be 3–4%. After two affected siblings, the recurrence risk rises to 10–13%, and in Northern Ireland, the risk may be as high as 20%. The risk for a woman with spina bifida to have an affected child is about 4%. There is some indication that there is an increased risk for NTDs among siblings of children who have other birth defects, such as cleft lip and palate.

A couple seen for genetic counseling had one normal son and had just delivered a stillborn infant with anencephaly. The shock was so great that they were sure that the risk for recurrence of the defect was very high. In their minds, they had only a 50% chance of having a normal child. They were relieved to discover that it was only about 3–4% and that prenatal diagnosis was available and could detect the majority of infants with NTDs, especially in women known to have previously had a child with NTD. Nurses should be sure to discuss the option of prenatal diagnosis with both members of such a couple, lest they disrupt their reproductive plans out of disproportionate fear of the recurrence of NTD. All such couples should be referred for genetic counseling in order to accurately determine their risk and to discuss with them the increased risk to other close relatives.

The most important aspect of NTDs currently is prevention. It was discovered first that recurrence of NTDs could be prevented by periconceptional supplementation of folic acid and vitamins, followed by the expansion of this to prevent first occurrences as well. Recommendations are for 0.4 mg. (400 µg) of folic acid for all women of childbearing age. The American College of Medical Genetics supports that but also recommends that women with a previous history of NTDs take 4.0 mg of folic acid daily, optimally starting three months before conception. There has been recent discussion about increasing the level of this recommendation.

Poor maternal nutrition in general also may contribute to NTD occurrence, as well as other birth defects such as imperforate anus, and dietary counseling that is ongoing and reinforced periodically should be done with females when they reach reproductive age.

Orofacial Clefts

The most common oral clefts are cleft lip, with or without cleft palate (CLP), and cleft palate alone (CP). The incidence for CLP varies in the population and is highest in Native Americans, Japanese, and Scandinavians. CP and CLP are considered to be genetically and etiologically distinct, and they may occur alone or with other anomalies. Over 340 syndromes that include CLP or CP have been recognized. Cleft uvula (1:80) and submucous cleft palates (1:1,000) are thought to represent incomplete forms of cleft palate. It also appears that congenital heart disease is prevalent in nearly 7% of all children with clefts, and so all children with clefts should be periodically evaluated with this in mind. It has been reported that children with CLP have short stature about four times more frequently than normal children when matched for age. Eventually catch-up growth should occur, particularly when nutrition is optimized and the cleft is repaired, unless the cleft is part of another syndrome. Growth velocity needs to be monitored. It is important that the infant with a cleft be evaluated fully in order to exclude chromosomal disorders and single gene defects such as van der Woude syndrome, in which the recurrence risk is high, or Gorlin-Goltz syndrome, in which the associated nevi may turn malignant. Preconceptional multivitamins including B_{12} and folic acid supplementation have been reported to reduce the recurrence risk of orofacial clefts by as much as 50%. Cigarette smoking during pregnancy appears to be a risk factor.

The appearance of a child with a cleft is shocking to the parent who is expecting a normal baby. They experience the same reactions most other parents experience for other birth defects: guilt, anger, denial, and concern. Parents have also stated that an orofacial cleft was not an anomaly that could be hidden from others. They often feel that the appearance of such an infant is caused by some indiscretion on their part and that now everyone else will also know that. Great sensitivity and skill are needed on the part of the entire professional staff immediately after the birth of the infant and throughout the hospital stay. Before leaving the hospital, contact should be arranged for the parents with the cleft palate team, who will ultimately be involved in the lengthy treatment and also with one of the cleft palate parent groups for support and in-hospital visitation. Referral may be made to the local home health care or community health agency for a home visit by a nurse. An immediate challenge is that of feeding the newborn with a cleft. It is important for the nursing staff to spend time helping the mother to feel comfortable feeding her infant because she will soon be assuming this responsibility alone. Infants with CLP or CP often cannot create adequate suction and may need a different type of nipple or occasionally a small plastic artificial palate. Breast-feeding may be possible, depending on the nature of the cleft. There are publications available to help the nurse advise the mother who wishes to do this, and mothers should not be discouraged. Infants should be held upright when fed to prevent choking and may need to be burped frequently, as they tend to swallow air. The infant may need 30 to 45 minutes or more to feed. Parents need to feel comfortable, the child needs nourishment, and both need to develop an emotional bond to one another. Many parent groups have individuals who come to the home and who have found various successful "tricks" for feeding. The American Cleft Palate Educational Foundation can supply addresses of the local chapter.

Early arrangements for genetic counseling are important because parents may hesitate to conceive a wanted subsequent child because of exaggerated fears of recurrence risk. Again, such risk depends on the extent of the defect and the number of individuals affected. Care must be taken to exclude the possibility of a syndrome. For example, when one child and no other family member has CP, the risk for recurrence is 2% and for CLP 2–6%. It is not uncommon for genetic counseling to be sought by an adult with CLP or CP. The risk for an affected parent and one sibling is about 1 in 10. Often such adults have experienced emotional trauma in their own life, which they attribute to the anomaly, and they may require more in-depth counseling. Three-dimensional ultrasonography of the fetal face may have future use in prenatal detection.

The total habilitation of infants with oral clefts is complex, often requiring multiple surgical procedures and other therapies, and is generally agreed to be best accomplished by a team. The early involvement of the family with such a team provides ongoing family support as well as other optimal therapy. Team members usually consist of professionals with specialties in pediatrics, plastic surgery, audiology, speech pathology, nursing, genetics, dentistry, orthodontia, otolaryngology, social service, and general surgery. Other specialists may include psychologists, nutritionists, and radiologists. My former practice group, the Central Illinois Cleft Palate Team, planned for and discussed the scheduled patients prior to seeing them. After meeting with the patient and family, each member recorded his/her impressions and findings. These were shared, and the plans were then altered accordingly, finalized, discussed with the family, and evaluated. Comprehensive, coordinated, and integrated multidisciplinary services are essential.

The current trend is to repair cleft lips as early as possible, almost always before 3 months of age. Many surgeons allow an infant to resume nursing 24 hours after cleft repair. Mothers can manually express breast milk for feeding during periods when the infant cannot nurse. A variety of procedures are used for CP closure, depending on the exact nature of the cleft and its extent.

During infancy and childhood, children with CLP have increased susceptibility to ear infections and frequently having hearing problems. Routine ear exams and testing should be done periodically and their importance explained to the parents. Hearing loss can also be responsible for speech distortion, and hypernasality is a frequent finding. There is a tendency for children with a cleft to develop speech later than usual, and therefore they may need some language stimulation, which parents can carry out in consultation with the speech pathologist. The hearing problems and discomfort may cause increased fussiness. Parents should be told that this may occur. The hearing and speech problems as well as appearance can contribute to psychological sequelae and problems needing counseling assistance for the client and family.

CHROMOSOME DISORDERS

Information about the structure and variation in chromosomes has been described in Chapters 2 and 4. Many fetuses with severe chromosomal abnormalities die prenatally or relatively soon after delivery, especially if the chromosomal defect is non-mosaic. Thus, only three trisomies (13, 18, and 21) are relatively common among live-born infants. Other trisomies and the monosomies are almost always seen only as mosaics that include a normal cell line, the assumption being that enough normal cells are present to be compatible with life. A variety of structural changes of every chromosome have been reported. Each individual one is extremely rare. The only autosomal ones that are relatively common (1:20,000 to 1:50,000) are cri-du-chat (5p–), DiGeorge/velocardiofacial syndrome, and Wolf-Hirschhorn syndrome (4p–).

The major autosomal abnormalities seen are:

- Trisomy 21 (Down syndrome);
- Trisomy 18 (Edwards syndrome);
- Trisomy 13 (Patau syndrome);
- Deletion 5p syndrome (cri-du-chat syndrome);
- DiGeorge/velocardiofacial syndrome;
- Wolf-Hirschhorn syndrome (4p–).

Among the sex chromosome disorders, the overall incidence is about 1 in 400 live births. The most common are:

- Turner syndrome (45,X);
- Klinefelter syndrome (47,XXY);
- 47,XXX (triple X);
- 47,XYY males.

In any of the trisomies, and especially Down syndrome, the actual error can be caused by either the presence of a free extra chromosome or an extra one that is translocated to another chromosome. In translocations, the chromosomal material of 47 chromosomes and therefore three copies of each gene are present instead of the normal two, but the chromosome count is 46. This illustrates one reason that a full chromosome analysis is necessary. The risks for recurrence are very different for translocations as opposed to free trisomies. For example, in Down syndrome, if one parent has 45 chromosomes and a translocation of chromosome 21 to chromosome 14, the gametes they produce can theoretically result in six possible combinations in a zygote, which are shown in Figure 9.2. In theory, the chance of each of these occurring is equal, and because three of the six outcomes result in nonviable offspring, the chances of a normal child, a balanced translocation carrier like the parent, or one with Down syndrome would each be one third. In practice, the distribution is observed to be different. If the female is the translocation carrier, then the actual observed risk is 10–15% for having a child with Down syndrome, whereas if the male is the carrier, it is 5–8%. The risk for having a normal-appearing child who, like the parent, is a translocation carrier is about 45–50%. In either case, the option of prenatal diagnosis should be explained to the parents. If both chromosome 21s are involved in the translocation, 45,XX,t (21;21) or 45,XY,t(21;21), then only Down syndrome offspring can result because the monosomic alternative is nonviable; thus, the risk in this type for parents to have a child with Down syndrome is 100%. Such parents should have genetic counseling that includes discussion of other reproductive options. Although more children with translocation Down syndrome are born to women under 30 years of age than over 30 years of age, assumptions as to cause can never be made. Chromosome analysis *must* be done. The degree of mosaicism, if present, can also act to modify findings and prognosis. For a karyotype illustrating the major autosomal and sex chromosome abnormalities, see Figure 9.3.

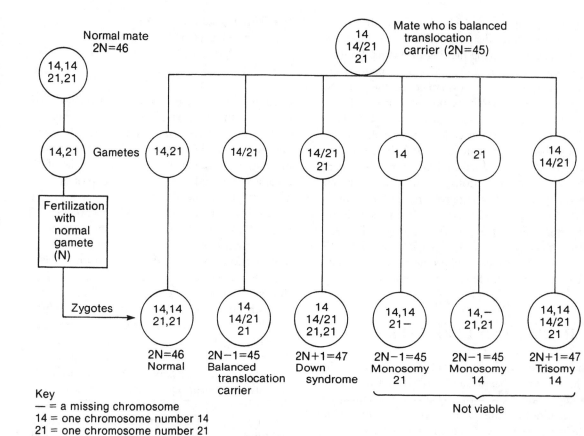

FIGURE 9.2   Possible reproductive outcomes of a 14/21 balanced translocation carrier.

In the severe autosomal anomalies other than Down syndrome, many affected individuals die relatively soon after delivery or in the first year of life because multiple, severe, life-threatening problems are present. Some, particularly those who are less severely affected or are mosaic, do survive, and parents often have angry feelings toward professionals who may have told them that their child would not live beyond a certain age. Thus, it is important to provide accurate information in a sensitive manner. One parent organization specifically for the rare chromosome disorders is the Support Organization for Trisomy 18, 13 and Related Disorders (http://www.trisomy.org). Down syndrome is described below. Information about the other autosomal chromosomal disorders is in Table 9.2.

Trisomy 21 (Down Syndrome)

First described as "mongolian idiocy" by Dr. John Langdon Down in 1866, Down syndrome is the most common chromosome abnormality in liveborns. It was the first chromosome abnormality associated (by Dr. Jerome Lejeune) with a specific chromosome—three copies of chromosome 21. Clinical features can vary greatly, as shown in Figure 9.4. There is no way, other than chromosome analysis, to tell if a free trisomy (about 95%), a translocation (about 5%), or mosaicism is present. About 90% of the time, the extra chromosome is of maternal origin. The type of chromosome abnormality is important in genetic counseling. The exact band responsible for the Down phenotype has been

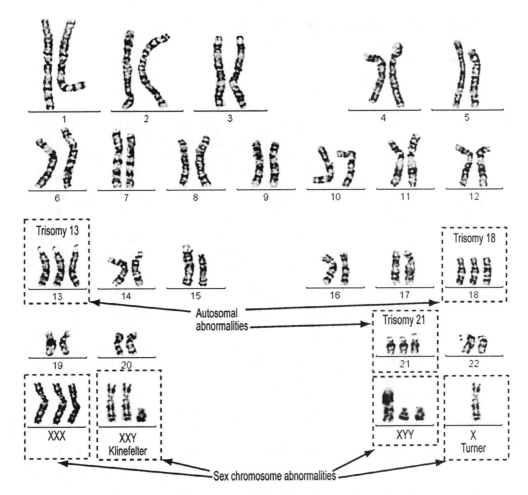

FIGURE 9.3   G banded karyotype illustrating major chromosome aberrations in a composite.

identified; the presence of the entire extra chromosome is not necessary in order to produce it. The karyotype of a patient with Down syndrome with a 14/21 translocation is shown in Figure 9.5.

Clinical features of Down syndrome include:

- Hypotonia, the most frequent early finding (infants may be floppy);
- Dysmorphic features, many of which are seen in a percent of normal people, including epicanthal folds, flat nasal bridge, upslanting palpebral fissures, and transverse palmer crease;
- Clinodactyly (incurved fifth finger);
- Wide spaces between first and second toes;
- Short stature;

- Short, broad neck;
- Protruding tongue with high arched palate;
- Brushfield spots of the eyes (light speckling of the edge of the iris);
- Intellectual disability, which may vary in degree;
- Congenital heart defects, especially atrioventricular septal defects, ventricular septal defects, and tetralogy of Fallot, which occur in 40–60%;
- Elevated risk for transient myeloproliferative leukemia in the newborn period and acute lymphocytic leukemia (ALL) in childhood;
- Gastrointestinal problems such as megacolon, celiac disease, and duodenal atresia;
- Otitis media and hearing impairment;

TABLE 9.2   Most Frequently Recognized Autosomal Chromosome Disorders

Chromosome Disorder	Incidence	Comments
Trisomy 21 (Down syndrome)		See text
Trisomy 18 (Edwards syndrome)	1 in 3,500 to 7,500 live births	Second most common live-born autosomal trisomy. Have three copies of chromosome 18 as free trisomy or translocation. About 10% survive past 1 year of age. Death is frequently from cardiopulmonary arrest. Clinical picture includes "rocker bottom" feet, mental disability, weak cry, poor sucking, failure to thrive, short sternum.
Trisomy 13 (Patau syndrome)	1 in 5,000 to 10,000 live births	Results from three copies of chromosome 13, either free or as translocation. Severe external malformations include cleft lip and palate, polydactyly, microphthalmia, absence of eyes, hand and nail deformities. Internal malformations include those of the heart, renal, and reproductive systems. May see "punched-out" scalp defect. Less than 10% survive the first year. A few survive into late childhood.
Deletion 5p (cri-du-chat syndrome)		Deletion of all or part of the short arm of chromosome 5. Very early hear catlike, mewing cry, low birthweight with mental and growth retardation, microcephaly, hypotonia, round face, poorly formed ears, respiratory and feeding problems, expressive language delay, self-injurious behavior. Many survive into adulthood depending on degree of deletion. IQ usually below 30 but may function at higher level.
Deletion 4p (Wolf-Hirschhorn syndrome)	1: 5,000 live births	Females more often affected. Deletion of certain region on the short arm of chromosome 4 (4p16.3), which may be submicroscopic. Includes microcephaly, intellectual disability, characteristic face with hypertelorism, wide nasal bridge, and congenital heart malformations.
DiGeorge/velocardiofacial syndrome	1 in 3,500 live births	Deletion in long arm of chromosome 22 (22q11.2). Typical clinical findings include conotruncal heart defects, palate abnormalities, learning, speech and language problems, hypotonia, T-cell abnormalities, thymus gland aplasia, or hypoplasia. At high risk for psychiatric disorders such as schizophrenia and depression.

- Ocular problems such as nystagmus, strabismus, glaucoma, and cataracts;
- Orthopedic problems such as scoliosis and hip dislocation;
- Thyroid problems, especially hypothyroidism;
- Hypogonadism in males and reduced fertility in females;
- In adulthood, a pattern of aging and neuronal degeneration similar to that seen in Alzheimer disease.

The severity of the disorder and the degree of developmental delay are not as evident in the infant as they later become, making it hard for many parents to accept the diagnosis. Many parents I have seen have believed that their child would eventually be normal. It takes time for the impact of the diagnosis to sink in and for realistic decision making to occur. Support is essential, and it should be suggested to the parents that they enroll their baby in an early intervention program as part of the effort to maximize their child's potential. Many persons with Down syndrome function at a higher social than intellectual level.

Persons with Down syndrome require regular childhood care such as immunizations and growth monitoring with standards appropriate to Down syndrome. In addition, special attention needs to be

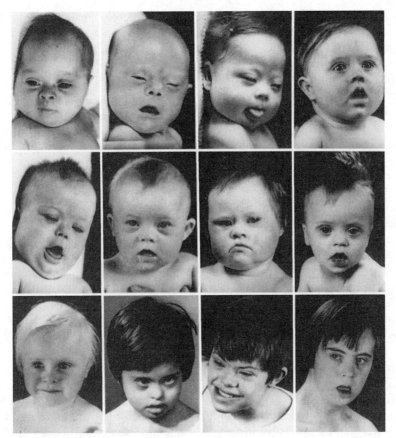

FIGURE 9.4   Photos of children with Down syndrome: A spectrum. From Tolksdorf, M., and Wiedemann, H-R. (1981). Clinical aspects of Down syndrome from infancy to adult life. *Human Genetics, (Suppl 2),* 3.

Translocation Down Syndrome

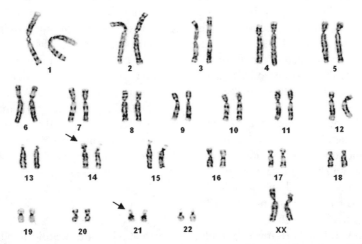

FIGURE 9.5   Karyotype of patient with Down syndrome caused by translocation of chromosome 21 to 14. Courtesy of Dr. Hana Aviv, Robert Wood Johnson University Hospital, New Brunswick, NJ.

paid to the eyes (for problems such as strabismus and myopia), to the ears (for otitis media and hearing loss), and thyroid function in addition to monitoring for heart disease, hematologic problems, orthopedic problems, gastrointestinal disorders, and others. Many believe that persons with Down syndrome are uniformly happy, friendly, and "good." While most tend to be, others can be stubborn, mischievous, and poorly coordinated, and about 10% have serious emotional problems. Families may require ongoing psychological support and counseling. Thus, persons with Down syndrome require ongoing medical treatment and, often, surgical procedures, which may be difficult for both the affected person and the family. Detailed guidelines for health management and for sports and activities have been developed by the American Academy of Pediatrics (2001). A wide variety of lay publications are available for families.

Males are usually infertile and have hypogonadism, whereas females can be fertile (although not frequently), and of those with free trisomy, about half of her offspring will have Down syndrome, and half will be normal. At one time, involuntary sterilization of a person with Down syndrome was almost routinely carried out in many institutions and is still on the books as law in some states, although rarely invoked. It is important to provide sex education appropriate to the developmental level of the person with Down syndrome. Socially acceptable sexual behavior should also be taught. Many parents need help in recognizing the sexuality of their adolescent or young adult. Appropriate contraceptive information and care should also be provided. Guidelines for help in teaching sexuality to persons with Down syndrome for both parents and professionals should be obtained. Adults with Down syndrome require care from clinicians who understand the syndrome and its manifestations and can provide sensitive, coordinated care.

Premature aging and development of early Alzheimer disease is a notable feature of Down syndrome. Mortality due to respiratory infection has been reduced, but can still be significant in the first few years of life. The rest live to about age 50 to 55 years, and about 45% of live-born infants survive to 60 years of age. The majority who do so are employed in some setting. It is only relatively recently that health professionals have addressed the prob-lems of adolescents and adults with Down syndrome. Examples of health promotional programs include those for weight control especially formulated for those with Down syndrome.

The Sex Chromosomes and Their Abnormalities

The sex chromosomes in humans are the X and the Y chromosome. Normal human females are 46,XX and normal human males are 46,XY. The X chromosome is believed to encode between 1,000 and 1,250 genes. As described in Chapter 4, daughters normally receive one X chromosome from their father and one from their mother. Sons normally receive their X chromosome from their mother and their Y chromosome from their father. In females, as discussed in Chapter 4, one of the two X chromosomes is inactivated within somatic cells, although few genes apparently escape and X inactivation can be skewed. The Y chromosome is one of the smallest and has relatively few genes.

Although nondisjunction gives rise to most of the sex chromosome abnormalities, neither 45,X nor 47,XYY is associated with increased parental age. The possible reproductive outcomes arising from meiotic nondisjunction at oogenesis and spermatogenesis are illustrated in Figure 9.6. First-division nondisjunction results in no normal karyotype, whereas second-division nondisjunction results in half normal and half-abnormal gametes and offspring.

Considering all the sex chromosome aneuploidies together, their overall incidence is about 1 in 400 live births. The most common sex chromosome variations are those in which there is a single extra or missing X or Y chromosome resulting in Turner syndrome (45,X), triple X (47,XXX), Klinefelter syndrome (47,XXY), or XYY (47,XYY). Those in which more Xs or Ys are added, such as tetrasomy or pentasomy X (48,XXXX; 49,XXXXX), are rare and intellectual disability is common. For sex chromosome variations, the most common mosaic conditions (some cells have a normal chromosome makeup while others do not) are 46,XX/47,XXY; 45,X/46,XX; 46XX/47,XXX; and 46,XY/47,XYY.

In general, those with mosaic sex chromosome abnormalities tend to show milder signs, and the degree tends to be related to the percentage of abnormal cells. The identification of persons with sex chromosome abnormalities often occurs at the fol-

Nondisjunction in oogenesis

Sperm	Ova					
	1st division nondisjunction		**2nd division nondisjunction**			
	XX	O	XX	O	X	X
X	XXX	XO	XXX	XO	XX	XX
Y	XXY	YO*	XXY	YO*	XY	XY

Nondisjunction in spermatogenesis

Ova	Sperm									
	1st division nondisjunction		**2nd division nondisjunction (if of X chromosone)**				**2nd division nondisjunction (if of Y chromosone)**			
	XY	O	XX	O	Y	Y	X	X	YY	O
X	XXY	XO	XXX	XO	XY	XY	XX	XX	XYY	XO
X	XXY	XO	XXX	XO	XY	XY	XX	XX	XYY	XO

* = non-viable

FIGURE 9.6 Possible reproductive outcomes after meiotic nondisjunction of sex chromosomes.

lowing points in the life cycle (examples are given in parentheses):

- Prenatally—due to prenatal cytogenetic diagnosis (all types)
- At birth—confirmation of prenatal diagnosis (all variations), clinical suspicion (45,X), or through newborn chromosome screening (all types)
- Childhood—due to establishing the cause of short stature (45,X) or speech or language disabilities (47,XXY)
- Adolescence—due to delayed development or absence of secondary sex characteristics (45,X; 47,XXY), delayed menarche (45,X), or short stature (45,X)
- Adulthood—due to fertility or reproductive problems (45,X; 47,XXY)

Mildly affected individuals, especially some with 47,XYY, 47,XXY, and 47,XXX or mosaics, may go unrecognized. Recently, a case report described the

first-time diagnosis of Turner syndrome in an elderly woman, important because of predisposition to certain conditions. Sex chromosome variations appear more frequently after the use of intracytoplasmic sperm injection, a method of assisted reproductive technology.

The four major sex chromosome variations (45,X; 47,XXX; 47,XXY; 47,XYY) are summarized in Table 9.3, and Turner and Klinefelter syndromes are

TABLE 9.3 Sex Chromosome Variations

Variation	Incidence	Comments
Turner syndrome (45,X)		See text
47,XXX (triple X)	1:850–1,250 live births	Extra chromosome usually of maternal origin. Tend to be tall; about one fourth may show mild congenital anomalies; some learning disabilities with IQs 10 to 15 points below siblings; may have some delay in walking, with clumsiness and poor coordination; language difficulties in receptive and expressive language; question of whether there is premature ovarian failure and early menopause. Are phenotypic females.
Klinefelter syndrome (47,XXY)		See text
47,XYY	1:840–1,100 live births	Are phenotypic males. In past had been called supermales, and in some cases were thought to be associated with criminal tendencies, but this is not the case. Show above-average height and are hard to distinguish from other males. May have some delayed speech; learning difficulties, especially in reading; difficulties with fine motor coordination; and low-normal to normal intelligence. Some behavioral difficulties may be related to low frustration threshold, immaturity, and impulsiveness, with childhood temper tantrums.

discussed below. The major sex chromosome disorders or variations are illustrated by karyotype in Figure 9.3. The point that the occurrence is no one's fault and could not be predicted or prevented should be reemphasized; genetic counseling should be recommended if not already done, and the availability of prenatal diagnosis for future parental pregnancies should be reemphasized. A level of anxiety and guilt is present to some degree in every family. It is also important to emphasize the gender identity of the person with one of these variations. They do not show any tendencies to homosexuality or lesbianism because of their chromosome constitution.

Turner Syndrome (45,X)

This monosomy is usually written as 45,X. The complete absence of the X chromosome occurs in about 50–60%, with the rest having various combinations of partial deletion, isochromosome formation, and mosaicism. In about 70–80% of the cases, the paternal X is missing. Chromosome analysis is necessary not only for diagnostic confirmation but also because about 25% of mosaic individuals can menstruate and because those (5–6%) with a XY cell line may be prone to malignancies such as dysgerminomas or gonadoblastomas. Persons with Turner syndrome are phenotypic females but have gonadal dysgenesis or streak ovaries.

Short stature is the most consistent feature, with an average untreated height attainment of about 144 cm (4′6″). Final height in those with Turner syndrome is influenced by other height-determining factors such as parental height and the extent of ovarian failure and cardiovascular status. The genes involved are located on the short arm of the X chromosome at Xp11.2-p22.1.

Many cases of Turner syndrome are detected at birth because:

- 60–80% show lymphedema of the hands and feet, which disappears shortly (see Figure 9.7);
- presence of a webbed neck is noted;
- coarctation of the aorta or another cardiovascular anomaly is found (25%).

In one case I saw, an alert delivery room nurse initiated chromosome study because of lymphedema. Prenatal detection is possible through chromosome analysis or sometimes through characteristics

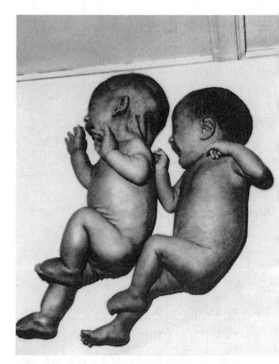

FIGURE 9.7.   Dizygotic twins. Note the lymphedema and extra nuchal skin in the twin on the left with Turner syndrome. Source: Nyhan, W.L., Sakati, N., (1976). *Genetic and malformation syndromes in clinical medicine.* Chicago: Year Book Publishers, Inc. Reprinted with permission.

revealed on ultrasonography. Other cases are detected in later childhood because of the child's short stature or at puberty, when secondary sex characteristics fail to develop and menstruation fails to occur (about 90%). Some are not detected until adulthood, when they are noted to have amenorrhea or infertility. The external genitalia and vagina remain infantile without hormone therapy. Only 1% have had children; most are infertile.

Common clinical features include:

- Short stature;
- Cubitus valgus (an increased carrying angle of the arms so that the arms turn out at the elbow);
- Broad "shield" chest with widely spaced nipples;
- Short neck;
- Low hairline;
- High narrow-arched palate;
- Short fourth metacarpals;

- Many pigmented nevi;
- Hypoplastic nails;
- Urinary tract anomalies (45–80% have some malformation such as horseshoe kidney);
- Cardiovascular anomalies, which occur in 20–44% with bicuspid aortic valve anomalies and coarctation of the aorta being most frequent, in addition to mitral valve prolapse and other anomalies;
- Nondevelopment of secondary sex characteristics, and amenorrhea;
- Infantile external genitalia and vagina without treatment;
- Infertility (affecting about 99%);
- Hypertension even without any accompanying cardiac or renal malformations;
- Primary hypothyroidism as well as antithyroid antibodies and Hashimoto thyroiditis;
- Other autoimmune phenomena, such as inflammatory bowel disease;
- Recurrent otitis media and a progressive sensorineural hearing loss, which may occur and should be evaluated;
- Ophthalmic disorders such as strabismus and ptosis;
- Developmental dysplasia of the hip, scoliosis later in life, and degenerative arthritis in the older individual;
- Cognitive defects in spatial perception and orientation, resulting in difficulties in telling left from right and reading maps, though intelligence is normal.

Detailed medical management may be found in Frías, Davenport, Committee on Genetics, and Section on Endocrinology (2003), Conway (2002), Saenger et al. (2001).

If untreated, the greatest problems reported by patients are short stature and the non-development of secondary sex characteristics. Early diagnosis, before cessation of bone growth, permits the use of recombinant growth hormone (GH) therapy often with oxandrolone, usually beginning at about age 9 or 10 years, to promote growth. This may be followed by ethinyl estradiol with or without progesterone to induce breast development, menstruation, and vaginal maturation. Growth velocity should be monitored, and specific growth charts for Turner syndrome should be used. It should be stressed that females with Turner syndrome have a feminine gender identity. If reproduction is desired, referral should be made to specialists in this area and to the Turner Syndrome Society (http://www.turner-syndrome-us.org).

Klinefelter Syndrome (47,XXY)

In 47,XXY, about 50% of the time, the extra X chromosome is of maternal origin, and about 50% of the time, it is paternally derived. Klinefelter syndrome is underdiagnosed. Most of the affected males are not ascertained until puberty, when incomplete development of secondary sex characteristics is noticed in the form of sparse body hair, gynecomastia, or small testes, which are discovered during a physical examination. Often the condition is not diagnosed until help is sought in adulthood for infertility. In adults, 47,XXY men may account for 14% of the cases of azoospermia. Some reports indicate an increase in the presence of minor congenital anomalies, especially clinodactyly. If multiple anomalies are present, these boys might be detected through chromosome analysis in infancy. Penile size is usually near normal in adolescence and adulthood, but may be small (below the 50th percentile) in children. Sexual functioning is normal. Although development of breast tissue may occur in normal male adolescents, it is more common and tends to persist in males with Klinefelter syndrome. In some patients, this gynecomastia is not seen until later in life. An increased risk of breast cancer and various germ cell tumors has been noted. Mammoplasty or, in some cases, prophylactic mastectomy is recommended for patients with persistent gynecomastia.

Clinical features include:

- Tall stature, with increased leg length;
- Overweight with fat distribution resembling that of the female, and sometimes an incomplete masculine body build;
- Decreased head circumference;
- Intelligence in the low normal range, but impaired coordination may give the impression of slowness;
- Speech and language delays, reading deficiencies, and poor spelling, plus difficulties in processing, retrieving, and storing information;
- Delayed walking and clumsiness;
- Personality impairment may exist in the form of passivity, unassertiveness, and shyness.

Although the timing of the use of testosterone therapy is a topic of debate, some therapists advocate its use in childhood to increase penile size, and most advocate therapy in late childhood to ensure normal pubertal development and prevent most of the behavioral problems. Therefore, it is important that adequate therapy be made available to such men so that problems of being different in appearance are minimized. In a long-term study, men with XXY tended to prefer noncompetitive outside physical activities such as sailing, camping, or fishing more often than sibling controls did.

Some other nursing points should be stressed to the individual and family:

- Males with Klinefelter syndrome have a male gender identity. Normality should be emphasized. They are not predisposed to feminine attributes or qualities, and there is no tendency to homosexuality (remember that the Y chromosome is male determining).
- Sexual adequacy is not impaired. Most 47,XXY males marry, and some (usually mosaics) can reproduce. If they are infertile, reproductive options such as adoption or artificial insemination can be discussed.

SINGLE GENE DEFECTS SEEN IN INFANCY, CHILDHOOD, AND ADOLESCENCE

Individually, the single gene defects usually result in inherited biochemical disorders that are each rare, but as a group, they impose a considerable burden on the patient, family, community, and society. The total reported incidence at birth varies from 1–2%, but accuracy is compromised by:

- The delayed appearance of mutant gene effects;
- Failure to accurately diagnose certain inherited disorders, especially in newborns, who die suddenly.

Consequently, their frequency is underestimated. About 25% are apparent at birth; more than 90% are evident by puberty. Lifespan is decreased in about 60%. The mechanisms of inheritance, gene action, and expression are reviewed in Chapter 4.

Inborn Errors of Metabolism

Most geneticists use the term *inborn error of metabolism* to describe a subgroup of about 300 inherited biochemical disorders that comprises those single gene mutations affecting known enzymes and metabolism. With a few exceptions, these are inherited in an autosomal recessive manner. Enzymes catalyze most reactions in metabolic pathways by acting on substrates in sequence. Some enzymes are conjugated (holoenzymes); that is, they consist of protein core (apoenzyme) and a cofactor (inorganic compound such as a metal ion) or a coenzyme (organic component such as vitamin, see Figure 9.8 top). Interruption of any of the steps in forming a functional coenzyme can lead to a nonfunctional holoenzyme as well and result in disease (e.g., methylmalonic acidemia can result from failure of coenzyme, vitamin B_{12} either to be absorbed or utilized). Replacement of the defective coenzyme effectively treats these disorders. Thus, metabolic dysfunction can occur because of alterations in the substrate, apoenzyme, cofactor, transport proteins, membrane receptors, or holoenzymes. A defect or deficiency of the needed substance at any stage of a metabolic reaction is referred to as a "block" and may be partial or total.

Consequences of Blocks in Metabolic Pathways

Specific consequences of a metabolic block depend on the pathway of which it is a part, but some general statements apply. A schematic representation of a hypothetical metabolic pathway is shown in Figure 9.8, bottom. From this diagram, it can be seen how a particular defect leads to various consequences or combination of consequences:

1. Lack of a functional transport carrier or membrane receptor protein means that a substance will not be able to get inside the cell (block 1) and will be excreted, lost, or accumulated in the wrong place, leading to ill effects. It may then not be available for participation in other reactions or pathways. For example, in cystinuria, the carrier responsible for transporting the amino acids cystine, lysine, ornithine, and arginine across the epithelial cell membrane in the renal tubules and in the intestinal wall is

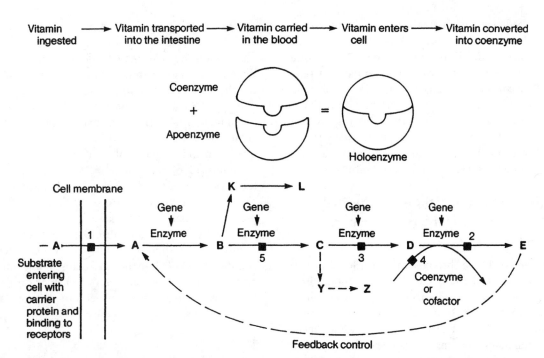

IGURE 9.8 (*Top*) Relationship between vitamins, coenzymes, apoenzymes, and holoenzmes. (*Bottom*) lypothetical metabolic pathway illustrating consequences of metabolic blocks A, B, C, D, K, L, Y, Z = ubstrates or precursors; ■ = block, E = product (see text for explanation).

defective; excessive amounts are excreted, and renal calculi often occur. Hartnup disease is another example of a transport disorder. Familial hypercholesterolemia is a receptor disorder, which is discussed in Chapter 10.

2. The substrate (D) immediately before the block (blocks 2 or 4) or a more distant precursor (A, B, or C) can accumulate. This substance may be toxic to the cell itself, interfere with other biochemical reactions, or give rise to systemic clinical manifestations. It may also be toxic because of the accumulation of the substrate or precursor itself (e.g., in Farber disease, ceramidase deficiency results in the accumulation of the lipid ceramide, causing joint swelling, stiff joints, psychomotor retardation, nodules, vomiting, hoarseness, and respiratory problems), or because such an accumulation (of substrate C) causes the opening of an alternate minor biochemical pathway (Y-Z), causing a product to be produced that normally is not, and it is this product that causes toxic signs and symptoms (e.g., in PKU, phenylpyruvic, and phenylacetic acid are formed and excreted in

the urine). In Figure 9.8, block 4 would prevent the availability of a needed cofactor.

3. The usual product (E) of the metabolic pathway either cannot be produced (blocks 1, 2, 3, 4, or 5) or is produced in inadequate amounts or defective form. Clinical effects can be seen due to its direct lack (e.g., lack of melanin in albinism caused by lack of tyrosinase); if it is needed as a substrate for a subsequent reaction, that reaction cannot occur, and the clinical manifestations may be somewhat removed from the original defect (e.g., lack of phenylalanine hydroxylase in classic PKU prevents the conversion of phenylalanine to tyrosine to dopa, and so melanin synthesis is diminished and persons with PKU have lighter hair and skin than their siblings).

4. Excess available substrate from the defective pathway (block 5) may be channeled to another normal pathway (B-K-L), causing overproduction of its product. This too may affect other reactions.

5. The usual product from the affected metabolic pathway may be functioning in a negative

feedback loop or other control mechanism (dotted lines from E to A), and thus, when not produced, fails to control production of some precursor in its own or another pathway (e.g., in congenital adrenal hyperplasia caused by the lack of 21-hydroxylase, cortisol production is decreased, so the hypothalamus responds by secreting more corticotropin releasing factor, causing increased adrenocorticotropic hormone [ACTH] by the anterior pituitary).

Clinical Manifestations of Inherited Biochemical Disorders in Newborns and Infants

In contrast to the chromosomal disorders and congenital malformations, most of the metabolic disorders show no gross anomalies at birth. Recognition of such disorders and their ultimate diagnosis is complicated by the fact that there are few precise clinical manifestations that can be considered diagnostic, and many defects of the same enzyme are due to alleles that take different clinical forms and may show a rapidly progressive severe infantile picture, a less severe later juvenile onset, or a milder adult form.

Clinical manifestations in the newborn and infant that should lead to further evaluation are shown in Table 9.4. Developmental assessment and signs and symptoms present in older children are discussed in Chapter 7. Dietary history is particularly important, because infants with certain metabolic errors do not exhibit problems until poorly tolerated food is introduced. Some infants develop symptoms of intolerance when they are switched from breast milk to formula because of changes in the protein composition. It is important to emphasize that early identification of an inherited biochemical disorder can allow for early treatment and eligibility for government-funded programs, family studies, genetic counseling, reproductive decision making, life planning, and, in subsequent pregnancies, prenatal detection and even in utero treatment. Because few symptoms are pathognomonic of a disorder and can be used for diagnosis, most require biochemical or deoxyribonucleic acid (DNA) testing for confirmation. Testing should be done for parents, and sometimes other family members if appropriate.

Because the newborn can respond to such illness in only a limited variety of ways, any history of the death of a sibling in infancy, even if a diagnosis was established, should be an indication for heightened observation and an increased index of suspicion for the nurse working with newborns and infants. Often the initial presentation is nonspecific, such as lethargy, poor feeding, failure to thrive, vomiting, irritability, or tachypnea. The major types of presentation may be thought of as those that lead to intoxication and often neurologic deterioration from accumulation of toxic compounds such as most of the organic acidemias; disorders that involve deficiency in energy production or utilization, often presenting with hypoglycemia such as hyperinsulinism or fatty acid oxidation disorders; seizures such as in vitamin-responsive seizures of various types; jaundice or liver failure such as fructose intolerance or tyrosinemia; and heartbeat disorders or cardiac failure suggesting mitochondrial fatty acid oxidation disorders.

CASE EXAMPLE

An extreme example of a missed metabolic disorder was the Stallings case. Patricia Stallings brought her 3-month-old son to an emergency room in St. Louis with symptoms that included vomiting and lethargy. When the laboratory reported finding ethylene glycol in his blood, suspicion of poisoning ensued, and the infant was placed in foster care. Another hospitalization for this infant occurred, and Stallings was accused of feeding him antifreeze. The infant died. She was tried for his murder and found guilty. By this time, she was pregnant again. When she had another son, a similar situation developed. Again, she was suspected of poisoning the second son. Alert geneticists read about the case and contacted legal counsel. This time the infant was diagnosed as having methylmalonic acidemia (MMA), a rare autosomal recessive biochemical disorder. After many twists and turns, Stallings was vindicated in the death of her first son, who was determined to have died from MMA, and she was released. Some cases of sudden infant death syndrome (SIDS) are known to be from inborn errors of metabolism, and increasingly this is investigated as a cause of death in these circumstances.

TABLE 9.4   Some Clinical Manifestations of Inborn Metabolic Errors in Newborns and Early Infancy

Sign/Symptom	Examples of Disorders
Overwhelming illness, may resemble sepsis	Propionate metabolism defects, MSUD, glycemia
Lethargy	Urea cycle disorders, galactosemia, MSUD, GM_1 gangliosidosis, Gaucher disease, orotic aciduria, nonketotic hyperglycemia
Coma	Urea cycle disorders
Convulsions	PKU, Menkes disease, Krabbe disease, MSUD, urea cycle disorders, infantile hypophosphatasia
Exaggerated startle reflex	Tay-Sachs disease
Hypotonia	Urea cycle disorders, Tay-Sachs disease, Menkes disease, glycogen storage disease II, acid phosphatase deficiency
Poor feeding	Propionate metabolism defects, GM_1 gangliosidosis, Menkes disease
Failure to thrive	Propionate metabolism defects, galactosemia, glycogen storage disease I, Gaucher disease, hypophosphatasia, glycogen storage disease II, Andersen disease, orotic aciduria, Menkes disease, severe combined immune deficiency
Eczema	PKU
"Sand" in diapers	Lesch-Nyhan syndrome
Candidiasis	Severe combined immune deficiency, propionate metabolism defects
Jaundice	Galactosemia, G6PD deficiency, α-1-antitrypsin deficiency, Crigler-Najjar syndrome, erythropoietic porphyria, hypothyroidism, pyruvate kinase deficiency
Vomiting	Urea cycle disorders, galactosemia, propionate metabolism defects, isovaleric acidemia, MSUD, PKU, fructosemia, Wolman disease, hypophosphatasia, Menkes disease, glycogen storage disease I
Cataract formation	Galactosemia, Hallermann-Strieff syndrome
Acidosis	Propionate metabolism defect, MSUD, isovaleric acidemia, oxoprolinuria, glutaric aciduria, pyruvate dehydrogenase deficiency
Enlarged abdomen	Propionate metabolism defect, MSUD, isovaleric acidemia, oxoprolinuria, glutaric aciduria, pyruvate dehydrogenase deficiency
Diarrhea	Galactosemia, Wolman disease, severe combined immune deficiency
Characteristic odors (e.g., of urine, sweat)	
Musty, mousy	PKU, tyrosinemia
Burnt sugar	MSUD
Cheese, "sweaty feet"	Isovaleric acidemia
Hops, dried celery	Oasthouse urine disease (methionine malabsorption)
Hypoglycemia	Glycogen storage disease Ia, galactosemia, MSUD, propionate metabolism defects, isovaleric acidemia, galactosemia

Note: Urea cycle disorders include carbamoyl phosphate synthetase I deficiency, citrullinemia, ornithine transcarbamylase deficiency, argininosuccinic aciduria, and argininemia.

MSUD = maple syrup urine disease. Propionate metabolism defects = methylmalonic acidemia, propionic acidemia, multiple carboxylase deficiency. PKU = phenylketonuria.

SELECTED GENETIC DISORDERS COMMONLY SEEN IN CHILDHOOD

Disorders following the inheritance patterns discussed in Chapter 4 that are important because of frequency or because they illustrate an important point are discussed next. Some, such as Marfan disease, may be recognized in childhood, adolescence, or adulthood and are discussed in Chapter 10.

Hemoglobin and Its Inherited Variants

The major normal adult hemoglobin (Hb A) is a tetramer composed of two alpha and two beta globin polypeptide chains that are associated with heme groups. Genes at different loci code for alpha (α) and beta (β) chains that contain 141 and 146 amino acids, respectively. The two pairs of genes that code for α chains are on chromosome 16, whereas the two pairs for gamma (γ) and one each for β and delta (δ) are all linked on chromosome 11.

During development, the embryo and fetus have different Hb chains present in order to meet their oxygenation needs. Zeta (ζ) and epsilon (ε) chains are the earliest synthesized and are usually found in embryos under 12 weeks. By 5 weeks of gestation, α, β, and γ synthesis begin. Major production of β chains coincides with the decrease in γ chain synthesis and does not reach its maximum rate until about 6 months after birth, when Hb F is less than 2% (Table 9.5). Therefore, any disorder that causes insufficient β chain synthesis is not usually manifested clinically until the infant is 3 to 6 months of age. Delta chain synthesis begins just before birth.

More than 400 inherited hemoglobin variants have been identified. There are two basic classes: those due to qualitative changes or structural changes, that is, an amino acid substitution or deletion in the globin part of the molecule as in Hb S or Hb C, and those resulting from quantitative changes, such as deficient globin synthesis as in the thalassemias (see Table 9.6). This latter group includes the hereditary persistence of fetal hemoglobin. The substitution of one nucleotide base for another, resulting in a different amino acid in one of the chains, may change the charge of the Hb molecule and its electrophoretic mobility, or it may be silent. Changes can alter such qualities as oxygen affinity (Hb Kansas), solubility (Hb S), or stability (Hb Torino), resulting in cyanosis or hemolytic anemia, but the majority show no manifestations unless a stressor is encountered, such as altered oxygenation, fever, or drug exposure (see Chapter 6).

Hb S, Hb C, Hb E, and Sickle Cell Disease

The disorders of sickling include sickle cell anemia (SS), sickle cell trait (SA), or compound heterozygous states such as for an association of Hb S and Hb C (SC disease). Both Hb S and Hb C result from the substitution of valine and lysine, respectively, for glutamic acid at position 6 of the beta chain. Both of these Hbs can form various combinations with other mutant Hbs and thalassemia (e.g., Hb Sβ thalassemia). The combination of these two alleles, or SC disease, results in a milder degree of hemolysis but with greater maternal and fetal complications in pregnancy and a longer lifespan than is found in sickle cell disease. Hb SC disease occurs overall in about 1 in 833 persons. One parent of a

TABLE 9.5   Composition and Description of Normal Hemoglobin

Chain Composition	Designation	Description	Percent in Normal Adult
$\alpha_2\beta_2$	Hb A	Major normal adult hemoglobin	97–98.5
$\alpha_2\delta_2$	Hb A$_2$	Minor normal adult hemoglobin	1.5–3
$\alpha_2\gamma_2$	Hb F[a]	Fetal hemoglobin	1
$\zeta_2\varepsilon_2$	Gower I	Embryonic hemoglobin	0
$\alpha_2\varepsilon_2$	Gower II	Embryonic hemoglobin	0
$\zeta_2\gamma_2$	Portland Hb	Embryonic hemoglobin	0

Note: Hb F exists in 2 forms: $\alpha_2\gamma_2^{136\,ala}$ = alanine at position 136 in the gamma chain and $\alpha_2\gamma_2^{136\,gly}$ = glycine at position 136 in the gamma chain

TABLE 9.6   Examples of Selected Hemoglobin Variants

Designation	Comment
Hb S	Point mutation in which valine is substituted for glutamic acid at beta chain position 6; reduced solubility of deoxy form
Hb C	Same as above but lysine is substituted for glutamic acid; trait (AC) found in 2–3% of American Blacks
Hb H	Tetramer of beta chains formed; impaired oxygen transport (see text)
Hb M Boston	Tyrosine substituted for histidine at alpha chain position 58; cyanosis, methemoglobinemia (see text)
Hb Barts	Tetramer of beta chains formed; impaired oxygen transport (see text)
Hb Chesapeake	Leucine substituted for arginine at alpha chain position 92; high oxygen affinity, polycythemia
Hb Constant Spring	Elongated alpha chain due to alpha-chain termination mutation; has 31 extra amino acid residues, slow synthesis; may resemble alpha-thalassemia clinically
Hb Freiberg	Deletion of valine at beta chain position 23; increased oxygen affinity; unstable Hb with mild hemolysis when exposed to sulfonamides
Hb Zurich	Arginine substituted for histidine at beta chain position 63; mild hemolysis when exposed to sulfonamides, unstable Hb

person with SC will have Hb S trait (SA), and one will have Hb C trait (AC). The incidence of Hb C trait in American Blacks is 2–3% and 17–28% in West Africa (see Chapter 3). Hb C disease is often asymptomatic despite mild to moderate hemolytic anemia, but abdominal and joint pain may occur with splenomegaly. Hb E is most common in Southeast Asia: the Hb E trait occurs in 15–30% of Southeast Asian immigrants to the United States, especially Cambodians and Laotians. It may also occur in American Blacks. Hb E disease is often asymptomatic except for mild anemia. Combinations of Hb E with thalassemias occur frequently in Southeast Asians, leading to more severe disease.

In sickle cell anemia, the basic defect is caused by the substitution of the amino acid valine for glutamic acid in the sixth position of the beta chain of the hemoglobin molecule, forming sickle cell hemoglobin (Hb S) instead of the normal adult hemoglobin (Hb A). This changes the charge of the hemoglobin molecule, resulting in a different electrophoretic mobility that can be detected. When this occurs in only one of the two chains, the individual is said to have sickle cell trait. An individual who receives two of these recessive mutant genes from his/her parents is said to have sickle cell disease. Approximately 7–9% of Black Americans have sickle cell trait. Individuals of Mediterranean ancestry (Greek, Italian, Arabic) also have a higher frequency of sickle cell than other population groups. It is believed that persons with sickle cell trait (SA) are normally asymptomatic but some may show exercise intolerance, especially at high altitudes. The chief reason to screen for sickle cell trait is to identify carriers so they can be counseled, and possibly to identify pregnant women who may be at higher risk for complications such as hematuria, urinary tract infections, and fetal distress at delivery. In sickle cell anemia itself, most of the symptoms arise from the vaso-occlusion resulting from red blood cell sickling. This sickling most often occurs in slow or reduced blood flow and in response to decreased oxygenation. Chronic hemolytic anemia, dactylitis (hand-foot syndrome resulting from bone necrosis and manifesting with soft tissue swelling), and acute bacterial infection, especially pneumonia and hepatosplenomegaly, occur around 6 months of age. Until this time, infants have protection due to the presence of high levels of fetal hemoglobin.

Periods of crisis occur that can be precipitated by stress. These are usually very painful, and result from sickling, stasis, and vascular occlusion. Many other manifestations occur, and the severity is variable. It is estimated that there is a death rate of 13–14% below 2 years of age, and as many as 50% used to die by age 20. Important therapeutic approaches such as hydroxyurea and comprehensive care in expert centers have markedly improved mortality.

Sickle cell anemia or SS disease may be detected as part of newborn screening programs (as discussed in Chapter 12), or be diagnosed in childhood. When diagnosis is confirmed, families should be taught about possible clinical manifestations and their complications. These can include overwhelming sepsis, painful sickle cell crises, splenic sequestration (abdominal distention with pallor and listlessness), dactylitis, leg sores and ulcers, symptoms such as paresis that might indicate a stroke, other neurological symptoms, and respiratory distress. Specialized care is available through comprehensive sickle cell centers, and these treatment programs are being expanded. Parents should be taught about symptoms needing attention such as those just mentioned and signs of infection, jaundice, and fever. Usually penicillin prophylaxis will be begun by 2 months of age. Children should receive the usual recommended immunizations. Hydration is important, and folic acid supplementation may be useful. Newer therapies such as hydroxyurea hold promise, Other routine health examinations include electrocardiogram, dental care, ophthalmologic examination, teaching on pain management, watching for gallstones, leg ulcers, and providing appropriate care as indicated. Pain control protocols should be evaluated, and parents should be able to contact their primary care provider or the sickle cell center to be sure treatment is adequate, because emergency room care for SS is often not optimal. For the adolescent, sports activities, pregnancy possibilities and risks, and contraception should be evaluated. For example, women with SS may be at higher risk for thrombosis when using oral contraception, and pregnancy may be riskier. The American Academy of Pediatrics (2002) has published health guidelines on sickle cell that have a list of resources for families.

The Thalassemias

Normally, α and β globin chains are produced i equal amounts. The thalassemias are a group of dis orders of Hb production that result from deficier or absent α or β globin chain synthesis. This chang in the rate of synthesis of one or more globin chair creates an imbalance. Those with a deficiency in th alpha chain are alpha-thalassemias and are mos prevalent in Southeast Asians, North Africans, an Blacks of African descent. The beta-thalassemias re sult from a reduced rate of synthesis of β globi chain and are most prevalent in populations bo dering the Mediterranean Sea, especially Italy, Greec Cyprus, and the Middle East. There are more tha 200 possible mutations. Within a given populatio a few mutations account for most defects. It is n unusual for a person to have thalassemia along wit a structural Hb variant or more than one type thalassemia. About 240 million people worldwid are heterozygotes for beta-thalassemia.

The most severe alpha-thalassemia is Hb Bar hydrops fetalis, in which there is complete absenc or inactivation of all four alpha genes, usuall through deletion. This is often denoted as --/--. N alpha chain synthesis occurs, and Hb Bart tetramers and Hb H comprise most of the Hb pres ent. Infants with the disorder are usually stillborn o die a few hours after birth. In Hb H disease, three o the four genes are absent (--/-α). Some normal H is produced, but the unstable Hb H causes he molytic anemia, splenomegaly, microcytosis, an impaired oxygen transport. In alpha-thalassemi trait, two of the four genes are absent (--/αα, calle α⁰ thalassemia, or -α/-α, called α⁺ thalassemia) and infants may have mild anemia with othe hematologic findings. In silent gene carriers, one o the four genes is absent (-α/αα), and there may b no signs except for slight microcytosis. It is impor tant to recognize the disorder to avoid mistreat ment for iron deficiency anemia and for accurat genetic counseling.

In beta-thalassemia, there may be a decrease synthesis of beta chains (β⁺) or no production (β⁰) In the homozygous state, beta-thalassemia is know as "thalassemia major." Although the clinical cours can vary, typically symptoms are not noticed righ after birth because of the presence of Hb F in th normal newborn. It is not until Hb A synthesi should be dominant that the manifestations are noticed. Hb F may persist as a compensatory mechanism, but it is not sufficient to prevent symptom development. Infants are pale and jaundiced, fail to thrive, have hepatosplenomegaly, and show prominent bones in the skull, spine, and face as the marrow hypertrophies. Long bone fractures ensue, and growth is retarded. The hemolytic anemia becomes so severe that transfusions are necessary; the frequent transfusions lead to iron deposition and therefore to cardiac and hepatic dysfunction and diabetes. Lung disease may also occur. Various approaches, such as iron chelation with desferrioxamine and other agents, have been used to remove the iron burden brought about by transfusion. One drawback is the need for injection and that discomfort and expense. Deferiprone is an oral agent used in some areas, but there are questions about safety and efficacy. More recently, fetal hemoglobin augmentation has been used as a transfusion alternative. Most severely affected persons die during adolescence or young adulthood from complications of the iron overload, especially in the myocardium. Bone marrow transplantation is sometimes done, and gene therapy holds promise. Population screening is common in Mediterranean countries such as Greece and Italy. When blood is being screened, among the major findings suggesting thalassemia are mean cell volume (MCV) less than 72–75 fL and microcytic anemia. Among the many other nursing implications of this disorder is the need to provide genetic counseling, including the option of prenatal diagnosis to the parents who are heterozygotes. They may function normally because one beta chain is normal while the other one is not. Nurses should be alert to the finding of an apparent anemia in persons of Mediterranean extraction for β-thalassemia and of Southeast Asian extraction for α-thalassemia.

Phenylketonuria and Hyperphenylalaninemia

The amino acid phenylalanine (phe) is essential for protein synthesis in humans. A complex reaction is involved in the hepatic conversion of phenylalanine to tyrosine (see Figure 12.3), and blockage causes elevations collectively refered to as hyperphenylalaninemias. These include transient hyper-

phenylalaninemia, persistent non-PKU hyperphenylalaninemia, classic PKU, and deficient tetrahydropterin biosynthesis that may result from impaired recycling of tetrahydropterin due to dihydropeteridine reductase deficiency. Hyperphenylalaninemia refers to phe levels above 2 mg/dl (120 μM) and may result from various mutations interfering with the conversion of phe to tyrosine, including phenylalanine hydroxylase (PAH) deficiency resulting in classic PKU and a mild non-PKU hyperphenylalaninemia. Therefore, several defects in different steps in the metabolism of phenylalanine or its cofactor can result in elevated phe. The most common of these forms is classic PKU, characterized by less than 1% of PAH activity. Variants account for about 10% of all cases, and more than 400 mutations of the PAH gene are known to result in classic PKU. Hyperphenylalanemia not resulting in classic PKU has different treatment approaches. It is important to rescreen infants who have positive early screening tests so that those with transient hyperphenylalaninemia are not placed on phenylalanine-restricted diets that could be harmful to them.

It is now rare to see a child manifest the full spectrum of symptoms resulting from classic PKU because of screening programs and prompt treatment, but occasionally an affected infant is missed. Therefore, PKU should not be automatically ruled out in infants manifesting signs and symptoms associated with the disorder. PKU is discussed in more detail in Chapters 5 and 12.

The overall incidence of classic PKU in the general population in the United States is approximately 1 in 11,000 live births; Irish and Scottish populations have an incidence as high as 1 in 5,000, and Black, Japanese, and Ashkenazi Jewish populations show an incidence as low as 1 in 100,000. Inheritance is by the autosomal recessive mode of transmission. The human *PAH* gene has been identified and mapped. Carrier detection and prenatal diagnosis of classic PKU are possible.

Lysosomal Storage Disorders

Lysosomal storage disorders is the terminology used to describe a group of about 50 genetic diseases that have in common the accumulation of certain metabolites within the cell organelle known as the lysosome. This accumulation is due to defective lysosomal enzyme activity or a genetic defect in a receptor, activator protein, membrane protein, or transport molecule. The abnormal deposition and storage of the particular substance can result in effects on the central nervous system as well as systemic manifestations. The individual disorders vary from the mucopolysaccharidoses such as Hurler disease; to the sphingolipidoses, which include the gangliosidoses such as Sandhoff disease and Tay-Sachs disease; glycogen storage disorders, such as Pompe disease; as well as mucolipidosis IV and Chédiak-Higashi syndrome. Collectively the incidence is 1 in 7,000–8,000 live births. The majority are inherited in an autosomal recessive manner with the exception of Hunter disease and Fabry disease, which are X-linked recessive, and Danon dis-

ease (glycogen storage disease IIb), thought to be X-linked dominant. These disorders are generally progressive and may vary in severity and expression. Many of these disorders have variant forms that may differ in age of onset (often with a severe form with infantile onset and less severe juvenile or adult forms, so that many patients first come to clinical attention as adults), clinical presentation, or disease course. Those who present as adults are often not diagnosed promptly. For example, a 38-year-old man with Niemann-Pick disease type C was misdiagnosed as having schizophrenia for 8 years, and a late adolescent male with Tay-Sachs disease was misdiagnosed with catatonic schizophrenia. Adult-onset Tay-Sachs disease can mimic Friedreich ataxia. Selected lysosomal storage disorders are summarized in Table 9.7. The mucopolysaccharide

TABLE 9.7   Characteristics of Selected Lysosomal Storage Diseases

Disorder	Enzyme Deficiency	Selected Characteristics (Infantile Form Unless Noted)
Fabry disease (diffuse angiokeratoma)	α-galactosidase A	Onset in late childhood, adolescence, or adulthood; telangiectasia, pain attacks, autonomic dysfunction, angina, EKG changes, paresthesia, lymphedema, hypertension, renal failure; death by middle age usual
Farber disease	Ceramidase	Psychomotor deterioration, subcutaneous nodules, failure to thrive, swollen joints, intellectual disability, hepatosplenomegaly, hoarseness, death
Gaucher disease	β-glucosidase	See text
Generalized gangliosidosis	β-galactosidase	Hepatosplenomegaly, skeletal abnormalities with dwarfism, joint stiffness, intellectual disability, cerebral degeneration, decerebrate rigidity, death
Krabbe disease	Galactocerebroside β-galactosidase	Irritability, convulsions, mental and motor deterioration, deafness, blindness, death
Metachromatic leukodystrophy	Arylsulfatase A	Hypotonia, quadriplegia, blindness, mental deterioration, megacolon, death
Niemann-Pick disease type A	Sphingomyelinase	Has many subforms; seizures, coronary artery disease, hepatosplenomegaly, failure to thrive, hypotonia, intellectual disability, death
Refsum syndrome	Phytanic acid oxidase	Peripheral neuropathy, cerebellar ataxia, retinitis pigmentosa, ichthyosis, deafness, cardiac arrhythmias (child)
Sandhoff disease	Hexosaminidase A&B	Muscle weakness and wasting, mental and motor deterioration, cerebellar ataxia, blindness, cardiomegaly, hepatosplenomegaly
Tay-Sachs	Hexosaminidase A	See text

Note: Each has one or more less severe forms with later onset. All are autosomal recessive except Fabry disease, which is X-linked.

disorders and Tay-Sachs disease are discussed next as examples.

Mucopolysaccharide Disorders (Mucopolysaccharidoses)

The mucopolysaccharidoses (MPS) are a group of lysosomal storage disorders that are characterized by the accumulation of glycosaminoglycans (GAG, or mucopolysaccharides). GAGs are long-chain complex carbohydrates that may be linked to proteins to form proteoglycans. They are present in ground substances and tissues such as cell, nuclear and mitochondrial membranes, cartilage, skin, bone, synovial fluid, umbilical cord, vitreous humor, and the cornea, where support is needed. They include chondroitin sulfate (SO_4), heparan SO_4, dermatan SO_4, keratan SO_4, and hyaluronan. When the specific lysosomal enzyme needed in degradation is defective, certain GAGs accumulate within lysosomes and are deposited, particularly in connective tissue, bone, viscera, the heart, the brain, and the spinal cord, giving rise to the particular symptom. There are at least seven distinct classification groups. Each has a pattern of deposition and urinary excretion of MPS that is valuable in diagnosis. These disorders are progressive and may show considerable variability in clinical severity.

The combined incidence of all the MPS disorders is 1 in 25,000 newborns. MPS I is usually classified into Hurler syndrome (most severe), Scheie (mild), and Hurler-Scheie, which is intermediate. It is believed that these are points on a continuous spectrum of severity. Hurler syndrome is one of the most frequently seen. Clinically, it is not usually detected until 6 to 12 months of age, although infants may have umbilical or inguinal hernias, a large tongue, and be unusually large. Usually the syndrome does not develop fully until well into the second year. Cardiac disease is very common, and cardiomyopathy may result in early death, even being a presenting symptom. Most affected children do not live past 14 years of age. A picture of a child with Hurler syndrome and characteristic features is shown in Figure 9.9. Enzyme replacement therapy using recombinant human α-L-iduronidase (Aldurazyme) has been used in treatment in mucopolysaccharidosis I, as has bone marrow transplantation and the combination of both. The following case illustrates many typical features.

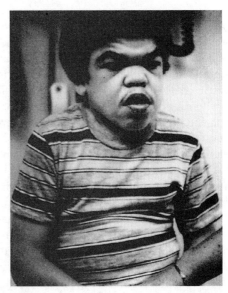

FIGURE 9.9   Boy with Hurler syndrome.

CASE EXAMPLE

A 22-month-old girl was referred to the genetic counseling center because of developmental delay and growth retardation. Examination revealed typical coarse facies, an enlarged tongue, kyphosis, hirsutism, and a protruding abdomen caused by an enlarged liver and spleen. Corneal clouding was noted. Her mother stated that the child had frequent colds and ear infections. The family history was negative; her 5-year-old brother was normal. Laboratory testing revealed findings characteristic of Hurler syndrome. The health care professional referred the family to genetic services. Included in the usual genetic counseling of the family based on the autosomal recessive inheritance was the information that prenatal diagnosis was available and could be used if another pregnancy was desired.

Tay-Sachs Disease

CASE EXAMPLE

The nurse in the well-baby clinic in the Williamsburg section of Brooklyn, New York, was talking to Ruth, the mother of a 7-month-infant girl, Sarah. Ruth is of Ashkenazi (Eastern European) Jewish descent. Ruth tells the nurse that she is concerned about Sarah because she had begun to sit up by herself but has seemed to lose this skill. In addition, she is having difficulty feeding Sarah. The nurse ascertains that Ruth and her husband, Stuart, had not undergone carrier screening for Tay-Sachs disease before or during pregnancy, and in reviewing the family pedigree and history, she notes that they are second cousins. The nurse during the physical examination sees a cherry-red spot on Sarah's fundus during ophthalmic examination. At this point, referral is made for more intense evaluation. Sarah is ultimately found to have Tay-Sachs disease. What would the nurse think about in terms of testing for the parents and in terms of the implications for the immediate and extended families?

Tay-Sachs disease is the best known of the lysosomal storage diseases. It is classified as a GM_2 gangliosidosis due to mutation of the *HEXA* gene encoding the α subunit of hexosaminidase A (Hex A), a lysosomal enzyme composed of alpha and beta polypeptides. At least 78 mutations in this gene have been identified. In the classic infantile form, the infant appears well except perhaps for an exaggerated Moro (startle) reflex. At 4 to 6 months of age, hypotonia, difficulty in feeding, and apathy begin. Motor weakness, developmental regression, and mental retardation follow. A cherry-red spot is noticeable in the fundus on ophthalmic examination, and blindness occurs by 12 to 18 months. Neurologic deterioration follows. Seizures, decerebrate rigidity, and deafness occur, with an eventual vegetative state. The head enlarges about 50%, and hypothalamic involvement may cause precocious puberty. Death is inevitable and typically occurs by 2 to 4 years of age, although a few children have survived to 6 years. Tay-Sachs is most common in Ashkenazi Jews and in French Canadians from eastern Quebec. Both juvenile and adult forms have been described. Those with the juvenile form may develop symptoms between ages 1 and 9 years. The availability of a screening test for carriers and its use among population subgroups has decreased the number of infants now born with Tay-Sachs disease.

Duchenne and Becker Muscular Dystrophy

The muscular dystrophies are a group of inherited muscle disorders for which the term *dystrophinopathies* is increasingly used. Duchenne muscular dystrophy (DMD) and Becker muscular dystrophy (BMD) are both X-linked recessive disorders that are allelic and result from different deletions in the dystrophin gene at Xp21.1. Mutation results in deficiency or defect of the functional gene protein product dystrophin. This cytoskeletal protein is located in the muscle membrane and is destabilized if dystrophin is deficient or altered resulting in lack of structural integrity of the muscle membrane. DMD is the most common (1 in 3,000–5,000 male births) and most severe. Initial common symptoms appear in early childhood, usually insidiously. These include:

- Delayed walking
- Abnormal gait, which is described as a duck-like waddle
- Toe walking
- Difficulty in climbing steps
- Protruding abdomen
- Tendency to fall
- Gower sign (a climbing up oneself to get up from the floor by pressing on the thighs)

About one third of these patients appear sporadically, with no previous affected relative. Unless there has been a previously affected child in the family, the diagnosis is often delayed.

Boys with DMD usually lose the ability to walk between 7 and 13 years of age and may become wheelchair dependent. It is important to keep them ambulatory as long as possible to prevent deformities and degeneration. Muscle weakness is progressive, with loss of function. The tendency for toe walking may lead to flexion contractures and forward hip tilt. Range of motion may help with these, but the child may benefit from braces. Death usually occurs in the second decade of life because of respiratory infection and insufficiency, progressing from trivial to severe. Death may be sudden and caused by myocardial insufficiency. Dilative cardiomyopathy leading to arrhythmias may occur and can be treated with angiotensin-converting enzyme (ACE) inhibitors and beta-blockers if indicat-

d. Congestive heart failure may occur. Boys with DMD are at increased risk for features of malignant hyperthermia when given anesthesia.

Once a child is diagnosed (today usually by DNA analysis and electromyography), female family members become concerned about their status as carriers. Females with an affected son and another affected male relative are obligate heterozygotes, but where there is only one affected male relative, carrier status is more difficult to ascertain. Some carriers (about 10%) manifest mild symptoms such as pseudohypertrophy of the calves or muscle weakness. Carrier identification today is usually by DNA testing. DMD has been suggested as appropriate for newborn screening; although treatment is not available, further affected children in a family might be avoided. Corticosteroids have been used for some effects, but the main hope lies in gene therapy.

BMD usually has its onset in adolescence. Ambulation is usual until about the age of 16 years. Affected males often survive into the fourth decade or later. Symptoms are similar to DMD but milder, often with exercise-related muscle pain. Usually the affected man becomes dependent on a wheelchair eventually. Dilated cardiomyopathy may occur that may necessitate heart transplantation. BMD usually shows the presence of muscle dystrophin, but it is abnormal in size and quantity. Carrier detection is possible.

Neurofibromatosis 1

First characterized in 1882 by von Recklinghausen, neurofibromatosis attracted attention because of publicity resulting from the movie and play *The Elephant Man* (although Joseph Merrick did not actually have neurofibromatosis). There are two major types:

- Neurofibromatosis type 1 (NF1), formerly called von Recklinghausen disease
- Neurofibromatosis type 2 (NF2), formerly called bilateral acoustic neurofibromatosis

NF1 has a prevalence of approximately 1 in 2,500 to 1 in 5,000. Both are autosomal dominant (AD) disorders with one of the highest new mutation rates known—about 50%. The *NF1* gene, identified in 1990, is located at chromosome 17q11.2 and codes for neurofibromin, a protein product involved in control of cell growth and differentiation with a tumor-suppressor function.

Despite widely variable clinical features and expression, diagnostic criteria have been established. For diagnosis, a person must have two or more of the following:

- Six or more café-au-lait spots over 5 mm (0.5 cm) in prepuberty and over 15 mm (1.5 cm) in postpuberty (the normal population usually has 0–3). The café-au-lait spots are not usually seen at birth but develop around 1 year of age and may fade in the elderly.
- Two or more neurofibromas of any time or one plexiform neurofibroma.
- Freckling in the axillary or inguinal regions.
- Optic glioma (tumor of the optic pathway).
- Two or more Lisch nodules (benign hamartomas of the iris).
- A distinctive bony lesion such as dysplasia of the sphenoid bone or thinning of the long bone cortex.
- A first-degree relative with NF1 by the previous criteria.

Other features may develop:

- Macrocephaly
- Short stature
- Spinal curvature (scoliosis or kyphosis)
- Hemihypertrophy
- Neural crest malignancies (e.g., pheochromocytoma)
- Hypertension
- Seizures
- Speech defects
- Learning disabilities, especially visual-spatial learning problems

Knowledge of possible manifestations forms the framework for diagnosis, treatment, and management. The severity of NF1 varies greatly. Even within a family, one patient may have only café-au lait spots, or axillary freckling, whereas another has macrocephaly, multiple neurofibromas, severe spinal curvature, learning disabilities, and hemihypertrophy. It is important to identify the person who has the gene from someone who has an isolated physical characteristic.

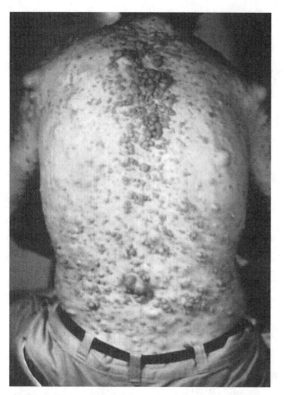

FIGURE 9.10   Multiple neurofibromas in a man with neurofibromatosis. Courtesy of Dr. Dorinda Shelley, Peoria, Illinois.

CASE EXAMPLE

In my own practice, I have seen several cases of NF1. One young woman sought genetic counseling regarding whether her 2-month-old son had inherited NF1. Her father had NF1 and had multiple neurofibromas on his body (see Figure 9.10). She had lost an eye to optic glioma and had macrocephaly, freckling, and hypertension. Interestingly, she did not regard herself as severely affected, believing that her father's manifestations would be harder to live with for her. Her son did show macrocephaly and one café-au-lait spot. Before all information was collected, she moved across the country, and was followed by a genetic counseling center there. I later learned that her son was indeed affected.

Nurses should be aware of the worsening o symptoms that occurs in puberty and pregnancy Patients should be advised to have at least an annu al physical examination because of the frequen progression to malignancy in the disease and to de tect complications. The Committee on Genetics o the American Academy of Pediatrics has publishec recommendations for health supervision with an ticipatory guidance for children with NF, as have Theos and Korf (2006). These recommendation include frequent ophthalmological examination evaluation of speech, neurodevelopmental progres and learning needs, examination for neurologic pathology, and skin lesions with changes.

Osteogenesis Imperfecta

Osteogenesis imperfecta (OI) is a genetic disorde of the connective tissue, with an incidence in th West of about 1 in 20,000 live births. It results from mutation in either the *COL1A1* or *COL1A2* gene that encode both chains in type I collagen. There are several classes of OI. Basically, OI is characterizec by connective tissue and bone defects including on or more of the following:

- Bone fragility and osteoporosis leading to fractures
- Blue sclerae
- Progressive bone deformities (including long bone curvature)
- Presenile hearing loss
- Dentinogenesis imperfecta (a dentin abnormality of the teeth showing opalescence and blue or brown discoloration)

There are other features as well:

- Hernias
- Joint hyperlaxity
- Elevated body temperature of one or two degrees F
- Heat intolerance, which may include difficulties with anesthesia
- Varying degrees of short stature
- Triangular face
- Large "tam-o'shanter"-shaped skulls

Variability in clinical expression is common, and type I may be mild enough so that it is missed altogether. Some individuals may suffer hundreds of fractures in a lifetime, whereas others suffer only one or a few, and still others have little bone fragility; some have little height effect, others are two to three standard deviations below the mean, and others are six or more deviations below the mean. Kyphosis and scoliosis are very common as the individual gets older.

OI is considered to be inherited in a autosomal dominant manner, although in some rare cases, autosomal recessive transmission apparently occurs. It may occur sporadically. Although the reason for growth deficiency is not fully understood, growth hormone for treating the short stature has been used in clinical trials. Bone marrow transplant to produce normal cells and gene therapy to suppress the dominant mutant allele may hold future treatment promise. Prenatal diagnosis is available. In those choosing to continue an affected pregnancy, cesarean section to minimize fetal trauma can be done, and arrangements for delivery in a specialty hospital should be made.

Those who are diagnosed in infancy present immediate problems and challenges to the new parents and the nursing staff. The simple act of lifting the child may cause bones to break. In diapering, the infant should never be lifted by the ankles but supported carefully in good alignment. The crib, and later the playpen, should be mesh and padded. All treatment tables should be padded. The infant can be most easily held or transported in an infant seat, on a padded piece of plywood, or on a pillow so that support is provided. Because of the ongoing body temperature elevation, light clothing should be used and water, or later juice, should be offered frequently. Infants with OI have the same need for physical contact and stimulation as other infants, but parents and others may be afraid to handle them because of fragility. The nurse should help the parents to learn to be secure in handling and help promote bonding as well as using stroking and touching. Those children with severe disease will have many hospitalizations. Nurses should be willing to listen to both the parents and the child, who usually become quite expert by early childhood in how movement can be best accomplished. At the time of diagnosis, one of the most helpful things that the nurse can do is to refer the family to one of the organizations for OI.

Before a diagnosis of OI is made, the parents of the infant who is sustaining fractures may be suspected of child abuse. Such an experience can be very traumatic for them. Radiologic confirmation of OI due to the presence of wormian bones, the types of fractures, the presence of blue sclera (although normal infants may have this as well) or dentinogenesis imperfecta, and a family history of OI or its signs and symptoms may help in establishing the true diagnosis, as will DNA testing. The potential for respiratory insufficiency due to instability of the ribs and infections is present. Coughing can result in rib fracture, and each fracture episode can increase deformity, further decreasing respiratory capabilities. Respiratory infections can be life threatening in infants and children with severe disease, and so measures should be directed at prevention and prompt treatment. Children may experience delay of developmental milestones, such as standing and walking, because of fear of fractures and pain. Newer approaches to therapy include using bisphosphonates to improve bone mass. Pamidronate may be used intravenously in severe forms and appears particularly useful when begun early. Oral bisphosphonates may be used in later therapy.

Pregnancy problems for the woman with OI may include respiratory problems, increased spontaneous fractures, increased awkwardness, and an increased susceptibility to hernias. Careful monitoring of the pregnancy is necessary, and cesarean section may be necessary due to the possibility of fractures in labor and delivery. Genetic counseling and prenatal diagnosis should be provided.

Cystic Fibrosis

"Woe to that child which when kissed on the forehead tastes salty. He is bewitched and soon must die." This folk saying from northern Europe as quoted by Welsh and Smith (1995) was an early reference to cystic fibrosis (CF). Today the picture is brighter. The median age for a person with CF to live is more than 30 years. CF is the most common semilethal genetic disease in Caucasians with an incidence of about 1 in 2,000 to 1 in 2,500 live Caucasian births. It is especially frequent in certain ethnic groups, such as the Hutterites in Alberta, Canada, where the frequency is 1 in 313. It is less frequent in American Blacks and Asian populations.

It is transmitted in an autosomal recessive manner. The frequency of heterozygote carriers in White populations is about 1 in 25, in Ashkenazi Jews about 1 in 29, in Hispanics 1 in 48, in American Blacks 1 in 65, and in Asians about 1 in 150.

The basic defect is a mutation in the *CFTR* gene on chromosome 7q31.2 whose product is the CF transmembrane conductance regulator. This protein is expressed in the membrane of epithelial cells that line such structures as the pancreas, intestines, sweat ducts, vas deferens, and lungs, influencing water balance and sodium transport. This protein is involved in chloride ion channel function (an ion channel is essentially a protein tunnel that crosses the cell membrane and changes conformation as it opens and closes in response to various signals) regulating and participating in transport of chloride and probably other electrolytes across epithelial cell membranes. Some *CFTR* mutations cause an abnormal protein to be produced or no protein production, but others cause defective regulators of, or conductors through, the CFTR ion channel or defective regulation of other channels. More than 1,000 *CFTR* mutations are known. The most common mutation (accounting for about two thirds across populations) is ΔF508del, a deletion of phenylalanine at position 508 that results in abnormal protein folding and lack of CFTR at the cell membrane. There are three other mutations that are particularly common—G551D, G542X, and R553X —all of which act in various ways to cause deficiency of CFTR. The degree of deficiency can vary. When *CFTR* function is 10% or greater, usually abnormalities are not seen. Thus, the specific mutation a person has can influence the clinical expression and course and can be useful when counseling a family.

Genotype-phenotype correlations are of interest in predicting both mortality and morbidity. Those who are most severe, with less than 1% of activity, usually have the full spectrum of involvement, including pancreatic exocrine deficiency, progressive pulmonary infection, and congenital absence of the vas deferens. Genetic testing is complicated because of the large number of *CFTR* mutations known. Most commercial tests look for 70, which should identify most of the common mutations. About 1% of persons with CF do not demonstrate known gene mutations, and about 18% show only one mutated gene despite symptoms. Because of variability in

pulmonary disease among those with the same *CFTR* genotype, a search has been done for other influences, both genetic and environmental. Environmental factors that were postulated to influence variability of phenotype included *Pseudomonas aeruginosa*, *Burkholderia cepacia*, tobacco use, and nutrition. CF modifier genes have also been suggested.

Generally a child will have the same mutation as his/her carrier parents so that prenatal testing for the mutations known to be carried by the parents is accurate. Diagnosis is still done sometimes by sweat testing, but genotyping, tests of pancreatic function, and using nasal potential-difference measurements are more common.

Many of the symptoms of CF result from the fact that in CF, mucus and serous secretions are abnormally concentrated, sticky, or dry, allowing blockage of ducts and other structures to occur. The most obvious systems affected are the respiratory and gastrointestinal and give rise to the most common symptoms, including progressive lung disease, sinusitis, pancreatic exocrine insufficiency (found in about 90% to some degree), which can lead to diabetes mellitus, and infertility in males. How the mutant gene manifests effects is being elucidated. It is believed that because of abnormal thickening, mucin from the pools in the lungs may protect the bacteria *P. aeruginosa* from the body's immune system. The salty secretions may also influence body defense. This may partly explain why people with CF are so susceptible to infections with *P. aeruginosa*.

A common presentation is in childhood with a persistent cough, often with colonization, and perhaps loose, bulky stools and failure to thrive. There is extreme variability in the severity of clinical illness and in the system involved. About 50% are diagnosed before 1 year of age. Those with milder disease or less common manifestations may not be diagnosed until adolescence or adulthood and frequently have previously been misdiagnosed as having asthma, celiac disease, or chronic bronchitis. Because aspermia is present in 95–98% of males with cystic fibrosis, infertility with azoospermia should lead the practitioner to include cystic fibrosis as a diagnostic possibility. Men seeking assisted reproduction by such techniques as intracytoplasmic sperm injection are now usually tested for CF status before the procedure is done; depending on results, further testing of their partner and counseling would be done. Females may have delayed puberty as well as decreased fertility. Various presenting manifestations may be seen in different age groups as shown in Table 9.8.

Advances in cystic fibrosis care and experience at specialized centers have allowed survival with good life quality into adulthood with a median age of survival of over 30 years currently. Management is dependent on the severity of disease, age of diagnosis, and degree of involvement of body systems. It is aimed at controlling and preventing respiratory infections; maintaining nutrition; minimizing unpleasant gastrointestinal effects; preventing and treating complications; and providing support, teaching, and counseling to the client and the family. Treatment may include postural drainage with chest percussion; antimicrobial therapy; diet therapy, including determining a diet to result in stabilization of pulmonary function and optimal growth,

TABLE 9.8   Various Presenting Signs and Symptoms of Cystic Fibrosis in Various Age Groups

Newborn

Meconium ileus	Intestinal atresia
Melconium plug syndrome	"Salty" taste

Infancy

Failure to thrive	Steatorrhea
"Salty" taste	Hypoproteinemia, anemia, edema
Rectal prolapse	Hypoprothrombinemia, hemorrhage
Heat prostration/dehydration	Rapid finger wrinkling in water
Frequent, bulky stools	Abdominal distention

Childhood

Frequent, bulky, offensive stools	Heat prostration/dehydration
Chronic secretory otitis media	Inguinal hernia
Intussusception	Hydrocele
Biliary cirrhosis, jaundice	Type 1 diabetes mellitus
Rectal prolapse	

Adolescent/Young Adult

Aspermia (males)	Chronic cough
Infertility	Bronchiectasis
Chronic cervicitis (females)	Glucose intolerance
Thick cervical mucus (females)	Type 1 diabetes mellitus
Cervical polyps (females)	Intestinal obstruction
Delayed secondary sexual development	Reactive airway disease, asthma
Poor growth/small for age	Acute pancreatitis

All Ages

Chronic cough	Sinusitis
Elevated sweat electrolytes	Clubbed fingers
Nasal polyps (especially below 16 years of age)	Recurrent pneumonia, bronchitis
Absence of vas deferens (males)	Bronchiectasis
Cor pulmonale	Sputum culture showing *Staphylococcus aureus* or *Pseudomonas aeruginosa*
Pancreatic insufficiency and malabsorption	Family history of similar symptoms, infant deaths, diarrhea
Presence of hard fecal masses in right lower quadrant of abdomen	

paying attention to energy expenditure, pancreatic enzymes, and fat-soluble vitamins; antiinflammatory therapy; use of bronchodilators and aerosolized substances such as rhDNase I (Dornase Alfa) and Pulmozyme (recombinant human DNase); and more drastic measures such as lung transplantation. Because use of high-dose pancreatic enzyme supplements can cause the complication of fibrosing colonopathy, it has been recommended that the daily dose should be below 10,000 units of lipase per kg. Gene therapy appears to hold great promise. Testing for status as a CF carrier in couples planning pregnancy, in those with a family history of CF, partners of persons with CF, and as a part of prenatal screening programs has rapidly become a standard of care. Newborn screening and widespread population carrier screening have not yet received national endorsement but are being done in many areas.

Although there is no known impairment of sexual performance or desire, most males with cystic fibrosis are sterile, and decreased fertility may be present in females due to thick cervical mucus. Menstrual problems and vaginal yeast infections due to antibiotic therapy are common, and the client should be referred to a gynecologist experienced in the care of patients with CF. Both females and males should be encouraged to consider alternative reproductive plans and options such as contraception, sterilization, adoption, and artificial insemination. Preconception counseling and family planning information is important in adolescence, and genetic counseling may also need to be provided. Pregnancy in cystic fibrosis women may be complicated because of pulmonary function changes and the increased cardiac work load. Couples contemplating having children should also be encouraged to consider the necessary increase in everyday work and activities.

Hemophilia

Hemophilia A (classical hemophilia) and hemophilia B (Christmas disease) are caused by deficiencies of coagulation factor VIII (antihemophilic factor) and coagulation factor IX, respectively. Their incidence is 1 in 4,400 to 1 in 7,500 male births. Hemophilia A results from a mutation on the gene located on Xq28, and hemophilia B results from mutations at Xq27; more than 2,100 are known. Both are transmitted in an X-linked recessive manner, and

about one third result from a new mutation with no prior family history. In such isolated cases without prior positive family history, it is important to determine if the mother is a carrier. Females at risk can have a determination of relevant factor activity, and those below the normal range confirm carrier status, but in those falling within the normal range, the possibility of the mother's being a carrier is not excluded. DNA testing may be useful in certain cases to detect carriers. Prenatal diagnosis for women who are known carriers has been accomplished.

The severity of clinical disease varies with the percentage of the blood level of factor present, ranging from those with little factor present and severe disease, to essentially normal coagulation efficiency at levels of 50% or higher. The availability of concentrated factor preparations such as cryoprecipitates, comprehensive care programs, and the use of therapeutic and prophylactic home infusions radically altered treatment, complications, and prognosis, allowing less disruption of family plans. However, those with hemophilia suffered a setback when human immunodeficiency virus (HIV) entered the blood supply, infecting thousands with hemophilia. The use of recombinant factor VIII and factor IX concentrates for home infusion is now the recommended type. Desmopressin, an antidiuretic hormone analogue, can be used to raise the factor VIIIC concentration in persons with mild hemophilia A. In addition to treatment, prophylaxis may be used several times a week through infusion to prevent bleeds. While long-term information is not yet available, this approach may be an option for some, permitting a young child even with severe hemophilia to have a normal life with few or no bleeds and few restrictions. Gene therapy is under investigation.

The major problem in hemophilia is hemorrhage into the joints and muscles; if not stopped, it can result in prolonged bleeding, leading to deformities and immobilization. These often occur spontaneously, that is, where no recallable injury has occurred, but which probably result from normal physiologic strains that are usually unnoticed. The most common sites are ankles, knees, wrists, and elbows. For parents of boys with hemophilia in the past, these were a constant overhanging concern, because their occurrence usually meant hospitalization and carried the risk of loss of function, nerve damage, deformity, the wearing of various orthopedic appliances, long school absences, and high costs.

Often parents were overprotective, but such spontaneous bleeds were not preventable until the advent of prophylaxis. Some boys notice a "bubbly" feeling at the site of the bleed before it is otherwise noticed. Most infants with hemophilia develop symptoms in the first year of life. They may first be noticed in the form of subcutaneous hematomas or easy bruising or even at circumcision, and may follow intramuscular injections or mouth injury. Often the parents are suspected of child abuse. The type of bleeding that occurs is slow, steady, internal bleeding as opposed to gushing from superficial cuts. Thus, the child with hemophilia is not usually going to "bleed all over the neighbor's carpet." Referral should be made to a comprehensive hemophilia center for care, and to hemophilia organizations.

Achondroplasia

Achondroplasia is a type of disproportionate dwarfism. It is transmitted in an autosomal dominant manner with complete penetrance and often occurs as a sporadic mutation (in about seven eighths of new cases). It is related to increased paternal age. Achondroplasia is due to mutation in the fibroblast growth factor receptor-3 gene (*FGFR3*) on chromosome 4p16.3. It can be recognized at birth but is not always. The limbs are short and the head is large, with a prominent forehead and mandible, a flattened area at the base of the nose, "trident" hands, and marked hypotonicity. Later, kyphosis and lordosis may develop. It is important to remember that there is no intellectual impairment. The mean height for females and males with achondroplasia is about 48 inches and 52 inches, respectively. More than 10,000 persons with achondroplasia live in the United States. The American Academy of Pediatrics has developed health supervision recommendations for persons with achondroplasia at various age ranges.

The Fragile X Syndrome

The fragile X syndrome is now considered one of the most common causes of mental retardation. First identified in males, it is now known that females are affected as well. The clinical signs are very subtle and become more obvious in later childhood and adulthood, although the presence of mental retardation may prompt chromosome studies and thus lead to earlier diagnosis. Fragile X syndrome is more common than originally thought, and the prevalence is estimated at approximately 1 in 4,000 males and 1 in 6,000 females.

Early indicators in infancy may be high birthweight, macrocephaly, frontal bossing, and a large anterior fontanelle, but it is difficult to detect in early childhood. Later, males with the fragile X syndrome generally have one or more of the following:

- Macroorchidism (enlarged testes which may not be seen until 8 or 9 years of age but are seen in 90% after puberty)
- Large, prominent jaw and forehead
- Large, low-set ears
- Large head circumference
- Hypotonia
- Flat feet
- Soft skin, which may become callused with biting, a self-injurious behavior sometimes seen
- High arched palate
- Aversion of gaze
- Strabismus
- Hyperextendible joints
- Mitral valve prolapse
- Hyperactivity
- Behavioral aspects such as autism, attentional deficits, sensitivity to sensations, hand flapping, mood lability, and tantrums
- Language and speech difficulties, including echolalia (repetition of words continuously at the end of the phrase) and talking inappropriately and incessantly about a single topic
- Intellectual disability to some degree in about 85%, with typical IQs of 20 to 70

Males who are premutation carriers are susceptible to the fragile X–associated tremor/ataxia syndrome (FXTAS), which develops in about 30% between 50 and 60 years of age (see Chapter 10). This syndrome is a neurodegenerative disorder with cerebral ataxia, dementia, parkinsonism, and peripheral neuropathies.

In females with the full mutation, approximately 50–67% have some mental impairment; it is severe in approximately one third. About one third have normal intelligence. Females with full fragile X often have learning difficulties and behavior problems that might suggest the diagnosis, such as attentional deficits, language problems, mathematical difficulty, excessive shyness, and social anxiety.

Facial features are similar to those of males. Fragile X premutation carrier females have a median age of menopause that is 6 to 8 years earlier than other women, and about one fourth have ovarian failure before 40 years of age. They may be at increased risk for lower bone mineral density.

The mutation resulting in fragile X syndrome results from an expansion of CGG trinucleotide repeats in the *FMR1* (fragile X mental retardation) gene located on the long arm of the X chromosome. Normal persons generally have 5 to 50 stable repeats at that site, and these are stable when they are transmitted to the next generation. In some families, this repeat is unstable and expands with each generation. The expanded CGG repeats leads to the shutting down of transcription of *FMR1* through methylation (explained in Chapters 2 and 4). Geneticists have distinguished four categories of these repeats, which can vary somewhat. These are shown in Box 9.5. Persons with the premutation were originally thought to be unaffected; however, older males with this number of repeats may have Parkinson disease, and females may have premature ovarian failure.

In general, when a male with a premutation passes it to his daughters, they are unaffected, but their children are at risk. The premutation must pass through the female in order for it to expand to a full mutation and be expressed clinically. This expansion is believed to occur during early development of the embryo. When there are more than 200 repeats present, methylation occurs, and the *FMR1* gene is not expressed. The *FMR1* gene encodes a protein (FMRP), which is expressed most in the brain and testes. To sum up inheritance, an unaffected transmitting male may pass on a premutation to all of his daughters (sons do not normally inherit their father's X chromosome). The daughters will be unaffected carriers themselves, as there has been no amplification of the premutation from their father during spermatogenesis. But during oogenesis, amplification of the repeats occurs to more than 200. The daughter's sons will therefore inherit a full mutation and be affected; their daughters inherit a full mutation and may show a spectrum of clinical expression because of X inactivation. If the premutation is at the lower end of the range there may be less of an increase in the size of the unstable sequence as it is passed through oogenesis. Thus, somatic features tend to be less noticeable than in males, but they can have full expression with characteristic features and profound mental retardation.

Molecular diagnosis is possible for diagnostic testing and prenatal diagnosis but has not been recommended for population screening at this time. Testing for fragile X syndrome should be considered for persons with intellectual disability, developmental delay, autism, a family history of fragile X, or undiagnosed intellectual disability. Prenatal diagnosis is indicated if the mother is a carrier. All testing should be accompanied by appropriate counseling. Other cytogenetic fragile sites have been identified. Fragile X and other sites have been proposed for newborn screening programs but are debatable because no curative treatment is available and the benefits would be mostly in terms of anticipatory guidance and life planning for the individual and genetic counseling, prenatal diagnosis, and reproductive options for the family.

Prader-Willi Syndrome

Prader-Willi syndrome (PWS) has been identified in 1 in 25,000 live births but this is believed to be an underestimate, and prevalence is believed to be 1 in 10,000–15,000 births. Genetically it results in any of several ways:

- Deletion of a critical portion of the normally inherited portion of chromosome 15 (approximately 70%)
- Maternal uniparental disomy (UPD, explained in Chapter 4) in which the child has inherited

---

BOX 9.5

CGG Repeat Size in the FMR1 Gene

CGG Repeat Size	Consequence
6 to 50–54	Normal
45 to 55	Gray zone or inconclusive, borderline; not a clear delineation
55 to 200 repeats	Premutation
More than 200 repeats	Full mutation (can be hundreds to thousands of copies)

two copies of at least the critical region of chromosome 15 from the mother (approximately 25%)
- A methylation defect (explained in Chapter 4) in chromosome 15, inactivating the critical region (approximately 5%)

PWS is interesting because it can arise through more than one genetic inheritance mechanism. It is an example of the clinical consequences of a specific type of imprinting and also UPD.

Clinical features include:

- Hypotonia in infancy, which can lead to hypoventilation and respiratory infection;
- Feeding problems and failure to thrive in infancy;
- Delay of developmental milestones;
- Characteristic facial features, including almond-shaped eyes, thin upper lip, downturned mouth, and mild strabismus;
- Hypogonadism, and delayed or incomplete puberty;
- In males, cryptorchidism, small testes, or hypoplastic scrotum;
- In females, hypoplastic labia minora and clitoris;
- Rapid weight gain between ages 1 and 6, with extreme food-seeking behavior and obesity.

Minor criteria include:

- Small hands and feet;
- Sleep disturbances such as apnea;
- Small stature;
- Hypopigmentation;
- Narrow hands.

The risk of recurrence depends on the genetic cause. PWS is challenging because of the extreme behavior manifestations and need for lifelong vigilance. Growth hormone has been used to successfully treat some children to improve growth and minimize obesity. A photograph of a child with PWS is shown in Figure 9.11.

Primary Immunodeficiencies

The primary immunodeficiencies occur in 1 in 2,000 to 1 in 10,000 live births. They are commonly

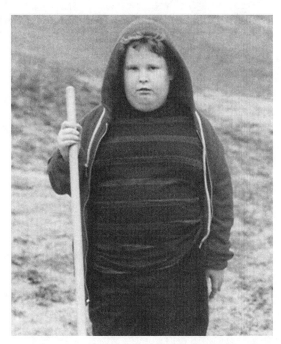

FIGURE 9.11.   Boy with Prader-Willi syndrome. Courtesy of Janalee Heinemann, Prader-Willi Syndrome Association, USA.

classified as shown in Table 9.9. Some of the primary immunodeficiencies have milder forms that become evident in later childhood rather than early. The following points should alert the nurse to consider the possibility of immune dysfunction or deficiency in an infant or child (although no one point is diagnostic by itself and may occur in other disorders as well):

- Increased susceptibility to infections, including increased frequency, severity, and duration.
- The development of complications, rare disease manifestations, or infections with organisms that are generally weak pathogens such as *Pneumocystis jiroveci* (formerly *carinii*).
- Frequent and severe upper respiratory infections in excess of the normal six to eight per year.
- Bronchitis, purulent otitis, tonsillitis, or sinusitis, eventually resulting in mastoiditis, draining ears, pnemonitis, bronchiectasis, or pneumonia.
- Osteomyelitis or meningitis.
- History of unusually severe childhood illnesses such as chicken pox.

TABLE 9.9   Examples of Primary Immunodeficiencies

Group	Disease Example	Comments
Defects in stem cell development with combined immuno-deficiency of both the cellular and humoral components	Adenosine deaminase (ADA) deficiency	Results in both cellular and humoral deficiency with recurrent infections and skeletal dysplasia. AR inheritance.
T-cell defects leading to defective cellular immunity	Purine nucleoside phosphorylase deficiency	Abnormal T-cell function. Neurological abnormalities and lymphoma development. AD inheritance.
B-cell defects leading to defective Igs and impaired humoral immunity	Bruton agamma-globulinemia	Agammaglobulinemia but intact cell-mediated immunity. Prone to bacterial infections and infection with *Giardia lamblia*. Tend to develop rheumatoid arthritis. XR inheritance.
Complement component disorders	Hereditary angioedema, deficiency of the C1 esterase inhibitor	Episodic recurrent episodes of edema of the skin with facial swelling and swelling of the upper respiratory and intestinal tract. The latter causes severe abdominal pain, vomiting, and diarrhea. Laryngeal edema can result in death. Can be triggered by trauma, stress, or infection. AD inheritance. See Chapter 6.
Phagocytic functional defects	Chédiak-Higashi syndrome	Defective mobility and bacteriocidal activity in neutrophils leading to recurrent infections, partial oculocutaneous albinism, photophobia, and nystagmus. Malignant lymphoma and leukemia develop. AR inheritance.

- Distended abdomen.
- Chronic diarrhea, with *Giardia lamblia* often being isolated from the stool.
- Skin rashes such as eczema and lesions.
- Malabsorption and vomiting.
- Persistent *Candida* infections of mouth, anal area, or mucous membranes.
- A family history of early deaths or severe courses of infection or consanguinity.
- An altered response to immunization. A normal response to live-virus vaccines usually indicates a normal cellular immune system.
- Failure to thrive leading to growth retardation.
- Delay of developmental milestones.
- Paleness, listlessness, and irritability.

In humoral deficiencies, the Gram-positive bacteria are usually responsible for infection, whereas in cellular immune deficiencies, the Gram-negative bacteria, fungi, viruses, protozoa, and mycobacteria are found more often.

Several of the known immunodeficiencies have distinctive features present in addition to the general ones described. For example, Job syndrome is known to occur most frequently in females with red hair, fair skin, hyperextendible joints, with eczema and recurrent cold staphylococcal abscesses occurring along with defects in neutrophil chemotaxis and high serum IgE levels.

Once the particular immunodeficiency is determined, genetic counseling services should be sought. Some types of deficiency are detectable through prenatal diagnosis. If the disease is detected in one sibling, the others should be screened in order to prevent complications that otherwise could be avoided and to detect siblings who are heterozygotes so that, when appropriate, they can benefit from genetic counseling and reproductive planning and also because some may have subtle immune system alterations.

Therapy varies according to the disorder. Infusions of purified human immunoglobulin (IVIG) may be used for certain combined immunodeficiencies and for agammaglobulinemias, for example. Because the mortality rate is very high for disorders such as severe combined immunodeficiency (SCID), bone marrow transplantation may be a viable alternative. One of the first trials of gene therapy was for adenosine deaminase (ADA) deficiency, and this promised hope for treatment in other conditions (see Chapter 5). However, gene therapy complications such as leukemia in some children receiving gene therapy for SCID and deaths have led to restrictions. One preventive measure is the widespread use of rubella vaccination to eliminate immunodeficiencies that develop secondary to in utero rubella infection.

Childhood Cancers

Cancer in childhood as related to genetics may be connected with a chromosome abnormality such as the increased frequency of ALL in children with Down syndrome, be a directly inherited type, or be secondary to a disorder conferring susceptibility such as xeroderma pigmentosa (see Chapter 10).

An example of a congenital anomaly that is associated with malignancy is cryptorchidism (undescended testes), which is found at birth in about 2–4% of full-term male infants and about 30% of premature infants. They may spontaneously descend by 1 year of age. The risk of malignancy in cryptorchidism is estimated at about 22 times that for normal testes, and about 10% of all males with testicular malignancy are or have had cryptorchidism. The risk for development of malignancy is about six times greater for abdominal than for inguinal testis, and if repair is done before 11 years of age, the risk for malignant development may return to normal. Otherwise, increased risk continues, and about 50% of these males have testicular dysgenesis.

While cancers are relatively rare in childhood, malignancies develop in about 1 in 600 children, and inherited tumors are part of the picture. Two of these, retinoblastoma and Wilms tumor, are discussed below. Another sequela of treatment for childhood cancer has been the risk of development of second cancers, particularly when the first was treated with radiation. Those who have survived germline mutational cancers appear more likely to develop second neoplasms in adulthood.

Retinoblastoma

In 1971, Knudson proposed a "two-hit" model for retinoblastoma development. Persons with the inherited form of retinoblastoma had a germline mutation that was present in all body cells. A second mutation (somatic) occurring in any developing retinoblasts leads to development of a retinoblastoma (see Figure 10.2). Thus, in some patients with the predisposing germline mutation, a second somatic mutation might never occur, and they would never develop retinoblastoma. In others, bilateral or multifocal tumors might arise due to one or more "hits." In the sporadic type of retinoblastoma, both of the mutational events are somatic and occur in the same retinoblast. This type of event is very infrequent. Each of these two mutational events affects the *RB1* gene (a tumor-suppressor gene) on a different parental chromosome so that the result is the inactivation of *RB1* within the cell. In some cases, the loss of function or loss of heterozygosity (LOH) results from a subsequent deletion of the chromosome that includes the region of the *RB1* gene, 13q14. In some cases, a parent-of-origin effect has also been described due to imprinting (see Chapter 4 and Figure 10.2).

Retinoblastoma results from loss of function (LOF) in the gene *RB1*, a growth suppressor. In the inherited type, a germline mutation results in every body cell containing a mutant and normal gene, RB1+/RB1−. At this point, there is a genetic predisposition for retinoblastoma. For a retinoblastoma to occur, a second somatic mutation of the remaining normal allele must occur within the retinal cell; it does in about 90–95% of those with germline mutations. Thus, about 90–95% of children with a germline *RB1* mutation develop retinoblastoma before 5 years of age. They are also at risks approaching 2,000 times that of the general population for developing osteosarcoma.

Retinoblastoma is a childhood tumor formed from the precursors of retinal rod and cone cells. In the United States, it occurs in approximately 1 in 15,000–20,000 births. As more individuals survive and reproduce, this frequency should increase. In general, persons with nonhereditary retinoblastoma have only one eye affected by one tumor. Persons with the hereditary type usually are affected bilaterally, but in about 15% of cases, only a unilateral tumor is seen due to chance alone or because another tumor has not yet developed. Hereditary tumors generally appear earlier than nonhereditary ones (mean ages of 12–15 and 24–30 months). Detection can be difficult because of early development. Parents may be the ones to report a "glint, gleam, glow, glare, flash or relection" in the child's eye or call it a "cat's" or "animal" eye. On ophthalmoscopic examination, a white or yellow-white pupillary reflex (leukocoria) suggests retinoblastoma and must be further investigated. Infants born to families in which there is a history of retinoblastoma should have a full retinal examination a few weeks after birth and then every two months. Strabismus is another common presenting sign. Treatment of unilateral tumors is generally by enucleation, possibly followed by chemotherapy. Sometimes radiation is used. Diagnosis of retinoblastoma is a devastating experience for parents and family and should be done in a caring, confidential, and sensitive manner, with more than one discussion taking place and the availability of support.

Nurses should realize that lack of a family history of retinoblastoma does not indicate that the tumor in that family is nonhereditary or due to a new mutation because of the possibility of nonpenetrance. Thus, evaluation of family members including careful history, chromosome analysis, DNA testing in appropriate cases, and clinical indicators will be components of genetic counseling. Children who have recovered from retinoblastoma should be followed to detect the occurrence of primary tumors developing in later childhood or even adulthood.

Wilms Tumor

Wilms tumor, an embryonal renal malignancy, represents about 6% of all pediatric cancers in the United States and has a frequency of about 1 in 10,000 children. It occurs in both hereditary and sporadic forms. About 4–5% have bilateral tumors and 1–2% have a family history of Wilms tumors. The first Wilms tumor mutant gene, *WT1*, encoding a zinc finger protein, is located on chromosome 11p13. It is expressed only in certain tissues. In some cases, there is an association with aniridia, genitourinary anomalies, and mental retardation (WAGR syndrome) associated with deletions of chromosome 11p13, and also with hamartomas and hemihypertrophy. Certain germline mutations in zinc fingers of *WT1* occur in Denys-Drash syndrome

(Wilms tumor, male pseudohermaphroditism, congenital nephropathy). Other gene sites exist. Those with Beckwith-Wiedemann syndrome (an overgrowth syndrome with gigantism, macroglossia, endocrine problems, and other anomalies) are at increased risk for Wilms tumor. These groups need careful evaluation, screening with ultrasound, and monitoring for early detection. In about half the cases, activation of the silent maternal *IGF2* (insulin growth factor) allele occurs, relaxing imprinting. Increased expression of *IGF2* leads to somatic overgrowth in Beckwith-Wiedemann syndrome and tumor predisposition. The familial forms (usually bilateral, possible family history) are inherited in an autosomal dominant manner with about 60% penetrance. For those with the sporadic form (usually unilateral tumors with no family history, associated defects or malformations), the recurrence risk for offspring is less than 1–2%. For a parent with a unilateral tumor or a sibling with bilateral tumors, the risk for subsequent children is estimated at 10%. These children are also prone to develop second tumors after treatment and may develop heart problems as a consequence of adriamycin therapy for Wilms tumor.

KEY POINTS

- Many of the genetic disorders are noticed in childhood, but some may not be.
- All members of a family including parents, siblings, grandparents, and others are affected by the birth of a child with a genetic disorder.
- Families affected by the birth of a child with a genetic disorder require many kinds of assistance and support.
- Birth defects may result from various causes.
- Nurses should be familiar with the most common genetic disorders of childhood.
- The nurse should refer the family of a person with a birth defect or congenital anomaly for genetic evaluation and counseling.
- Provision of expert health care and continuity of care with a "health care home" is especially important for children and families with a genetic disorder.
- Health care for children with genetic disorders needs to include transition into adulthood.

10

Adult Health and Illness and Medical-Surgical Nursing

Two major categories of genetic disorders are particularly important in this specialty:

1. Single gene/inherited biochemical disorders, which may first be manifested in adulthood, such as Huntington disease.
2. Common or complex diseases that generally result from the contribution of several genes and environmental factors. Some of these may also exist in rare single gene forms, such as cancer.

In addition other single gene disorders may exist in alternative forms, one of which can be a mild form that becomes evident in adulthood. Increasingly, persons with "childhood" genetic disorders such as cystic fibrosis and congenital heart disease are living into early and middle adulthood. This can present unique care challenges because health care practitioners specializing in adults may not be experienced in managing these disorders, and relatively little may be known about how these genetic conditions interact with the normal process of aging. The sex chromosome disorders such as Turner syndrome, Klinefelter syndrome, triple X syndrome, and XYY syndrome are often not diagnosed until adolescence or adulthood but may be detected in childhood. They are therefore considered in Chapter 9.

In this chapter, six inherited genetic disorders that most commonly are manifested in adulthood—Huntington disease, autosomal dominant polycystic kidney disease, Marfan disease, Gaucher disease, and hemochromatosis—will be discussed as will adulthood effects of premutation carriers of fragile X syndrome. The common diseases of cancer, cardiac disease, emphysema, diabetes mellitus, and Alzheimer disease are also discussed.

SINGLE GENE INHERITED BIOCHEMICAL DISORDERS TYPICALLY MANIFESTING IN ADULTHOOD

Examples of inherited biochemical disorders due to mutation in a single gene are discussed here. In each case, the mutant gene is present at birth and could be detected at any time including prenatally, but the usual signs and symptoms are not usually manifested until adulthood.

Huntington Disease

Huntington disease (HD) is a progressive, degenerative, incurable disease of the nervous system. It is inherited in an autosomal dominant manner. Described by George Huntington in 1872, HD was earlier known as "chorea." It is believed that some of the women burned as witches in Salem, Massachusetts, in the 1690s had HD. For many years, the famous folk singer Woody Guthrie was erroneously believed to be an alcoholic rather than a person who had HD. Symptoms do not usually appear until age 35 years or over. Before deoxyribonucleic acid (DNA) testing, until the age of 70 years, one could not be said to be absolutely free of the disorder. HD occurs in 1 in 10,000 persons.

The mutant gene for HD, *IT15* (interesting transcript 15) is located on chromosome 4p16.3. It encodes the protein huntingtin, whose function is still unknown. This gene normally contains repeating triplets of CAG. CAG repeat lengths of approximately 10 to 35 are seen in people without HD. In HD, the unstable repeats expand (see Chapter 4). These can be detected with the appropriate testing. CAG repeat lengths of 26 and below are considered normal, 27 to 35 are considered mutable normal alleles that could have effects in the next generation, 36 to 39 are considered to have the HD allele with reduced penetrance, and 40 or more are considered to be HD.

HD is often not diagnosed until symptoms have progressed somewhat, even though, in retrospect, it becomes apparent that signs were present earlier. HD encompasses motor, cognitive, or emotional impairment. It may begin with subtle behavioral changes such as forgetting, inattention, irritability, impaired judgment, poor concentration, hypochondriasis, personality changes, and carelessness about hygiene. Symptoms such as slurred speech or unsteady gait can lead to arrest for alcoholism (known patients should wear medical identification). Promiscuity or an increased sexual drive may occur, resulting in increased numbers of descendants at risk. Over a period of as much as 10 to 20 years, the patient progressively deteriorates, showing increased tremor. Eventually he or she becomes bedridden and develops swallowing difficulties, choking, and the loss of bladder and bowel control. These families are under great stress not only because of the condition of their family member but also because of the uncertainty for others to develop it.

Before identification by gene testing was possible, a counselee who was a member of a family at risk for HD stated that every time she forgot an item or spilled something, she wondered if this was the beginning of her own disease. Some persons have even changed their family name and relocated to avoid stigmatization because of HD in the family. Presymptomatic or predictive testing for HD is available for affected families. Confirmatory testing can establish the diagnosis in someone with suggestive signs or symptoms. Issues relating to this are discussed in Chapter 5.

Autosomal Dominant Polycystic Kidney Disease

Autosomal dominant (adult) polycystic kidney disease (ADPKD) is a systemic disorder that has its manifestations usually noticed in adulthood, although renal cysts may begin in the fetus. Its frequency is 1 in 1,000. The renal cysts increase in both size and number and damage the kidney, but loss of function usually is not seen until the 30s or 40s. By age 50 years, about half of all patients develop renal failure, and about half have end-stage renal disease by 60 years of age. Penetrance is considered invariable by 70 years of age. Other symptoms and complications can be pain, infection, and hypertension. Polycystic liver disease may be manifested and affects women more severely than men. Hormonal influences such as pregnancy, birth control pills, and postmenopausal estrogen use are associated with more severe polycystic liver disease. Intracranial aneurysms occur more frequently in persons with ADPKD than the general population. ADPKD accounts for approximately 5% of all cases of end-stage renal disease.

There are at least three forms. Mutation of *PKD1* (on chromosome 16p13.3) coding for polycystin-1 is most common and accounts for about 85%, while mutation of *PKD2* (on chromosome 4q21-23) coding for polycystin-2 is milder and accounts for 10–15%. Direct DNA testing for these mutations can be done presymptomatically to see if the person inherited one of the mutant genes for ADPKD or to confirm diagnosis in someone with symptoms. An advantage of presymptomatic testing in persons at risk for inheriting a mutant ADPKD gene is that they can practice good diet habits and keep their blood pressure under control. Testing does not predict time of onset or severity of disease.

Hemochromatosis

CASE EXAMPLE

Malcolm, age 50, has been complaining of vague symptoms such as fatigue, weakness, arthralgia, and weight loss, but these had not been investigated in depth previously. To these, he has added loss of libido and impotence and also is complaining of mild dyspnea. As part of the workup, serum ferritin levels were done and found to be elevated. Genotyping was then done, and Malcolm was diagnosed with hereditary hemochromatosis. Other family members decided to be tested. One of his sisters does not have any *HFE* mutations, but the other has two mutant alleles as Malcolm does. What can each sister be told about her risk to develop hereditary hemochromatosis? What considerations are there for their children? Malcolm is now on a phlebotomy regimen and can expect no further complications from other organ damage. What kind of education can be provided to Malcolm?

Hemochromatosis is a very common autosomal recessive disorder with a frequency of 1 in 200 to 1 in 400 and a carrier frequency of 1 in 8 to 1 in 10 in White populations; it is most frequent in those of Scot, Irish, and English descent. The gene that is most commonly mutated in classic hereditary hemochromatosis, also known as hemochromatosis type 1, is located on chromosome 6 (6p21.3) and is designated *HFE*. Most North Americans have a mutational change known as C282Y, which substitutes tyrosine for cysteine at position 282 of the HFE protein, and most of the rest have H63D mutations. Normally all dietary iron is not absorbed; of the 15–20 mg of iron present in the average U.S. diet, males and reproductive-age females absorb 1 mg and 2 mg, respectively. Not all persons with the mutated gene show symptoms. When hemochromatosis is manifested, iron overload develops. Laboratory tests include iron saturation of serum transferrin (fasting) of 45–50% or higher in females and 60% or higher in males, and serum ferritin in which values over 200 ng/mL in premenopausal females and above 300 ng/mL in males and postmenopausal females are very suggestive. Confirmation of the genetic status is often by genotyping for *HFE*.

Men may show more serious disease than women, probably because of the physiological loss of iron due to menstruation and pregnancy in women. Iron is deposited in the liver, joints, heart, pancreas, and endocrine glands. The usual initial symptoms are somewhat vague: lethargy, weakness and abdominal and/or joint pain. Later, loss of libido, dyspnea, cardiac complaints, liver disease, diabetes mellitus, arthritis, skin pigmentation, and hypogonadism and infertility may be seen.

Homozygotes for hemochromatosis are relatively common among those with diabetes mellitus or arthritis and should be looked for. Hemochromatosis has been suggested for population screening because of the potential for prevention of damage, but despite the high population frequency, questions are raised about the natural history, effective timing, and type of interventions and other issues such as penetrance and actual disease development.

Treatment is relatively straightforward: lifelong phlebotomy of 500 mL of blood, usually weekly initially and then every 3 to 4 months, depending on iron levels and tolerance. If early treatment is not initiated, cirrhosis, liver failure, portal hypertension, carbohydrate intolerance, and diabetes may occur, as may cardiomegaly and dysfunction and arthopathy. It has been suggested that hemochromatosis is so common because it once conferred some type of selective advantage. For example, heterozygous women might have a reproductive advantage because of less likelihood of iron deficiency anemia, and for both men and women, survival in times of starvation might have been enhanced. Vitamin C supplementation can increase iron

---

BOX 10.1

Nursing Pointers in Hemochromatosis

- A high index of suspicion should be maintained for those with vague signs and symptoms typical of hemochromatosis, especially in the most at-risk ethnic and age groups.
- Treatment is lifelong, and need for adherence must be stressed.
- Patients should not use iron supplements unless there is a specific reason for doing so, and they should read labels of foods as well as vitamin supplements to avoid excess iron intake.
- Vitamin C supplementation should be limited.
- Eating raw oysters should be avoided.
- Alcohol consumption should be limited.
- Biochemical and genetic testing is available for family members.
- Referral for genetic counseling may be appropriate.

overload, as can supplemental iron. In addition, persons with hemochromatosis are susceptible to infection with *Vibrio vulnificus*, a bacterium present in raw oysters that thrives in iron-rich blood and organs; deaths have occurred from ingestion. In Africa, iron overload is correlated with heavy consumption of beer brewed in nongalvanized iron containers. Some teaching pointers include those shown in Box 10.1.

Marfan Syndrome

Marfan syndrome is an autosomal dominant disorder that is extremely pleiotrophic (multiple phenotypic effects from a single gene). It is very variable in expression. Some persons with Marfan syndrome are detected in childhood or adolescence, often because of height. Others remain undetected until adulthood. One case in our genetic clinic came to the light when a mother brought her son to the clinic for celiac disease follow up (they were new to our clinic). When we looked at the mother, we believed she had Marfan syndrome. We were able to follow-up on that suspicion and confirmed Marfan syndrome. We then referred her to a cardiologist, who detected aortic dilatation requiring medication. Recognizing the syndrome probably prevented sudden cardiac complications.

Marfan syndrome is believed present in about 1 in 5,000–10,000 persons but may be more frequent and underrecognized; 15–30% represent new mutations, meaning that others in the family do not have this mutant gene. The major defect is a mutation of fibrillin, a glycoprotein in the extracellular matrix that regulates transforming growth factor-β (TGF-β). The defect is in the fibrillin gene, *FBN1*, on chromosome 15q21.1. It has also been found that mutations in genes encoding these TGF-β receptors can result in individuals with symptoms similar to Marfan syndrome. Mutations of the gene can occur, leading to variable clinical expression. For example, a particular mutation is associated with the severe neonatal form. Among the characteristic features are skeletal findings including tall stature compared to normal family members, pectus excavatum (hollow chest) or pectus carnitum (pigeon chest), reduced upper- to lower-segment ratio, arm span that may be greater than the height, scoliosis, joint hypermobility, and arachnodactyly (long, spider-like hands and long thumbs). Other features are ectopia lentis (dislocated lens), strabis-

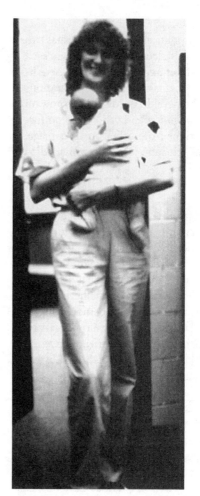

FIGURE 10.1   A woman with Marfan syndrome.

mus, and other ocular findings; aortic dilatation, dissecting aneurysms of the aorta, mitral valve prolapse, and other cardiovascular manifestations; and other findings. Marfan syndrome is the major reason for dissecting aortic aneurysms in persons under 40 years of age. A woman with Marfan syndrome is shown in Figure 10.1.

Because of their tall stature, it is not unusual for persons with Marfan syndrome to be athletes. Flo Hyman, the 6′5″ Olympic volleyball team member, and various high school and university basketball stars have died suddenly due to ruptured aortas from Marfan syndrome. Sports that may injure the eye or head can result in eye injuries. Thus, it is important that the school nurse be sure that athletes have adequate sports physicals, and if Marfan syndrome is present that a full diagnostic examination is done, including echocardiography, a slit lamp examination by an ophthalmologist, and others, deending on the symptoms. Often prophylactic beta-drenergic blockade such as propranolol or atenolol s prescribed. Activity needs modulation, and pregnancy poses increased risks needing close supervision depending on the person's cardiac status.

Gaucher Disease

Gaucher disease is a lysosomal storage disorder caused by deficiency of glucocerebrosidase and accumulation of glycosylceramide (glucocerebroside) that occurs in three forms: type 1, the visceral form that is usually chronic, often first appearing in adulthood; type 2, an acute neurological form often appearing in infancy; and type 3, a subacute neurological type often appearing first in childhood. It affects 10,000 to 20,000 Americans. In contrast to many of the other disorders in this category, the adult form is the most prevalent, accounting for about 80% of cases. Inheritance is autosomal recessive, and multiple alleles may cause mutations, with five mutations responsible for about 97% of the disease alleles among Ashkenazi Jews. A particular mutation, 1448C, occurs as a polymorphism in northern Sweden, leading to type 3 disease. Another specific mutation, 1226G, leads to mild type 1 disease in homozygotes; such individuals often are undetected unless revealed in the course of family or population studies. A rare perinatal-lethal type has been described, and is often associated with hydrops fetalis. In adult type 1, which is non-neuronopathic, Gaucher cells with accumulated glucosylceramide infiltrate the spleen, liver, and bones. Patients may first experience nonspecific symptoms such as fatigue, easy bruising, and enlarged abdomen with hepatosplenomegaly. Eventually bone fractures, infarctions and necrosis, pain, thrombocytopenia, anemia, and infection occur. The pain may be nonspecific and migratory, with episodes lasting 1 to 3 days.

The age of onset is variable, ranging from birth to 80 years but commonly first presents in adulthood. Some may be asymptomatic entirely, and others may not develop disease manifestations until they are in their 50s, in which case all of their children will already have inherited one mutant gene. Therapy for Gaucher disease can include treatment of symptoms, bone marrow transplantation with stem cells, and enzyme therapy with alglucerase or imiglucerase. Treatment is expensive. Detection of carriers and prenatal diagnosis is possible. It has a high gene frequency in Ashkenazi Jews, with a carrier frequency of about 7%. Population screening in this group for both carrier status and disease can be done, but accurate genetic counseling that includes prognosis can be difficult because of variability in expression.

Fragile X Premutation Carriers

Fragile X syndrome is a disorder due to expansion of trinucleotide repeats and is explained in Chapters 4 and 9. Elderly male premutation carriers may manifest the fragile X–associated tremor/ataxia syndrome (FXTAS) which consists of parkinsonism, intention tremors, cerebellar ataxia, autonomic dysfunction, peripheral neuropathy, and weakness in the legs and cognitive decline, plus short-term memory loss and executive function deficits. Female premutation carriers have also been identified, and it is believed that effects in these older women may be more subtle, including premature ovarian failure. It is believed that about one third or more of all male carriers will develop FXTAS over time. Progression is variable. An implication of the identification of FXTAS is that those older people who manifest ataxia and intention tremor should be screened for the *FMR1* mutation even in the absence of a positive family history. FXTAS came to be identified when mothers of children with fragile X syndrome spoke about their own fathers (premutation carriers) who were experiencing tremors and gait problems. Testing for older men and women for premutations may be indicated in those showing neurological symptoms, as well as for women with premature ovarian failure.

Other Genetic Disorders Manifesting in Adulthood

Many of the single gene disorders have forms that first appear in adulthood. In these cases, with severe infantile forms, and moderate juvenile forms, the adult form tends to be milder. An example was the case of a 38-year-old man who was misdiagnosed with schizophrenia for 8 years but actually had Niemann-Pick disease type C, an autosomal recessive neurometabolic disorder associated with chorea, ataxia, seizures, and other signs most common in childhood. Some cases of early stroke (below 50 years of age) are mitochondrial disorders that have stroke as a feature, such as MELAS (mitochondrial encephalopathy, lactic acidosis and stroke-like episodes), which can present in childhood, adolescence, or adulthood. Persons with Leber hereditary optic neuropathy (LHON), another mitochondrial disorder, typically present in their 20s or 30s with sudden and painless central visual loss and central scotoma. Other symptoms may include headache at onset, cardiac conduction defects, and dystonia with lesions in the basal ganglia.

COMMON/COMPLEX DISEASES OF ADULTHOOD

The common (complex) diseases have long been observed to "run in families." The genetic contribution to the common or complex diseases is of particular interest to medical geneticists because of the potential for early identification of susceptible individuals followed by targeted interventions that might prevent the disease, prevent or ameliorate complications, or allow initiation of early treatment. In general, the common diseases refer to disorders that are frequent in the population and that are not, in large part, attributable to single gene mutations. A subset of most of the common diseases may be due to single gene mutations, especially cases with an early age of onset, but for most of them, causation appears due to multiple gene mutations and environmental influences (multifactorial inheritance is described in Chapter 4). These may include coronary disease, cerebrovascular disease, diabetes mellitus, cancer, and emphysema.

The genetic contribution could be one or two major genes in combination with minor ones; several minor ones with additive effects; several genes, some with protective effects; or other combinations. Environment could be internal or external and includes dietary components, exposure to infectious agents or toxins, exercise, temperature extremes, sunlight exposure, radiation, and the internal milieu. There may be many susceptibility factors for a given condition, and these may vary in different populations. Susceptibility may not necessarily mean disease development, so some persons with the mutant gene may develop the condition, and others may not.

In some instances, forms of a multifactorial common disorder may be inherited as a single gene

Mendelian disorder. These tend to have an earlier age of onset, be normally infrequent in younger individuals (an example is the occurrence of an adult type tumor in a child), or, in the case of cancers present with multiple primary neoplasms. An example is a subtype of type 2 diabetes mellitus: maturity-onset diabetes of the young (MODY).

A major problem that plagued early investigations of the genetic component in common disorders was the way in which the disease was defined. For example, when colon cancer was not looked at globally but, for example, was considered as colon cancer with extreme polyposis, then it was possible to identify the *APC* gene mutation on chromosome 5. In order to look for the genetic components in common disorders, a variety of methods have been used. These may, in some instances, look at the genome of affected persons in specific populations or use mathematical and genetic modeling or may rely on genetic mapping and whole genome scans. Below, the genetic contributions to heart disease, cancer, emphysema, Alzheimer's disease, and diabetes mellitus are considered.

Heart Disease

Coronary heart disease is the leading cause of death in most industrialized countries. In some cases, a single gene mutation results in direct heart disease either alone (e.g., long QT syndrome, discussed below) or as part of other genetic syndromes (e.g., Marfan disease, discussed earlier). In regard to heart disease in adults, some rare gene mutations result in heart disease, while in other cases, one or more genes are believed to lead to susceptibility to coronary disease, which is ultimately influenced by environmental factors. It is possible for many gene mutations to have coronary involvement as an indirect end result. For example, mutant genes may affect conditions that contribute to cardiac risk factors such as obesity, diabetes mellitus, and hypertension. Genes may also influence response to therapy for cardiovascular disease. Early heart disease is more likely to have a strong genetic component than heart disease that develops in middle age or later and may be due to mutations in single genes. Besides congenital heart disease (discussed in Chapter 9), the major categories of heart disease that are caused by or heavily influenced by genetics are the diseases due to

- Hyperlipidemia and atherosclerosis;
- Cardiomyopathies;
- Disorders of rhythm.

Disorders of Lipid Metabolism

As the Vytorin commercial goes, "Cholesterol comes not just from your footlong frank but also your Uncle Frank," recognizing both the dietary and genetic influences. Genetically determined defects and deficiencies of lipoprotein components alone or in combination, and their transport and metabolism, have been related to the risk for the development of coronary artery disease (CAD). Both established and emerging cardiovascular risk factors are known. Examples of emerging ones are small, dense low-density lipoprotein (LDL) levels, metabolic syndrome, and homocysteine levels. Numerous conditions have been identified as risk factors for coronary artery disease. The major ones are elevated total or low-density lipoprotein cholesterol (LDL-C); decreased high-density lipoprotein cholesterol (HDL-C); family history of myocardial infarction or sudden death in male or female parents or siblings before 55 years and 65 years, respectively; male gender aged 45 or above; female gender aged 55 or above; diabetes mellitus; obesity; cigarette smoking; and hypertension. Other factors that affect lipoproteins include high-fat diets, stress, sedentary lifestyle, liver disease, renal disease, certain medications, and excessive alcohol intake. The association between hyperlipidemia, the process of atherosclerosis, and (CAD) is generally accepted. Some characteristics have been noted for genetic susceptibility for CAD that would then allow stratification into familial average-, moderate-, and high-risk categories. (See Scheuner, 2003, for details.) Based on the risk category, early detection and prevention approaches could be designed. Genetic susceptibility characteristics are shown in Box 10.2.

Categories of single gene disorders causing hyperlipidemias and thus CAD include defects in the apolipoproteins (apo) (e.g., apo B deficiency leading to classic abetalipoproteinemia), receptor defects (e.g., LDL receptor disorder leading to familial hypercholesterolemia), enzyme defects (e.g., lipoprotein lipase deficiency), and defects in transfer proteins (e.g., cholesteryl ester transfer protein deficiency). Aside from those with single gene defects, hyperlipidemia is not a single disorder; it exists as

> **BOX 10.2**
>
> ### Cardiovascular Genetic Susceptibility Characteristics
>
> - Early onset of CAD (below 55 years of age for men and below 65 years of age for women)
> - Involvement of multiple vessels with atherosclerosis
> - Angiographic severity
> - Two or more close relatives with CAD
> - Female relatives with CAD
> - Presence of related disorders in close relatives such as diabetes or hypertension
> - Presence of multiple CAD risk factors in affected family members such as diabetes, hypertension, insulin resistance, or the prothrombin G20210A mutation
> - Absence of established risk factors in family members with CAD such as hypertension or smoking (Scheuner, 2003, p. 273)

various types, each with its own causes, manifestations, and profiles. In the general population, plasma lipid levels are modulated by the interaction of environmental factors within the boundaries set by genetic determinants. Environmental factors such as diet act on the person with a single gene disorder affecting lipoprotein, gene-gene interactions, and thus the degree of expression. Blood lipid levels are a continuous curve in the general population and are influenced by age and sex. Some genetically determined lipid disorders resulting in coronary diseases are listed in Table 10.1.

Because of their solubility properties, dietary lipids such as cholesterol and triglycerides are transported in the blood mainly in the form of complex macromolecules called lipoproteins. These molecules often consist of a core of nonpolar lipids, a surface layer of polar lipids and apoproteins (apo). Each class of lipoprotein contains triglycerides (esters of glycerol and long-chain fatty acids), cholesteryl esters (esters of cholesterol and long chain fatty acids), free cholesterol, apoproteins, and phospholipids combined in different proportions. Each component in the system has some control, as do

TABLE 10.1   Examples of Genetic Lipid Disorders

Name	Inheritance Pattern	Prevalence	Remarks
Familial combined hyperlipidemia	AD	1–2:100 to 1:200	May cause 10–20% of all premature coronary artery disease. Found in 11–20% of survivors of myocardial infarction under 60 years of age; lipoprotein phenotype varies; presence of elevated total cholesterol and/or elevated triglycerides in several members of same family; combination of total elevated cholesterol and elevated triglycerides; basic defect unknown; may involve upstream transcription factor.
Familial defective apolipoprotein B-100	AD	Heterozygote 1:500–700	Caused by mutations in apoB-100. Delaying clearance of blood LDL. Elevated LDL cholesterol, tendon xanthomas.
Familial dysbetalipoproteinemia	AR	1:5,000	Mutations in apolipoprotein E gene resulting in deficiency. Most common variant is E2/E2 genotype; may be other factors involved; elevation of VLD remnants in blood, xanthomas. Seen in adulthood usually.
Familial hepatic lipase deficiency	AR	Rare	Moderate hypertriglyceridemia; may have xanthomas, premature coronary disease.
Familial hypercholesterolemia (FH) IIa	AD	Heterozygote 1:500; homozygote 1:1,000,000	LDL receptor deficiency or defect (see text).
Familial hypertriglyceridemia	AD	1:500	May not be expressed until person is in his/her 20s or 30s; 5% of survivors of myocardial infarction had disorder; basic defect unknown; VLDL and triglycerides are elevated; episodes of abdominal pain with or without pancreatitis are frequent; eruptive xanthomas can occur; often hypertension, diabetes mellitus, insulin resistance, hyperuricemia are present. Relationship to coronary artery disease is not as strong as other diseases.
Lecithin cholesterol acyltransferase (LCAT) deficiency	AR	1:1,000,000	Mutations in the LCAT gene can result in classical LCAT deficiency or in fish-eye disease. Both have low HDL. Classical deficiency LCAT patients may show renal disease, corneal opacities, and occasional xanthomas. Fish-eye disease patients show corneal opacities that may be seen early in childhood.
Tangier disease	AR	Very rare	Mutations in ATP-binding cassette (ABCA 1) gene with severe deficiency of HDL-C cholesterol, ester accumulation in liver, spleen, tonsils, peripheral nerves. Signs/symptoms include orange-colored tonsils, hepatosplenomegaly, and peripheral neuropathy. Rectal mucosa may have fatty deposits.

other factors such as hormones, cholesterol intake, and metabolic alterations. The components, enzymes, and cell surface receptors are involved in the regulation of lipid levels.

Familial Hypercholesterolemia (FH)

FH is an autosomal dominant (AD) disorder due to mutations in the LDL receptor gene on chromosome 19p. These mutations cause defects in functioning or reduction in number. FH was the first genetic disorder shown to cause myocardial infarction (MI). Goldstein and Brown received a Nobel Prize in 1986 for their work on understanding this disorder. Because it is an autosomal dominant disorder, both heterozygotes and homozygotes are affected. In the United States, the prevalence of heterozygotes and homozygotes is 1 in 500 and 1 in 1 million, respectively making it a very common genetic disorder. Among survivors of MIs, the frequency of heterozygotes has been estimated at 1 in 20.

The result of the gene mutation is reduced numbers of LDL receptors or defective ones, depending on which mutant allele is present. This results in the decreased ability or inability of LDL-C to bind to its cell surface receptors. LDL-C therefore cannot enter the cell to be degraded in adequate amounts. It accumulates in the plasma and is deposited in abnormal sites such as the arteries (causing atheromas and atherosclerosis), the soft tissue of the eyelids, the cornea (arcus cornae), the tendons, elbows, ankles, and knees. Tendon xanthomas (fatty deposits resembling bumps) of the dorsum of the hand and Achilles tendon may be very painful and are characteristic. They are not usually seen in the heterozygote before 20 years of age. The finding of such xanthomas on physical examination should alert the practitioner to the need to determine the cause. In heterozygotes, LDL-C levels are about three times normal; in the homozygote, they may be 6 to 10 times normal.

The heterozygote is exposed to the effects of premature and accelerated atherosclerosis even in early childhood. Whether to institute vigorous therapy at an early age is debatable because myelination of the central nervous system is not complete until about 6 years of age, and LDL-C is important in the

delivery of lipids to the tissues. For male heterozygotes, the typical age of onset of coronary heart disease is 40 years of age, and by 60 years, 85% will have had an MI as compared to 15% for males without the mutant gene. For females, the typical age of onset is 55 years of age, and by 60 years, 50% will have a MI as compared with a 10% risk in unaffected females. Both the heterozygote and homozygote may also have peripheral or cerebral vascular disease.

The homozygote is much more severely affected. By 4 years of age, most patients will have developed planar yellow-orange xanthomas at the knees, buttocks, elbows, and hands, especially between the thumb and the index finger, as well as tendon xanthomas and arcus cornae. MI, angina pectoris, and even sudden death usually occur in the homozygote between 5 and 20 years of age. MIs have been reported as early as 18 months. Few live past 30 years, and death may occur in childhood. The statins are a mainstay of therapy, but different LDL receptor mutation genotypes can result in varying responses to therapy. For both the heterozygote and homozygote, diet therapy alone will not lower lipid levels to the normal range, but may be used as adjunctive therapy. The most promising approach is gene therapy.

Gene testing and screening by molecular methods for the defective gene is possible. The practicality for generalized screening is limited at this time because there does not yet appear to be a small number of mutations responsible for the defect in a vast majority of affected persons or a testing technique that will detect enough mutations to be useful and meet screening test criteria. Such screening is somewhat controversial, especially for infants and children. Targeted or cascade testing is being done, however, particularly within at-risk families. Reasons include the potential for blood relatives to benefit from lifestyle modifications, closer monitoring, or more aggressive lipid-lowering therapy depending on the specific mutation, family pattern of disease development (FH tends to have similar patterns within families), and their lipid levels and other parameters. Nursing points related to genetic factors in hyperlipidemia and coronary disease are in Box 10.3.

BOX 10.3

Nursing Points Related to Genetic Factors in Hyperlipidemia and Coronary Disease

- Be alert for a genetic component in young persons with hyperlipidemia and CAD, particularly those with MIs who may first be noticed in the coronary care unit.
- Ascertain the family history for lipid-related problems and sudden deaths of persons who have been diagnosed with coronary disease, especially if early onset.
- Be aware of those who have the highest risk for cardiovascular disease based on assessment of genetic risk factors.
- Close blood relatives of persons having a coronary disorder at an early age may need to be referred for plasma lipid analysis and other testing such as DNA analysis.
- Be alert for the signs and symptoms of hyperlipidemias—xanthomas, abdominal pain of unexplained origin, fatty food intolerance, and so on—and refer such individuals for appropriate evaluation.
- Realize that some symptoms associated with hyperlipidemia such as xanthomas and arcus cornae can occur in persons with normal lipid levels.
- Encourage the reduction of secondary risk factors in persons with hyperlipidemia such as cigarette smoking, sedentary lifestyle, obesity, excess alcohol consumption, stress, and high-carbohydrate diet, and also encourage these in their blood relatives.
- Use or develop specific programs for risk reduction that are based on the person's culture, health belief system, and individual motivational factors in order to maximize success and that take into account the degree of risk (average, moderate or high) that they may have based on familial and genetic risk factors, as well as lifestyle factors.
- Before a person begins therapy for hyperlipidemia, check to see that secondary disorders (i.e., diabetes mellitus) or contributing factors (i.e., oral contraceptives) have been ascertained, substituted for, or corrected, if possible.
- Optimal health for the particular individual should be a basic goal.
- Any therapy for hyperlipidemia is usually based on the assumption that treatment will be long term.
- Recognize that the ongoing use of medications that are unpleasant to take or have unpleasant side effects may result in the client's failure to adhere to the treatment plan. Techniques for ways to minimize any unpleasantness should be shared and periodically reviewed with the client and family, The compliance literature should be used for ideas on ways to maximize the client's adherence.
- Assess the client's current food and alcohol intake and medication use.
- Recognize that not all persons who adhere to a low-cholesterol, low-fat diet can lower their plasma lipids by dietary means alone.
- For those who are on a lifelong dietary regimen, be able to refer them to a variety of cookbooks and hints for the use of food substitutes.

Cardiomyopathies

Cardiomyopathies are diseases of the heart muscle that may be primary or secondary to other inherited disorders such as glycogen storage disease II. Classification is usually in the following categories: hypertrophic, dilated, restrictive, and unclassified cardiomyopathy. The cardiomyopathies are believed to be responsible for about 2% of sudden deaths.

Hypertrophic Cardiomyopathy

The prevalence of hypertrophic cardiomyopathy (HCM) in the general population is about 1 in 500. The mode of transmission is autosomal dominant. Genetic heterogeneity is prevalent. The pattern of phenotypic expression may be influenced by other modifying genes and environmental factors. HCM results from genes that encode cardiac sarcomere proteins that are essential for heart muscle contraction. One of the most important is the cardiac troponin T gene on chromosome 1q (CMH2). Certain mutations are more frequently associated with varying outcomes, and genotype-phenotype correlations are of great interest. Clinicians should be alert for the possibility of these gene mutations in HCM occurring in middle-aged or elderly patients so that clinical or genetic screening can be accomplished in their families. In families with known HCM, clinical surveillance may need to be continued throughout adulthood.

HCM is characterized by left ventricular hypertrophy. It has been the most common cause of sudden death in children and adolescents, especially in athletes. Sometimes sudden death is the initial presentation. Until then, the person had no recognizable symptoms. For others, there can be varying degrees of clinical severity, including a slow, relatively benign course. The most common initial complaints in the 50% who present with symptoms are chest pain, dyspnea, mild exercise intolerance, and syncope. Atrial fibrillation may develop in about 10–25%. In those without symptoms, detection usually occurs during a routine physical exam such as for a school athletic physical or electrocardiogram (ECG). Further exploration such as a transthoracic echo Doppler examination and studies to detect ventricular function and so on is necessary in those with a suggestive family history. Outcomes vary and include sudden death, heart failure with congestive features, and atrial fibrillation and its consequences. Treatment depends on manifestations. Both surgical and nonsurgical approaches are used for septal reduction. An automatic implantable cardioverter defibrillator may be needed to prevent sudden death. Molecular techniques can be used for gene testing and will identify about 60–70% of those with HCM. Presymptomatic testing is possible. If a family member has been diagnosed with HCM as a result of sudden death, screening of children or adolescents may be warranted so that preventive measures may be taken. The nurse should be alert to this when taking family histories. In families with multiple affected members, adolescents, even if symptom free, may be wise to avoid strenuous athletics.

Dilated Cardiomyopathy

Dilated cardiomyopathy (DCM), which occurs with a prevalence of 36.5 per 100,000, is a chronic heart muscle condition characterized by dilatation and impaired contractility of the left or both ventricles. It may result from genetic causes or from viral or toxic or metabolic agents, alcohol use, immune dysfunction, or idiopathic causes. Men are more frequently affected. There is a usually a long period in which the person has no symptoms and the disorder remains unrecognized. The typical age of onset is 20 to 50 years. The most frequent presentation is end-stage heart failure manifested by exercise intolerance, exertional dyspnea, and chest pain. Sometimes the enlarged heart or ECG abnormalities are detected during a routine examination. Conduction abnormalities may be frequent. Nearly 30% of relatives of persons with DCM have ECG abnormalities. Ventricular dilatation may lead to impaired systolic contraction, congestive heart failure, and sudden death. The heart is increased in weight. Mendelian inheritance is seen in about 25% of cases. Inheritance is most commonly autosomal dominant, but autosomal recessive, mitochondrial mutation, and X-linked recessive inheritance have been described. Some gene mutations have been identified, including those in cardiac actin (15q14), desmin (2q35), and δ-sarcoglycan genes (5q33-34), and loci have been linked to the AD form, including CMD1D (chromosome 1q32), CMD1G (2q31), and CMD1B (9q13-22), as well as locations on other chromosomes. In some cases, DCM is associated with other features such as sensorineural hearing loss (6q23-24). DCM frequently accompanies both Duchenne and Becker muscular dystrophy (see Chapter 9). Treatment includes weight control, restricted sodium intake, ACE inhibitors, digitalis, diuretics, anticoagulants, beta-blockers, and other medications depending on symptoms and need. DCM is the major indication for heart transplant at present.

Arrhythmias

Primary disorders of the cardiac electrical system resulting from genetic abnormalities include primary rhythm disturbances. Certain gene variations may also increase the risk of arrhythmias resulting from treatment with certain medications and are thus significant for treatment choices. The actual prevalence of dysrhythmias due to genetic causes is underestimated.

The best-described arrhythmia is the long QT syndrome (LQT), a cardiac arrhythmia showing a prolonged QT interval on ECG. It can present with syncope, ventricular fibrillation, and sudden death. Unexplained cases of near-drowning have revealed families with inherited LQT, and women with hereditary LQT are at risk for untoward cardiac events in the postpartum period, which may be prevented prophylactically by using beta-adrenergic blockers. LQT is genetically and phenotypically heterogenous. The genetically transmitted form is caused by mutations in genes encoding ion channels. Mutations in genes of at least seven loci are implicated in LQT, and three forms are well delineated. These are mutations in potassium channel genes, *KCNQ1* or *KVLQT1* (LQT1) (described below), *HERG* or *KCNQ1* (LQT2); and in the sodium channel gene *SCN5A* (LQT3). Inheritance may be autosomal dominant or, more rarely, autosomal recessive or the result of nongenetic causes. The autosomal recessive form of LQT1 is known as the Jervell and Lange-Nielsen syndrome and is associated with congenital sensory deafness as well. LQT has been reported in up to 1% of children with congenital deafness, and so ECG screening should be done in children with congenital deafness. The AD type of LQT1 has been called Romano-Ward syndrome. Mutation in the potassium channel gene *KVLQT1* may cause both of these, as well as play a role in normal hearing.

LQT consists of recurrent syncope with abnormal myocardial repolarization and sudden death, usually from ventricular arrhythmias. Occasionally an affected person presents with seizures. Persons with the gene may be asymptomatic when detected. On ECG, prolongation of the QT interval is seen. Genetic testing can identify those who possess the known genes. In addition, untoward events tend to be gene specific. For example, persons with LQT1 tend to experience cardiac events during exercise, those with LQT2 with arousal-type emotions even such as a sudden loud noise, and those with LQT3 without arousal, often occurring during sleep. Those whose ethnicity is Asian or Pacific Rim may be particularly susceptible to these events. Treatment varies but may include beta-adrenergic blockers even for those who are asymptomatic. In addition to education about preventive medication, certain drugs can precipitate torsades de pointes in people with LQT. These include cardiac and noncardiac drugs. Examples of such drugs are chlorpromazine, pentamidine, and procainamide.

Other Conditions

Other conditions with a genetic component may also result in heart disease. For example, there is a type of hereditary cardiomyopathy resulting from amyloid deposition that may lead to sudden death. This type results from a variant in transthyretin (a serum carrier protein) and is particularly common among Blacks. Elderly Black patients with heart disease of undetermined etiology should be tested for transthyretin amyloidosis. Alterations in the renin-angiotensin system may be related to heart disease. A particular genotype of the ACE gene, DD, has been associated with a susceptibility to both myocardial infarction and CAD probably because of aberrant blood pressure regulation. The use of ACE inhibitors may be useful in prevention.

Aging and Alzheimer Disease

With the rapid growth of the population 85 years and above, the study of aging has intensified. The influence of genetics on biologic aging can be considered in relationship to length of life or longevity, patterns of aging, the aging process, and maximum lifespan. The search for specific aging genes has resulted in interest in disorders with a known genetic basis that have some of the characteristics of aging. These include conditions such as Down syndrome (discussed in Chapter 9) and rarer genetic syndromes such as progeria, Werner syndrome, and Cockayne syndrome. These were formerly thought to represent actual premature aging syndromes, but on closer study this proved not to be true.

Various dementias are not necessarily a consequence of aging. Dementias may accompany aging, however. One of these, Alzheimer disease (AD), is the fourth leading cause of death in the United

States and the most common cause of dementia in older persons. There are other types of dementia, and Picks disease (frontal lobe atrophy) is believed due to a single AD gene in about 20% of cases. The lifetime risk of developing AD is 15% in the general population. AD is characterized by dementia involving personality changes; memory loss; deterioration of cognitive functions such as language, motor skills, perception, and attention with neuronal cell loss; deposition of senile plaques; and neurofibrillary tangles in the cerebral cortex. There may also be associated symptoms such as depression, emotional outbursts, gait disorders, seizures, incontinence, and sexual disorders. The deposition of plaques and tangles also occurs in normal aging but not in the number and extent seen in AD. The plaques are largely composed of beta-amyloid, a peptide derived from the beta-amyloid precursor protein (APP). AD is genetically heterogeneous. Cases of AD may be early onset (60–65 years of age or below) or late (above 60–65 years). To date, four gene defects have been associated with AD. Three genes whose defects cause familial AD are inherited in an autosomal dominant manner. One gene (a specific form of the *APOE*) appears to be a susceptibility gene, and between 15% and 50% of all cases of AD may be accounted for by this genotype. These are shown in Table 10.2.

A specific genotype for apolipoprotein E (APOE), a lipoprotein involved in cholesterol metabolism and synthesized in the brain, is associated with susceptibility to late-onset AD. The *APOE* gene has at least seven allelic forms, ε1–ε7. Persons with two alleles of ε4 have a higher risk (5- to 10-fold or more) of developing amyloid deposition and AD than those with one or no alleles. The ε4 allele may also be associated with a faster progression to AD and an earlier age of onset. The ε2 allele may have a protective effect by lowering the risk and increasing the age of onset. These findings have implications for genetic testing, drug treatment, and preventive drug compounds that might mimic the action of *APOE* ε2. This is not necessarily a direct relationship since persons without the ε4 allele may develop AD, and those with it may not. Thus it is a risk factor.

Genetic testing for the *APOE* genotype could be for confirmatory diagnosis of a person who already has symptoms of dementia or for those who are asymptomatic and at risk (predictive or presymptomatic testing). The issue of clinical testing for the *APOE* genotype has provoked various statements regarding genetic testing for APOE for predictive screening in asymptomatic persons because the *APOE* ε4 allele is also found in persons without AD and is not found in many with AD. A major issue with susceptibility testing for late-onset AD disease is the associated uncertainty of the meaning of the results. Even if the individual in question learns that he/she does not possess the ε4 allele, he/she may still eventually develop AD. And those at higher risk for the development of AD because they do possess the ε4 allele may not develop AD. Opinions vary on the utility of genetic testing for those who are already symptomatic. Some believe that it might be a valuable adjunct to diagnosis, while others recommend conservatism in such use.

Emphysema and Alpha-1-Antitrypsin Deficiency

CASE EXAMPLE

Harold is a 27-year-old man of Swedish ancestry who has come to the clinic with a complaint of some dyspnea on exertion, along with a

TABLE 10.2 Genes Associated with Alzheimer Disease

Type	Chromosome	Defective Gene	Approximate Age of Onset (Years)
AD1—early onset, familial	21	APP	43–62
AD2—late onset, familial and sporadic susceptibility	19	APOE, ε4	Over 55
AD3—early onset familial	14	PS1 (presenilin-1)	29–62
AD4—early onset familial	1	PS2 (presenilin-2)	40–88

chronic but mild cough. He smokes cigarettes occasionally and recently has begun volunteering as a firefighter. On taking his family history, the nurse notes that one sister died in early childhood of "liver disease." After various tests, results show expiratory airflow limitation; notably, the forced expiratory volume in 1 second (FEV1) is 33% of the predicted value. This combined with the history provides the basis for testing for alpha-1-antitrypsin deficiency. Harold is found to have PI*ZZ. Refer to this case as you read below, and think about future life planning for Harold.

Emphysema or chronic obstructive pulmonary disease may be due to genetic or nongenetic factors. An association has been made between alpha-1-antrypsin (AAT) deficiency and an inherited form of emphysema as well as childhood cirrhosis. AAT is a serine proteinase inhibitor (serpin) that is mainly synthesized by the liver and is rapidly released into the plasma. The small molecular size of AAT allows it to leave the plasma and easily enter other body tissues and fluids, where it is widely distributed. When proteolytic enzymes such as elastase are released from cells after events such as tissue injury, AAT inhibits their activity and therefore protects organs such as the liver and lungs against damage.

AAT is synthesized under the direction of a gene known as Pi (for protease inhibitor) that is located on chromosome 14 (14q32.1). The Pi system demonstrates much genetic variability; more than 100 alleles coding for different molecular variants have been identified. According to standardized nomenclature, the designations in Box 10.4 are commonly used, although some use PI instead of Pi.

AAT variants may be classified as normal, deficient, null, or dysfunctional. The most common normal allele is Pi*M. The most common normal phenotype is Pi MM and is associated with a 100% serum level of AAT. There are subtype variants of M, such as M1, M2, M3, and others, which differ in amino acid sequence but appear to function normally, and there are other normal non-M variants. There are two important deficient variant alleles: Pi*Z and Pi*S. These may be present in the heterozygous state (PiMS, PiMZ, PiSZ) or the homozygous state (PiSS or PiZZ). Thus, there are varying degrees of AAT deficiency. The Pi*Z allele is the one most commonly associated with clinically significant effects of low serum AAT levels.

AAT deficiency occurs in 1 in 1,600 to 1 in 2,000 live births in White North American and Northern European populations and less frequently in Southern European and other populations. It is particularly frequent in Sweden, where it is included in newborn screening programs. It is estimated that PiZZ is present in 1 in 40,000 to 1 in 100,000 Black Americans and was originally thought to be infrequent in Asian populations. More recent epidemiological studies among various geographic and ethnic groups in 58 countries indicate that there are at least 3.4 million persons with deficiency alleles (PiSS, PiSZ, PiZZ) and 116 million carriers (PiMS and PiMZ) worldwide. AAT deficiency affects persons in all racial subgroups. AAT deficiency is underrecognized; only about 5% of persons with some degree of deficiency are identified. The inheritance mechanism is autosomal recessive with codominant expression of each gene on the basis of both the quantity and activity of the enzyme present.

Clinical expression of AAT deficiency commonly occurs bimodally in relation to age: in infancy or childhood manifested by symptoms of liver disease or in early adulthood manifested by pulmonary symptoms and, more rarely, liver disease. Clinical expression also depends on the genotype, the degree of AAT deficiency, and modulating factors such as cigarette smoke exposure. The most information is known about PiZZ. It has been estimated that of all infants born with PiZZ, 80% will eventually develop emphysema, 10% will suffer from childhood cirrhosis, and the rest will not show any overt clinical disease.

In some AAT-deficient individuals, liver disease may not be found until late childhood or adolescence, when patients present with abdominal distention caused by hepatosplenomegaly or portal

---

BOX 10.4

Pi Nomenclature

- Pi*M, Pi*S, Pi*Z, etc. for alleles at the Pi locus
- Pi*MM, Pi*MS, etc. or simply PiMM or PiMS or MM, MS for phenotypes
- Pi*M/Pi*S, Pi*M/Pi*Z, etc. or Pi*MS or Pi*MZ for genotypes

hypertension and esophageal variceal hemorrhage. Latent hepatic dysfunction in middle-aged and older adults has been found is some cases to be due to AAT deficiency. The older adult may present with hepatitis, cryptogenic cirrhosis, and/or hepatocellular carcinoma. Patients in older age groups with liver disease should be tested for AAT deficiency. Patients over 40 years of age with AAT deficiency should have periodic liver function assessment.

The association of AAT deficiency with chronic obstructive pulmonary disease (COPD), particularly emphysema, has been extensively validated. Emphysema caused by AAT deficiency usually involves the basal regions of the lung. Onset is early, often beginning in the late 20s or early 30s. Before age 40, 39–60% of Pi ZZ individuals develop COPD, as do 85–90% by 50 years of age. Even in clinically asymptomatic individuals, abnormalities in lung function can be detected early. The first symptom is usually dyspnea on exertion, followed by cough and recurrent pulmonary infections with severe expiratory airflow limitation and typical findings associated with emphysema. By adulthood, it is possible for a Pi ZZ individual to have both liver abnormalities and COPD. The detrimental effects of smoking in the Pi ZZ individual have been firmly established. The onset of COPD occurs approximately 15 years earlier in Pi ZZ individuals who smoke and decreases life expectancy. Smoking also leads to an early permanent loss of tolerance for exercise. As in liver disease, sex plays a yet unknown type of protective role. Adult Pi ZZ females who are nonsmokers are the least likely to develop pulmonary disease, and adult Pi ZZ males who smoke are the most likely. Other disorders such as panniculitis, a rare inflammation of subcutaneous fat, with bumps and necrosis, as well as some autoimmune disorders, may be seen.

For those with severe damage from emphysema, lung transplantation may be an option. For less severe circumstances, therapy may be directed at treating the symptoms of emphysema or liver disease. Antioxidant therapy may be useful. Augmentation therapy of weekly intravenous infusions of exogenous AAT (Prolastin) can have side effects but generally shows good results. Use of recombinant AAT preparations is also possible and avoids risks of plasma-derived product. Gene therapy aimed at the lung or liver to correct AAT deficiency may be a future option. Administering AAT by inhalation of

---

BOX 10.5

Nursing Points in Education in AAT Deficiency

- Emphasize the importance of not smoking for both the individual and for those living with the affected person because of the danger of second-hand smoke.
- Emphasize avoiding alcohol and other agents toxic to the liver, including certain medications.
- Counsel on the need to avoid respiratory irritants at home and on the job.
- At the appropriate time, teach affected females to avoid oral contraceptive agents, and provide information on other contraceptive measures.
- Emphasize the need for early recognition and treatment of any respiratory infection including vaccination for pneumococcal infections and other respiratory pathogens as indicated.
- Note the need to maintain physical activity to promote cardiovascular fitness without exhausting the individual.
- Be alert for symptoms of COPD, liver disease, and glomerulonephritis in the AAT-deficient person.
- Note the need to maintain good nutritional status and its relationship to immunocompetence and health. What constitutes good nutrition and elements of any special diet should be included.
- Provide career guidance and planning to select a job in which individuals will not be exposed to such known lung irritants as grain, cotton and other fibers, coal dust, wood dust (as in sawmills), and hair sprays or to any chemical industry in which they might be exposed to hepatotoxins or noxious chemical irritants.
- Note the desirability of choosing a permanent place of residence that is low in pollution and grain dust if this is possible.
- Genetic counseling should include the availability of prenatal detection for future pregnancies.

aerosolized AAT is considered experimental, but it holds promise.

The nurse should be clinically alert for the possibility of AAT deficiency in adults and children with COPD and liver disease, as some cases will have this genetic cause. It is not possible to predict along what path a specific individual with AAT deficiency will develop or how severe the disorder will be. All individuals with neonatal jaundice or childhood liver disease should have their AAT status determined by Pi typing. Some points nurses can use in patient and family education are shown in Box 10.5.

The practice of industrial or preemployment screening for AAT-deficient individuals has positive and negative points for the occupational health nurse to consider. Although current employees may benefit from placement in a position that is of lower risk and from the institution of other health-promoting measures as previously described, job discrimination can also result, thus limiting the advancement of a person who possesses the mutant gene. It may even cost some people their jobs because of the potential of developing emphysema and other associated conditions. A major problem lies in the uncertainty of the magnitude of the risk of clinical disease for heterozygous individuals. At the present time, widespread general population screening has not been recommended. Detailed genetic testing recommendations have been given by the American Thoracic Society/European Respiratory Society (2003).

Diabetes Mellitus

Diabetes mellitus (DM) is not a single disease but "a group of metabolic diseases characterized by hyperglycemia resulting from defects in insulin secretion, insulin action, or both" (American Diabetes Association, 2006 p. S43). The classification is shown in Table 10.3. The two major types, type 1 (formerly called insulin-dependent diabetes mellitus, or IDDM) and type 2 (formerly called noninsulin-dependent diabetes mellitus, or NIDDM) are quite different in genetic and clinical aspects. *Impaired glucose tolerance* (IGT) and *impaired fasting glucose* (IFT) are terms used to describe the state between normal and diabetic. They are considered risk factors for future diabetes, not clinical diseases. In addition, the diagnostic criteria for diabetes mellitus have been revised, and a fasting glucose concentration of 109 mg/dl is now defined as the upper limit of "normal," resulting in more individuals being classified as diabetic. Gestational diabetes, one of the classifications, is discussed in Chapter 8.

DM is an important cause of morbidity, mortality, and health care costs. In the United States, in 2005, the National Institute of Diabetes, Digestive and Kidney Diseases (NIDDK), National Institutes of Health, estimated that the prevalence of cases of DM was about 20.8 million, about one third of which were believed to be undiagnosed. Of these, about half were type 2. Additionally, DM results in complications such as cardiovascular disease, hy-

---

TABLE 10.3   **Classification of Diabetes Mellitus**

  I. Type 1 diabetes
      A. Immune mediated
      B. Idiopathic

 II. Type 2 diabetes

III. Other specific types of diabetes mellitus
      A. Genetic defects of β-cell function (example: MODY2)
      B. Genetic defects of insulin action (example: type A insulin resistance)
      C. Diseases of the exocrine pancreas (example: cystic fibrosis)
      D. Endocrinopathies (example: hyperthyroidism)
      E. Drug- or chemical-induced (example: pentamidine)
      F. Infections (example: congenital rubella)
      G. Uncommon forms of immune-mediated diabetes (example: stiff-man syndrome)
      H. Other genetic syndromes sometimes associated with diabetes (example: Down syndrome)

IV. Gestational diabetes mellitus

Source: Adapted from the American Diabetes Association (2006).

pertension, blindness, kidney disease, and nerve damage. DM is more frequent in certain ethnic and racial groups. The highest known prevalence is in the Pima Native Americans in Arizona (35–50%) and the Naruans (a Pacific Island group). In such populations, type 2 DM may result from a single major gene rather than multiple ones. Among the U.S. population at age 65 years, the prevalence is 33% in Hispanics, 25% in Blacks, and 17% in Whites.

Evidence for genetic contribution to DM comes from twin studies, sibling studies, migration studies, population studies, genetic and molecular techniques such as linkage analysis, DNA techniques including mapping and genome scans, the identification of genetic markers and variations, and the association with certain HLA types (see Chapter 3). The propensity to develop diabetes-related complications such as nephropathy, cardiovascular disease, neuropathy, and retinopathy is also believed to have a genetic component

Although genetic disorders that have impaired glucose metabolism as a component are comparatively rare when considering all known causes of DM they are important because they underscore the fact that known gene mutations at different sites can all result in the same end point. This is true regardless of the pathogenetic mechanism involved—whether it is insulin deficiency due to pancreatic degeneration or to hyperglycemia resulting from production of an abnormal proinsulin molecule. There are more than 60 genetic disorders that have glucose intolerance, DM, or hyperglycemia as components, with a variety of inheritance patterns. These include such diverse disorders as leprechaunism (an autosomal recessive disorder characterized by elfin facies, intellectual disability, and insulin-resistant DM), Mendenhall syndrome (an autosomal recessive disorder characterized by insulin-resistant DM), pineal hyperplasia (skin problems, hirsutism, and phallic enlargement), disorders affecting the pancreas such as cystic fibrosis or hemochromatosis, as well as disorders of the adrenal and pituitary glands. Many drugs and chemicals are also known to promote glucose intolerance and frank DM. The extent of their ability to cause damage may be influenced by the genotype (genetic makeup) of the person exposed to the agent, as well as to external factors.

Type 1 Diabetes Mellitus

Type 1 DM (T1DM) has two subtypes: immune-mediated diabetes and idiopathic diabetes. Few persons with T1DM fit into the idiopathic category, which has a strong, inherited component. The immune-mediated category results from autoimmune destruction of the pancreatic beta cells, which leads to the absolute extinguishing of insulin secretion. Exogenous insulin is therefore eventually necessary for control. T1DM usually, but not invariably, has its onset before the age of 40 years (considered before 30 by some), with a peak between 5 and 15 years of age, and often another less-defined peak at age 20–35 years. It was formerly referred to as juvenile diabetes, although now it is evident that about half of the cases are recognized above 20 years of age. Obesity is rarely present.

T1DM is considered to be multifactorial in that both genetic and environmental factors are necessary for expression (see Chapter 4). The genetic component is generally considered to be polygenic, in which many genes each contribute a susceptibility effect. Some believe that a few major genes rather than many minor genes determine this susceptibility. Data from twin studies show a concordance rate of 30–50% in monozygotic twins, with lower rates in dizygotic twins and siblings. To date, several chromosomal areas have a well-established association with T1DM. These are the HLA region, which is the major histocompatibility complex in humans (see Chapter 3) on chromosome 6 (6p21) in the histocompatibility region, and the insulin gene region on chromosome 11 (11p15); the putative genes are called *IDDM1* and *IDDM2*, respectively. It is estimated that *IDDM1* contributes 40–60% and *IDDM2* contributes about 10% to the familial inheritance of T1DM. Another putative gene, *IDDM6*, has been located on chromosome 18q21. The insulin gene region includes a region of variable number of tandem repeats (VNTR) that flank the insulin gene. The VNTR region is believed to have a role in modulating insulin gene expression. The variations in number, presence, location, and sequence of elements within this area are associated with susceptibility to T1DM. There are many other possible candidates for T1DM susceptibility loci, which have been designated with putative *IDDM* numbers.

A search for an association between HLA and T1DM was reasonable because of previously determined associations between HLA and other diseases sharing chronicity, unknown etiology, and autoimmune components as features. HLA is fully discussed in Chapter 3. Within the HLA region, more than 90% of White persons with T1DM express the serologically determined HLA DR3 (DQA1*0501 and DQB1*0201) and/or DR4 (DQA1* 0301 and DRQB1*0302), with the highest risk being for those who are heterozygous for DR3 or DR4. But these antigens are also present in persons who do not develop it. Thus, possession of these antigens alone is not sufficient to cause T1DM. Alleles distinguished by molecular means suggest that combinations of *DQA1* and *DQB1* alleles, especially *DQA1*0501-DQB1*0201/DQA1*0301-DQB1*0302*, confer even higher susceptibility in all ethnic groups. Various combinations confer varying degrees of susceptibility in different ethnic and racial groups. Of particular interest is the finding that some combinations of HLA alleles appear to be protective in regard to T1DM, particularly *DQB1*0602*. As is the case with other disorders associated with particular HLA types, not all persons with the susceptible HLA type develop diabetes. HLA DR3 or HLA DR4 are present in about 90% of persons with T1DM.

The nature of the nongenetic or environmental contribution to T1DM is believed to be most important in early childhood, and perhaps even in utero. Some of these putative modifiers or triggers are the early introduction of artificial milk (cow's milk) and solid foods to infants under 3 months, viral infections (especially rubella, mumps, and coxsackie virus), toxic exposures, maternal-fetal blood group incompatibility, and conditions that increase stress on the beta cells such as a cold climate, puberty, pregnancy, and rapid growth or low vitamin D intake.

Type 2 Diabetes Mellitus(T2DM)

T2DM is defined as ranging from predominantly insulin resistance with relative insulin deficiency to a predominantly insulin secretory defect with insulin resistance (American Diabetes Association, 2006). T2DM was formerly referred to as adult-onset diabetes, as it usually begins after age 40 years. In contrast to T1DM, T2DM is predominantly a result of genetic predisposition or causes. The number of adults with T2DM has risen rapidly and has been called an epidemic. T2DM is genetically het-

erogenous. A few rare single gene defects that affect small subgroups of those with T2DM have been identified such as the MODY defects, and defects in genes encoding glucokinase, insulin, the insulin receptor, and in the mitochondria. In the majority of affected persons, it is considered to be polygenic or multifactorial—caused by a number of genes and influenced by other factors such as obesity and exercise. Some genes may be primary and others may be related—for example, those that predispose to obesity. In some cases, T2DM susceptibility genes may be population specific.

In early twin studies, 90–100% of identical twin pairs were concordant for T2DM with lower concordance in dizygotic twins and siblings. Because these twin studies were largely concerned with persons in the middle to older age group who had been living apart for a number of years, any environmental factor would have to have exerted its influence in the early years of life when they shared a common environment.

Genetic Defects of β-Cell Function

This category includes the following:

- MODY (discussed below).
- Mitochondrial DNA mutations.
- Others such as the inability to convert proinsulin to insulin or the production of mutant insulin molecules with impaired receptor binding. Each of these is inherited in an autosomal dominant (AD) pattern with relatively mild impaired glucose metabolism.

MODY consists of several types of AD single gene conditions with high penetrance in which DM develops at a young age (usually before age 25 years, and often in the first decade of life) but in which insulin is not usually required. It is considered by some to be a subtype of T2DM, and some feel that the term *MODY* should not be used but rather *autosomal dominant T2DM*. At least six gene mutations can result in MODY. The major one consists of mutations in the hepatocyte nuclear factor (HNF)1α on chromosome 12q24 known as MODY3. Genetic counseling differs for persons in this category, and it is important to have a correct diagnosis.

Observations of persons with DM who had an affected parent revealed that they more frequently had affected mothers than affected fathers, and DM is frequently associated with certain mitochondrial diseases. This suggested that mtDNA mutations (see Chapter 4) might play a role in DM. The first identified association of a specific point mutation in the mtDNA (A3243G, an A to G mutation in mtDNA at position 3243 in the tRNA) with deafness and diabetes is known as MIDD (maternally inherited diabetes and deafness). Since then, other point mutations and deletions in mitochondrial genes have been described in connection with diabetes mellitus.

Cancer

The contribution of genetic mechanisms to cancer development and metastasis continues to be elucidated. About 10% of all cancers are believed to be inherited directly. However, genetically determined individual differences that can determine susceptibility to cancer when exposed to a given environmental trigger may be important in whether cancer eventually develops in a much larger proportion of individuals. The genetic component can be through a gene directly causing cancer, a precancerous condition, or a susceptibility to environmental agents that can result in cancer. As an illustration of the last, there are many polymorphisms in the cytochrome p450 enzymes. These enzymes metabolize polycyclic aromatic hydrocarbon compounds found in cigarette smoke. Persons with specific variants of the cytochrome p450 enzymes metabolize these compounds differently from others and have increased lung cancer rates. Thus, some people are more susceptible to lung cancer when exposed to cigarette smoke because of their genetic makeup.

The understanding of cancer development has been difficult because the term *cancer* includes at least 100 different forms of disease that we collectively call cancer. Further, a particular cancer may exist in both a hereditary and nonhereditary form, with the basic causative processes being similar. The development of cancer is thought to be a multistep process with a necessary first step being a mutation in the genetic material. This first mutation could be a hereditary one occurring in all germline cells, in which case the mutation would be in all body cells, or the mutation could be somatically acquired in

one or more cells, and passed to descendants of that cell(s) but not be inherited by the next vertical generation (from parent to child) through the gonads. As a second step, an environmental agent could then cause mutations again in one or more somatic cells. In the case of somatic changes, genetic changes may occur in the tumor cell and not be reflected in the germline and are not known to affect future generations. Therefore, all cancer is a genetic disease in one sense, although the genetic change may not be heritable or passed to another generation. An illustration using retinoblastoma is shown in Figure 10.2.

Mutations in three classes of genes appear to be the most important in triggering cancer:

- Proto-oncogenes
- Tumor-suppressor genes
- DNA damage recognition and repair genes, including DNA mismatch genes

It is also possible that other mutations might predispose individuals to cancer. For example, genes that alter the metabolism of potentially carcinogenic agents in the environment or food, that have an impact on a cell-binding site for oncogenic viruses, or that alter the tissue response to hormones or drugs might provide the initial susceptibility for another cancer-causing event to act on. Mutant genes may also allow tumor cells to attract and develop a blood supply, thus influencing metastasis. Knowledge of these can suggest treatment approaches that interfere with this process. Some known inherited rare single gene disorders result in cancer, and some forms of cancer are directly inherited.

These three classes of genes—proto-oncogenes, tumor-suppressor genes, and DNA repair genes—have normal cellular functions. Proto-oncogenes are normally concerned with the regulation of cell growth, differentiation, division, senescence, and apoptosis. Each oncogene appears to code for a protein that is involved in signal transduction from the cell membrane receptors to the nucleus or have a function in growth factors and their receptors or nuclear proto-oncogenes (such as in the *MYC* family), and transcription factors. When allelic mutations generate variant oncogenic forms of proto-oncogenes, these become known as oncogenes.

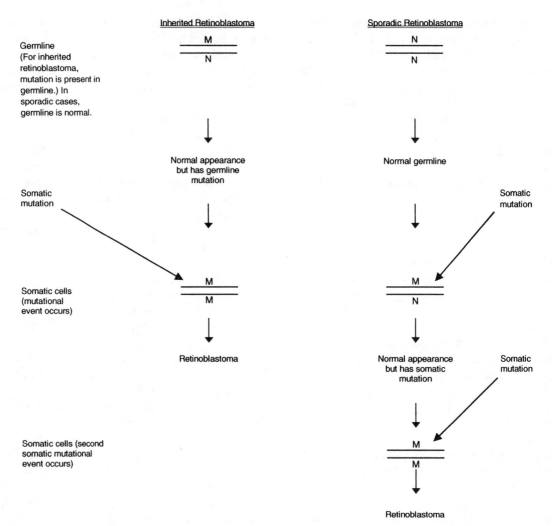

FIGURE 10.2   Two-hit theory of retinoblastoma. M = mutation; N = normal. *Mutation* can refer to alteration in gene or a chromosomal deletion.

Oncogenic alleles can be activated as a result of specific chromosome abnormalities or by other mechanisms. The activation of oncogenes has been likened to a jammed accelerator in a car. Tumor-suppressor genes (formerly known as anti-oncogenes) are inhibitory to cell growth and division. These genes are involved in complex interactions that integrate stimulatory and inhibitory messages internally and externally and govern the regulation of the cell cycle that includes protein synthesis, rest, DNA replication, and mitosis. Less is known about tumor-suppressor genes than oncogenes. The best-known tumor-suppressor gene is *p53* (sometimes known as *TP53*), which is the most common mu-

tated cancer gene known so far. When functioning normally, *p53* suppresses genes that are involved in the stimulation of growth and activates genes involved in the control of growth, differentiation, and apoptosis (the process of programmed cell death). Another is *p16*, also known as *CDKNZA* which, when mutated, is associated with multiple primary melanomas and pancreatic cancer in some families. DNA damage repair genes normally do just that: act in ways to repair damage that occurs to DNA either during replication or because of external mutational events. These are also known as DNA mismatch repair genes because they detect DNA sections that do not match.

Nurses should be alert for suggestions that a person with cancer may have an inherited form through the family history, health history, or physical assessment (see Box 10.6).

Single Gene, Constitutional Chromosome Disorders, Congenital Anomalies, and Cancer

At least 200 of the known single gene disorders are associated with neoplasia development. Some hereditary disorders associated with cancer are shown in Table 10.4. The single gene disorders can be divided into those in which the cancer itself is considered to be an inherited trait and genetic syndromes that predispose to malignancy. In the preneoplastic conditions, the initial abnormality is not malignant itself, but the risk of cancer development is greatly increased because of the inherited predisposition.

Constitutional chromosome disorders are those in which chromosome abnormalities are present throughout the body cells, not just in one or a few types of tissue. A few are known to be associated with an increased risk of cancer. The best known of these is Down syndrome, described in Chapter 9.

BOX 10.6

Clues That Cancer Is Inherited

- The occurrence of adult-type tumors in a child
- Occurrence of the cancer at an unusually young age for that cancer (germline tumors generally appear earlier than those due to sporadic causes)
- Two or more unusual cancers in the same person or close relative
- Cancer occurring in the less usually affected sex (e.g., breast cancer in the male)
- Recognition of a specific syndrome or genetic disease in a person that may predispose to cancer (such as Peutz-Jeghers syndrome predisposing to gastrointestinal and other cancers)
- Bilateral tumors in paired organs
- Multiple premalignant or malignant tumor presentations
- Multiply affected family members

The rate of acute leukemia in patients with Down syndrome is 16 to 30 times the rate found in normal individuals of the same age, and its onset is earlier. Acute nonlymphocytic leukemia (ANLL) predominates in children with Down syndrome in contrast to other types of leukemia in non–Down syndrome children of the same age group. A form of megakaryoblastic leukemia develops in about 10% of newborns with Down syndrome, and of those who recover, about 25% will develop acute megakaryoblastic leukemia, usually by 4 years of age. The reason for the association of leukemia and Down syndrome remains unknown, but one speculation is that a general cell sensitivity to transformation or induction into malignancy may be present.

In Turner syndrome (described in Chapter 9), there may be mosaicism with both a 45,X and a 46,XY cell line. In individuals with the Y chromosome line, the risk of the development of a gonadal malignancy such as dysgerminomas or gonadal blastomas ranges from 15% to 30%. Thus, it is important to identify patients with a Y chromosome cell line. Periodic examination and monitoring to detect early malignant changes is vital.

The cancer most associated with anomalies appears to be Wilms tumor (often associated with WAGR syndrome and Beckwith-Wiedemann syndrome), which are discussed in Chapter 9. An example of a congenital anomaly associated with malignancy is cryptorchidism (undescended testes), which is found at birth in about 2–4% of full-term male infants and about 30% of premature infants. They may spontaneously descend by 1 year of age. The risk of malignancy in cryptorchidism is estimated at about 22 times that for normal testes, and about 10% of all males with testicular malignancy are or have had cryptorchidism. The risk for development of malignancy is about six times greater for abdominal than for inguinal testis; if repair is done before 11 years of age, the risk for malignant development may return to normal. If not, increased risk continues, and about 50% of these males have testicular dysgenesis. Interestingly, about 25% of tumors in patients with unilateral cryptorchidism develop in the descended testicle. Approximately 4% of males with cryptorchidism have close relatives who are also affected, and it is believed that the disorder is inherited in a multifactorial way. Nurses should stress the importance of early repair to the parents in order to prevent cancer development.

TABLE 10.4   Some Hereditary Disorders Associated with Cancer

Disorder	Inheritance Mode	Other Features
Ataxia telangiectasia	AR	More common in Mediterranean populations. Chromosome instability that predisposes to malignancies such as lymphoreticular malignancies. Sensitive to radiation. Telangiectasia, growth restriction, progressive cerebellar ataxia, immune defects.
Bloom syndrome	AR	Chromosome breaks and rearrangements. Short stature; high pitched voice characteristic facies including prominent nose and ears, long, narrow face, butterfly rash, and small jaw; may have intellectual disabilities, lung problems, immune deficiency, and high risk of cancer usually in the 20s.
Cowden disease (multiple hamartoma syndrome)	AD	Breast fibrocystic disease and cancer, goiters and thyroid cancer, meningioma. Papules on face, especially nose, eyes, mouth; other skin lesions such as vitiligo and café-au-lait spots; polyposis in GI tract.
Fanconi anemia	AR	Chromosomal instability disorder with radiation hypersensitivity. Increased incidence of lymphoid malignancies, aplastic anemia.
Hereditary mixed polyposis syndrome	AD	Colorectal polyps including atypical juvenile polyps adenomas with early adenocarcinoma of the colon and/or rectum. Not firmly established.
Juvenile polyposis	AD	Multiple juvenile polyps of GI tract, adenocarcinoma of colon, and other GI lesions may be seen. Usually presents under 10 years of age, but can be seen into early adulthood.
Muir-Torre syndrome	AD	Adenocarcinoma of gastrointestinal tract such as colon and duodenum and genitourinary sites and skin lesions, including basal and sebaceous cell carcinoma and adenoma. Rare.
Multiple endocrine neoplasia (MEN)	AD	
Type 1 (Wermer syndrome)		Parathyroid hyperplasia, pituitary tumors, pancreatic islet cell tumors, peptic ulcer disease.
Type 2A (Sipple syndrome)		Parathyroid hyperplasia, pheochromocytomas, medullary thyroid cancer.
Type 2B		Pheochromocytoma; mucosal neuromas; medullary thyroid cancer; characteristic facial appearance with hypertrophied lips; Marfanoid appearance; enlarged nerves of GI tract and megacolon; skeletal abnormalities.
Peutz-Jeghers syndrome	AD	Melanin pigmentation of oral mucosa, face, lips, fingers and toes; diffuse polyposis and cancer of any region of GI tract, especially the small intestine, ovary, testes.
Turcot syndrome (many are FAP variants; some are not)	AD	Primary nervous system tumors such as cerebral giomas, colon adenomatous polyps of colon carcinoma.
von Hippel–Lindau syndrome	AD	Development of multiple tumors including pancreatic cysts and cancer; renal cell cysts and carcinomas, pheochromocytomas, retinal angiomas, cerebellar hemangioblastomas, carcinoma, pancreatic cysts, and adrenal tumors.
XY gonadal dysgenesis	X-linked recessive	Dysgerminoma.
Xeroderma pigmentosa	AR	Defect in nucleotide excision repair. Severe skin effects from ultraviolet light. Skin cancer, melanomas, eye damage.

AD = autosomal dominant transmission. AR = autosomal recessive transmission. GI = gastrointestinal.

Childhood Cancers

A number of cancers generally make their first appearance in childhood. While they often have a substantial genetic component, they also have a noninherited form. Retinoblastoma and Wilms tumor are discussed in Chapter 9.

Cancer in Families

The aggregation of cancer in families has long been a subject of interest. The reasons for such aggregation are not always clear, apart from the known inherited syndromes and tumors. The occurrence of more than one neoplasm in a family can occur simply by chance because of the frequency of neoplasias in the population; it could represent common exposure to environmental factors, either chemical or infectious; or inherited genetic susceptibility can be the cause. Genetic factors can contribute to both familial susceptibility and the single occurrences of cancer in smaller families. Families may also show a specific inheritance pattern for certain cancers that are not shown to be heritable in the population at large. Careful family evaluation of each patient presenting with a cancer may help to clarify contributing genetic factors. The formation of the National Cancer Registry with regional centers to keep track of individuals with familial predispositions to various cancers has been implemented in some places to promote medical counseling as well as surveillance, and individual tumor registries exist. However, some see this as an invasion of privacy and violation of confidentiality.

Li-Fraumeni Syndrome

One of the primary ways to collect information about families can be through a detailed family history. This should include a history of benign neoplasms and birth defects. When meticulously followed up by someone who is trained in the specific information to collect, this can result in identification not only of the type of genetic transmission operating for that family but also of new relationships and understandings. An example is the circumstances that led to the eventual elucidation of the Li-Fraumeni syndrome.

Li described the investigation of a family that began in Massachusetts with the hospital admission of a child with rhabdomyosarcoma. A family history revealed acute leukemia in the father and unknown cancers in other relatives. Interviews with parents led first to Arizona, where a high frequency of cancers was noted in relatives of the father. Relatives lost to contact were located by means of old family and courthouse records, and family members in Ohio were located. In this branch of the family, 5 of 10 persons had died with cancer. Hospital pathology and mortality records were used to establish and confirm diagnoses. A high proportion of this family's neoplasms were sarcomas and breast cancer, most cases being diagnosed before age 35 years. This experience led these investigators to review the histories of children treated for rhabdomyosarcoma nationally and ultimately led to the uncovering of excessive soft tissue sarcomas, breast cancers, and multiple primary neoplasms occurring together in several families.

Li-Fraumeni syndrome is a rare autosomal dominant inherited disorder occurring in about 1 in 50,000, in which the affected person develops tumors by young adulthood. The most common are breast cancer, soft tissue sarcoma, brain tumors, osteosarcoma, leukemia, and adrenocortical carcinoma. In later life they may develop lung, prostate, pancreatic, colon, and stomach cancer, melanoma, and lymphomas. Multiple and successive tumors often occur. Thus, this should be looked for during health evaluations. Most affected individuals have germline mutations in the p53 tumor suppressor gene (*TP53*), located on chromosome 17p13, or the Checkpoint kinase 2 gene (*hCHK2*) located on chromosome 22q12.1. The latter activates protein kinase in response to DNA damage, preventing cell cycle progression. Genetic heterogeneity is present. Observations of the Li-Fraumeni families allowed some elucidation of the effects of p53 inactivation and its involvement in a variety of human cancers.

Breast and Ovarian Cancer

More than 215,000 new cases of breast cancer are diagnosed each year in the United States, and about 1 million worldwide. Males account for less than 1% of all cases. Breast cancer was one of the cancers in which a hereditary component had been postulated early and its presence in blood relatives cited as a factor increasing risk, particularly if it occurred in a woman's mother, sisters, or aunts. A family history of breast cancer in a close blood relative such as a mother, sister, or aunt and breast cancer in the family occurring before age 50 years denote increased risk. Breast cancer may be associated with another syndrome such as Cowden syndrome (see Table 10.4), be associated in syndromes with other cancers, or occur alone. The risks in the general population for breast cancer and ovarian cancer are about 11% and 1.6%, respectively.

BRCA1 and BRCA2 mutations are believed to be responsible for about 5–10% of all breast cancer and about one third each of the hereditary breast cancers. Other genes as described above, some with low penetrance, may confer susceptibility to breast cancer. Some of the genes involved in breast cancer development are still unknown. Birth prevalence of BRCA1, BRCA2, and p53 mutations has been estimated at 1 in 476, 1 in 667, and 1 in 5,000, respectively. Issues of testing for cancer are discussed later in this chapter.

Ovarian cancer is the fifth most common cancer and the most common cause of death from gynecological malignancy in women. At least 90% are sporadic; the rest are believed due to inherited susceptibility. Hereditary ovarian cancer is often associated with hereditary breast cancer as part of a syndrome or together and may occur with hereditary nonpolyposis colon cancer, discussed later in this chapter. The association of ovarian cancer with BRCA1 and BRCA2 mutations is discussed in the following section. As is seen in breast cancer, some of the gene mutations resulting in susceptibility to ovarian cancer are as yet unknown.

BRCA1 *and* BRCA2

BRCA1 and -2 normally function as tumor-suppressor genes. Germline mutations of BRCA1 are associated most with breast and ovarian cancer, but both male and female carriers have elevated risks for colon cancer, and males are at increased risk for prostate cancer. Thus, persons who carry these mutations are more likely to develop cancer. They may develop cancer at an earlier age, develop cancer in both breasts or ovaries, or have more than one type of cancer such as breast and ovarian cancer in the same person. Over 900 mutations are known in the BRCA1 gene on chromosome 17q12-21. Within families, usually the same alteration in BRCA1 occurs. Both BRCA1 and BRCA2 mutations are particularly prevalent in certain population groups, especially Ashkenazi Jewish women; among women with ovarian cancer, the hereditary proportion may approach 50%. In BRCA1 mutations, a

particular alteration, 185delAG (deletion of an adenine and guanine), is prevalent in Ashkenazi Jewish women. Approximately 1% of them carry this mutation. Another alteration in BRCA1, 5382insC (insertion of a cytosine), is also prevalent.

BRCA2 is located on chromosome 13q12-13. Multiple mutations are also seen in BRCA2. More than 900 mutations are known. A particular mutation of BRCA2, 6174delT (deletion of a thymidine), is common in Ashkenazi Jews, and 1 in 40 Ashkenazi Jews has one of the three most common mutations of BRCA1 or BRCA2. In Iceland, most familial breast and ovarian cancers are associated with BRCA2 rather than BRCA1, and a particular mutation, 999del5, excessively occurs in Icelanders. There may be an association between the risk and the mutation location. Further studies will add to this information and make counseling more accurate.

What is the risk of developing various cancers in persons with mutations in BRCA1 and BRCA2? For females carrying the mutated BRCA1, the lifetime risk of developing breast and ovarian cancer has been variously estimated. These estimates have changed with experience and because of differences in populations studied. It is expected that these risks will be altered as new information is forthcoming, and so recent information should be consulted. Other genetic factors, some unknown, appear to influence risk. The lifetime risk for a woman with a BRCA1 or BRCA2 mutated gene to develop breast cancer has been variously estimated at 50–85%. More recent studies tend to the lower end of these ranges. The risk of prostate cancer in male carriers of BRCA1 and BRCA2 mutations is increased fourfold, and the risk of colorectal cancer is increased fourfold for both males and females. Men with BRCA2 mutations have an estimated 6% risk of developing breast cancer. The lifetime risk for a woman with a germline BRCA1 mutation to develop ovarian cancer is approximately 16–44%. Women with BRCA1 mutations have a 25–30% risk to develop breast cancer in the contralateral breast within 10 years of an earlier breast cancer diagnosis. For woman with BRCA2 mutations, the lifetime risk of ovarian cancer is estimated at 10–27%. At this time, genetic testing can be done for the major known mutated alleles but not for 100% of all possible mutations.

The BRCA1 and BRCA2 genes are inherited in an autosomal dominant manner. Thus, a daughter of man or woman with a mutated gene has a 50% chance of inheriting that gene mutation. However, just inheriting the gene does not mean the person will definitely develop cancer. It is not possible to predict which gene carriers will develop cancer, and if so, which types, and which will not. Some women who have early breast cancer even with a positive family history do not have a *BRCA1* mutation, and some do have this mutation without a strong family history. Developing cancer at a young age was found to be important in prediction, however. Other genetic and nongenetic risk factors also play a role and should be accounted for in individual risk assessments such as young age at menarche, a body mass index above 35, and high intake of dietary fat. Thus, developing appropriate guidelines for which women should be offered population-based genetic screening and testing for *BRCA1* or *BRCA2* remains challenging. Preimplantation genetic diagnosis is now available in most of Europe for testing for susceptibility to certain cancers including possession of *BRCA1* and *BRCA2* mutations (Braude, 2006).

Colorectal Cancer

Colorectal cancers are the third most common cancer in the United States; over 145,000 persons developed these cancers in 2005. Colorectal cancer may be sporadic or due to germline genetic mutations that can lead to cancer development in varying degrees of frequency. The most frequent directly inherited conditions associated with colorectal cancer are familial adenomatous polyposis (FAP) and hereditary nonpolyposis colorectal cancer (HNPCC, also known as Lynch syndrome). Relatively recently, an autosomal recessive condition resulting in mutations in the *MYH* gene resulting in multiple adenomatous polyps and colon cancer has been recognized. *MYH* is a base excision repair gene. Other relatively rare single gene disorders may be associated with colorectal cancer, as shown in Table 10.4.

FAP is a relatively rare type of autosomal dominant condition caused by germline mutation leading to inactivation of the adenomatous polyposis coli *(APC)* gene located on chromosome 5q. *APC* is a tumor-suppressor gene that functions as a regulatory gatekeeper for colorectal epithelial cells. When mutated, hundreds to thousands of colon tumors develop and can progress to malignancy. Penetrance is about 100%. It accounts for about 1% of all colon cancers. A variety of mutations may occur. A

particular *APC* mutation, 11307K, has been found in about 6% of Ashkenazi Jews tested, thus indicating one population in which targeted population screening would be useful at this time. Multiple colon polyps are common and are shown in Figure 10.3. Polyps can be seen as early as 8 years of age but typically occur in late adolescence or young adulthood. Gardner syndrome is a variant of FAP but tends to have a wider spectrum of extraintestinal findings, such as desmoid and soft tissue tumors and osteomas. Congenital hypertrophy of the retinal pigment epithelium (CHRPE) is a common extracolonic manifestation in FAP. Other extraintestinal manifestations include dental and skeletal anomalies, hepatoblastoma, adrenal carcinoma, and papillary thyroid cancer. An attenuated variant of FAP may be seen in which the adenomas are fewer, with a later age of onset of malignancy.

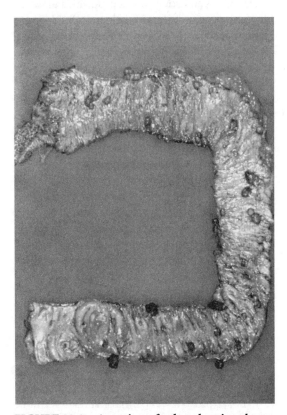

FIGURE 10.3   A section of colon showing the carpeting of polyps as seen in familial adenomatous polyposis. Courtesy of Dr. John Murphy, Southern Illinois University School of Medicine, Springfield, IL.

HNPCC is more common. It represents about 6–10% of all colon cancers and is believed to have a frequency of 1 in 200 to 1 in 2,000. Five different gene mutations have been implicated to account for about three-quarters of HNPCC. These are inactivating germline mutations in various DNA mismatch repair genes. The most frequent are MLH1 (chromosome 3p) and MSH2 (chromosome 2p). Others are MSH6, PMS1, and PMS2. These genes are involved in DNA mismatch repair: they recognize, excise, and repair mismatched sequences on newly replicated DNA. After the initial germline mutation that is inherited, in some cells, the other gene copy is inactivated by a somatic mutation, and the result is genetic instability that allows initiated cells to progress rapidly to cancer. Microsatellite instability is seen in tumor tissue. Penetrance is about 70–80% so that 20–30% of those with the mutation may not manifest cancer.

HNPCC is autosomal dominant, with a predilection for proximal colon cancer location and an early age of onset. The chance for developing colorectal cancer is up to 75% by 65 years of age. There is also increased cancer risk in other organs, especially the endometrium of the uterus, ovaries, stomach, small intestine, pancreas, brain, upper urinary tract, and hepatobiliary. For women, there can be up to a 40–60% risk of developing endometrial cancer and a 5–15% chance of developing ovarian cancer. There are various clinical criteria for HNPCC that were developed after the original stringent Amsterdam criteria that are known as the Amsterdam II criteria, the Modified Amsterdam criteria, and the Bethesda criteria developed especially for use in small families.

Prostate Cancer

Prostate cancer is the most common cancer in men in the United States and accounts for about 40,000 deaths per year. About 10–15% of cases are believed to result from mutated genes. BRCA2 mutations have been shown to be responsible for an increased risk for early-onset prostate cancer, as have BRCA1 mutations to a lesser degree, and 2% of men with early-onset prostate cancer have shown germline BRCA2 mutations. Black males appear to have a higher rate than White, Hispanic, or Asian males in the United States. Another potential susceptibility gene is the hereditary prostate cancer 1 locus (HPC1) on chromosome 1q24-25. At this time, no associated gene mutations are identified that have as direct and strong association as BRCA1 does with breast cancer. In persons at risk for BRCA1 and BRCA2 mutations or by virtue of family history of prostate cancer, it would be beneficial to institute screening for prostate cancer at an earlier age than the general population, probably at age 40 years, using a serum prostate-specific antigen test in addition to digital rectal examination.

Malignant Melanoma

There are over 60,000 new cases of invasive melanoma in the United States each year. It is the fifth leading cancer in males and sixth in females. Familial malignant melanoma is believed to account for about 10% of all cases of malignant melanoma. Two susceptibility gene mutations have been identified: CDKN2A (cyclin-dependent kinase inhibitor 2a) on chromosome 9p21 and CDK4 on chromosome 12q14. The risk for developing melanoma if the person possesses a susceptibility gene has been estimated at 50% by 50 years of age but is influenced by exposure to ultraviolet radiation including sunlight and modifying genes such as variants in the melanocortin-1 receptor gene (MRC1R). Risk factors include family history of melanoma and patient history of multiple or dysplastic nevi, as well as host characteristics such as red hair, freckling, and fair skin. Certain variants of MC1R are most prevalent in individuals with those characteristics.

Chromosome Changes and Genetic Influences in the Leukemias, Lymphomas, and Other Cancers

Specific nonrandom chromosome changes have been reported in most of the leukemias and lymphomas. In the case of the solid tumors, this information has been slower to emerge due to technical problems. The chromosome changes may involve gain or loss of a whole or part of a chromosome, translocations, inversions, or other changes alone or in combination. In many cases, the genes associated with these chromosome changes and their expression profiles are now being elucidated. The major result of chromosome aberrations is usually protooncogene activation, often because the gene for a T-cell receptor or antigen receptor gene or immunoglobulin is relocated near it or because a fusion gene is created that may encode and affect transcription factors. The fusion protein created appears to be particularly important in solid tumor development. These fusion proteins are considered tumor-specific antigens and may eventually be therapeutic targets.

Chromosome aberrations in relation to leukemia and lymphoproliferative disorders can be used for the following:

- Diagnosing—for example, demonstrating a clonal chromosome aberration in a myeloproliferative disorder such as polycythemia vera can aid in distinguishing it from a nonneoplastic reactive proliferation
- Following the natural history of a disorder—for example, to predict blast crisis in chronic myelogenous leukemia (CML)
- Establishing a prognosis—for example, in AML, a chromosome 16 inversion or a t(8;21) translocation is associated with a relatively good prognosis, while the t(9;22) translocation appears to carry a poorer outcome
- Selecting and monitoring chemotherapy for efficacy and resistance—for example, in adult ALL, t(1;9) carries a poor prognosis, also in ALL, patients with t(15;17) are being treated with retinoic acid while those with t(8;21) and inv 16 are being treated with high-dose cytarabine
- Predicting or establishing remission or exacerbation—early relapses can be detected by looking for certain cytogenetic abnormalities and additional therapies begun

A full discussion of cytogenetic changes in cancer is beyond the scope of this chapter.

More than 90% of patients with CML have a specific chromosome marker in bone marrow cells, known as the Philadelphia (Ph) chromosome. Ph represents a translocation of genetic material from chromosome 22 to chromosome 9, noted as t(9;22). The shorter chromosome 22 is referred to as the Ph chromosome. As a consequence of this translocation, the proto-oncogene ABL (Abelson murine leukemia virus), normally on chromosome 9, is moved to chromosome 22 within the breakpoint cluster region, BCR, forming a BCR-ABL fusion gene and product that has increased tyrosine kinase activity. The new gene relationship is detected even in CML without detectable cytogenetic rearrangement. The t(9;22) is also seen in about 15% of cases of ALL, rarely in AML, and in about 5% of cases of

acute nonlymphocytic leukemia (ANLL). This molecular information about CML led to the development of a pharmacological treatment, imatinib mesylate, which is a BCR-ABL tyrosine protein kinase inhibitor. In CLL, gene expression profiling revealed that expression of a gene ZAP-70 distinguished those who had relatively stable disease from those with progressive disease requiring early treatment with 93% accuracy.

Another example of well-described chromosomal rearrangement is in Burkitt's lymphoma, a B cell malignancy. Three major translocations are seen. One, t(8;14)(q24;q32), is found in 75–90% of cases. The result of the t(8;14) translocation is to move the MYC gene to the site of the gene for the heavy chain of immunoglobin (Ig), resulting in activation of the oncogene.

Assessment of Risk, Detection, Genetic Testing, Prevention, and Counseling in Cancer

The major significance of finding inherited types of cancer or cancer susceptibility lies in the possibility of prevention, early detection and diagnosis, the chance to consider personal plans and affairs, choice of treatment plans, and establishing prognosis. For example, persons who have BRCA1 and have cancer in one breast need to consider the appropriate detection and prophylactic strategies because of the tendency for multifocal tumors and the development of cancer in the contralateral breast.

Considering whether a person or family should be referred for genetic risk assesment and counseling often begins with initial assessment for those who might be at increased risk for hereditary susceptibility for ovarian, breast, or colon cancer by the primary care provider. The family history, discussed in Chapter 7, is often a source for identifying those who should be referred for more expert risk assessment and/or genetic counseling. Guidelines are in place in various health provider groups to help the clinician determine who should be referred. Genetic testing and counseling may take place within the genetics clinic, the cancer clinic, the familial cancer clinic, or cancer site–specific clinics. The primary risk assessment, education, and counseling are often done by a cancer nurse specialist trained in genetics or by a genetic counselor trained in familial cancer. Probabilities of carrying the mutant BRCA1 gene under varying histories and findings have been developed. The risk for actually developing cancer when carrying a mutant gene such as *BRCA1* or *BRCA2* is not yet fully elucidated, as discussed above. However, a person who has a gene mutation and does not develop cancer can transmit the mutation to his/her offspring, who could or could not develop cancer themselves even if the parent did not.

Here are illustrative case examples:

CASE EXAMPLE 1

Joyce is a 60-year-old woman who had been diagnosed with breast cancer and successfully treated. In talking to the nurse, she remarks that her mother had had breast cancer, as had her sister and an aunt. She has three daughters and one son who are apparently in good health. She is thinking of seeking genetic testing to determine if she carries a mutant gene for cancer susceptibility. What are appropriate responses by the nurse? What questions and issues should be considered?

CASE EXAMPLE 2

Ellen is 30 years old and has been diagnosed as carrying a *BRCA1* mutation. She has two sisters, Brenda and Barbara; one brother, Thomas; and three aunts. She tells you that she plans to tell one sister, Brenda. She does not plan to tell Thomas, because "he's a man," or her other sister, Barbara, because "I don't speak to her." What are some issues to be discussed? Why? Sometime later, Brenda comes in and tells you how relieved she is that she was negative for the *BRCA1* mutation. She also says, "Now I don't have to worry about getting breast cancer." What are some possible responses by the nurse? Why?

Genetic testing for cancer, like other genetic testing, should take place within the context of adequate and appropriate culturally competent education, counseling, and access to prevention, surveillance, and treatment options. It may begin with the identification of an at-risk person or family, found because of careful history taking over three generations and clarification of findings (for example, an aunt's "female" cancer may be cervical and

not ovarian) that necessitate medical records and pathology reports if obtainable. Sometimes a person who has already been diagnosed with a cancer such as breast cancer will want genetic testing because he/she wants to know if he/she has a mutation such as *BRCA1* or *BRCA2* that could be inherited by descendants, be present in other blood relatives who might have increased risk, as well as know his/her risk for developing a second cancer. The nurse should be able to explain, clarify, and interpret the information at a level that the client can understand and that is culturally sensitive and appropriate, free from any coercion, and to evaluate that understanding. All persons have the right not to choose genetic testing. If testing is likely to be informative, clients should have the right to choose to be tested. Some cancer genetics programs have as a component genetic counseling that includes calculating the risk for a person to carry a gene mutation for cancer before recommending testing based on clinical examination, pathology if relevant, family history, and so on. Specialized computer models may be used to do this. Some recommend that the risk be above a certain cutoff in order to recommend genetic testing. Should clients have the right to choose genetic testing whether or not they are assessed as being at an increased risk for an inherited susceptibility to cancer?

Some of the elements that should be addressed, and could be included in informed consent before a person decides to participate in genetic testing for cancer, are essentially the same as those discussed in Chapter 5, and not all will be repeated here. The person may also want to ascertain the extent of insurance coverage for the laboratory, counseling, education, and medical services, including prophylactic tests and surgery, if desired and indicated. Particularly important elements are risks of passing on the mutation to children and the meaning of the risks; what disclosure they might consider for other family members, why this can be important, and who will they tell (if anyone) about the test results; and provision for referral for periodic surveillance, testing, or treatment after testing.

Who should be tested for genetic cancer predisposition? Uncertainties also exist in who is a candidate for testing. A woman with a mother who developed breast cancer at age 70 years may seek testing but is not very likely to be a carrier of *BRCA1* mutation (although she could be). Likewise, the absence of one particular gene mutation does not mean that there is no susceptibility to breast or ovarian cancer. Moreover, a negative test does not mean a zero risk; the risk then becomes that of the population risk. The American Society of Clinical Oncology (ASCO) offered recommendations for indications for genetic testing for cancer susceptibility in 1996, which it updated in 2003. It recommends that genetic counseling and testing be offered when "1) the person has personal or family history features suggestive of a genetic cancer susceptibility condition; 2) the genetic test can be adequately interpreted; and 3) the test results will aid in diagnosis or influence the medical or surgical management of the patient or family members at hereditary risk of cancer" (p. 2398). It goes on to say that genetic testing should be done with pre- and posttest counseling that includes possible risks and benefits of early detection and prevention strategies. Because of the rapid evolution of knowledge and testing in regard to genetic testing for susceptibility to cancer and variations and limitations in models, it does not set numerical thresholds for recommending genetic risk assessment but states that "evaluation by a health care professional experienced in cancer genetics be relied on in making interpretations of pedigree information and determinations of the appropriateness of genetic testing" (p. 2398). As part of this, the society recommends that "practitioners recognize indications for genetic cancer predisposition testing, where testing is part of established or evolving standards of care for risk assessment and management." It goes on to say that this "includes families with features of well-defined hereditary syndromes and individuals with very early onset disease or specific rare tumors suggestive of possible genetic hereditary predisposition" (pp. 2398–2399). Examples of the first group would include FAP and von Hippel–Lindau disease. ASCO (2003) recommends better regulatory oversight and quality assurance for laboratories involved in genetic testing and believes that the "health care provider's obligations (if any) to at-risk relatives are best fulfilled by communication of familial risk to the person undergoing testing, emphasizing the importance of sharing this information with family members so that they may also benefit" (p. 2403). It states that case law is not yet developed in regard to the "duty to warn" and that there are differences when the relatives are also patients of the health care provider. What is the obligation of a person to notify their relatives who may be at risk?

Various criteria have been used to establish the diagnosis of HNPCC, which was discussed above. In the original Amsterdam criteria, now seen as very stringent by some, the following are included: the presence of histologically verified colorectal cancer in at least three relatives (including a first-degree relative of the other two), cases that span at least two successive generations and with the diagnosis of at least one of the colorectal cancers before 50 years of age, and the elimination of known polyposis syndromes to make the diagnosis. In the more liberal Bethesda criteria, clinical diagnosis criteria include the Amsterdam criteria, persons with two types of HNPCC-related cancers, persons with colon cancer and a first-degree relative with colon cancer and/or HNPCC-associated extracolonic cancer and/or adenoma with the cancer at under 45 years of age and adenoma at under 40 years of age; persons with colon or endometrial cancer under 45 years; persons with right-sided colon cancer with a histologic undifferentiated pattern under 45 years of age; persons with signet-ring-cell-type colon cancer under 45 years; and persons with colonic adenomas before age 40 years. Family history still remains an important means of identifying HNPCC.

Ethical Issues Surrounding Predictive and Presymptomatic Genetic Testing for Cancer

The ethical dilemmas seen in genetic testing for cancer have commonalities with other types of medical testing, genetic testing and screening, prenatal diagnosis and presymptomatic testing such as for Huntington disease (see Chapters 5 and 8) and will not be repeated here. One of the differences lies in the nature of cancer: the varying surveillance and treatment options and the varying outcome possibilities. Issues such as privacy, confidentiality, insurability (although disclosure of a negative test could be to the individual's benefit), possible employment discrimination, stigmatization, possible interference with family relationships, and the impact on marital and reproductive decisions are discussed in Chapters 5, 12, and 13. There have been fears that women who are at risk will abandon surveillance methods such as mammograms after a few negative ones, being lulled by false security. Another aspect has centered around access for high-risk women who cannot pay for testing and testing for those who can pay but may be deemed at low risk. The latter may be comparable to those who seek prenatal diagnosis because of anxiety, and many consider this to be a legitimate reason. The testing of children in genetically at-risk families for cancer has been controversial. In some cases, the benefits to be derived are clearer than in others, and the family's own beliefs and experiences are important. For example, a child who does not have an *APC* mutation in FAP families would be spared annual colon examinations that might be started at 11 years of age or earlier. Other concerns center around the child's ability to understand the procedure, the implications of what may be found, and the capability of giving informed assent.

Prevention and Surveillance

Once a person is determined to be at risk by virtue of possessing a gene mutation known to be implicated in cancer development, a program of surveillance and of therapeutic preventive interventions can be implemented. For example, the recommendations for women with *BRCA1* or *BRCA2* mutations would include more than the usual recommended monthly self-breast examination. These women would be advised to have an annual mammogram and breast examination by an experienced practitioner beginning by age 25 years. This may be alternated with an MRI at the alternate 6 months. There is some controversy regarding mammography for several reasons, such as radiation exposure sensitivity in those with certain gene mutations. For ovarian cancer surveillance, women should have transvaginal ultrasound and a pelvic examination every 6 to 12 months and a blood test for cell surface glycoprotein markers in the serum such as CA125 every 6 to 12 months for early ovarian cancer detection beginning at age 25 years. For women with *BRCA1* and *BRCA2* mutations, among the choices are prophylactic mastectomy or oophrectomy with or without hysterectomy at about age 35 years or older. There are many aspects to consider with these options, including that tissue left behind could become malignant and that they still might develop one of the other associated cancers for which detection is not being pursued as aggressively. Men with *BRCA* 1 or 2 mutations should be alert for any breast mass or change.

Some centers are investigating the use of chemoprevention through such agents as tamoxifen and raloxifene to prevent breast cancer. Aromatase in-

hibitors such as anastrazole are of interest currently in preventing breast cancer development. Birth control pills may decrease the risk of ovarian cancer. Women with breast cancer gene mutations may want to avoid perimenopausal exogenous estrogen and follow a low-fat diet. Men and women should also have a rectal examination every year, a fecal occult blood test by age 40 years and over, and colonoscopy every 3 to 5 years. Males should have a prostate exam yearly and a prostate-specific antigen test every year after 50 years of age.

Persons who are at risk for colorectal cancer by virtue of being a first-degree relative of a person with FAP, or for Gardner syndrome, should have a flexible sigmoidoscopy at 10–12 years of age or earlier if indicated by family history. If no polyps are detected, this should be repeated every 1–3 years (if a germline mutation is present). For HNPCC, it is recommended that colonoscopy be done at about 20–30 years of age or 5 years earlier than the age at which the index patient was diagnosed. It is recommended that those at higher risk should have full colonoscopy to the cecum every 1 to 3 years. Women with these mutations should be screened for ovarian cancer by transvaginal ovarian ultrasonography and CA-125 and annual surveillance for endometrial cancer by endometrial aspirate beginning at age 25–30 years. Eventually, testing may be done on DNA of cells shed in feces. In terms of general health promotion, at-risk patients might also practice dietary modification such as a low-fat, high-fiber diet and pharmacologic measures such as nonsteroidal anti-inflammatory drugs that might modify risk by reducing the number and size of adenomas in FAP but do not provide complete protection. Some patients may elect to have prophylactic subtotal colectomy. Data on hysterectomy and bilateral salpingo-oophrectomy are lacking, but this option is available, preferably by 35 to 40 years of age. Diet modifications (low fat, high fiber, fruits and vegetables) and lifestyle modifications (exercise, not smoking) are suggested but are not proven to prevent cancer development. The psychological issues that accompany prophylactic surgery may have some similarities to those observed following mastectomy, hysterectomy, or colectomy for nonfamilial cancers and are discussed in detail in other texts.

KEY POINTS AND QUESTIONS FOR DISCUSSION

- What are some of the difficulties in associating single gene mutations with common or complex disease states?
- What is the difference between inherited cancer and inherited susceptibility to cancer?
- What are some points to include when discussing negative BRCA1 and BRCA2 tests with a 30-year-old woman?
- A man who has had two colonoscopies because he was at increased risk for colorectal cancer because of preexisting HNPCC tells you that he plans to stop this prophylaxis since he has tested negative each time. What would your response be, and why?

- Some genetic diseases are first manifested in adulthood although the mutant gene is present prenatally.
- Taking a correct family history over 3 generations may provide indications that a common disorder has a genetic basis in a given person or family.
- The nurse in the coronary care unit is talking with the wife of a 34-year-old man recently admitted with a myocardial infarction. The wife mentions that her husband is frightened because his father died of a "heart attack" at 32 years of age. What are the appropriate next steps for the nurse and why?

11

Psychiatric and Mental Health Nursing

The genetics of cognitive abilities, mental functioning, social attitudes, psychological interests, psychiatric disorders, learning disorders, behavior, addiction, mood, and personality traits have long been of interest to geneticists. This interest has been complicated by the complexity of brain function as well as the social, ethical, legal, and political implications of research in this area. Also complicating study is the tendency for such conditions to be too broadly defined, thus perhaps diluting the possible gene associations. For example, it is more fruitful to look for a specific type of genetic variation connected with a more narrowly defined communication disorder such as expressive, mixed, phonologic, and so on rather than the broadly used term. The contribution of genetic factors to the major types of mental illnesses such as schizophrenia and the mood or affective disorders (including major depressive disorders and bipolar disease) have been investigated.

The observations that disorders affecting mental health and behaviors tend to run in families is claimed as support for all of these theories. Biological families tend to share their genes, their cultural heritage, and their living environment, which includes similar exposure to pathogens, diet, stressors, toxins, dynamic family interactions, patterns of behavior, and other parameters. There has been increasing support for investigation into the contribution of genetic factors in mental illness and behavior. For example, a major workshop on schizophrenia recommended that major efforts be concentrated on looking for predisposing genes. Disorders known to be due to a single gene error

(e.g., Lesch-Nyhan syndrome), uniparental disomy (e.g., Prader-Willi syndrome), or a chromosomal variation (e.g., Klinefelter syndrome) can have effects manifested in terms of behavior. There has been increasing recognition of patterns of behavior that accompany some genetic disorders, and the term *behavioral phenotype* has been applied to these. These can provide genetic leads to areas for further exploration of chromosome and gene areas that may be responsible for certain behaviors. Many of the genetic disorders can be modified by their external environment, so that behavioral effects may or may not be apparent (e.g., phenylketonuria when phenylalanine is restricted). In multifactorial disorders, a model for the interaction of genes and environment is already present. It is realistic to expect that genetic factors are at least in part responsible for the etiology of the major psychoses, with the question being to what extent. It is also likely that in some relatively rare families, the abnormal phenotype such as schizophrenia may be determined by a single gene error, whereas in others, a different gene may confer a susceptibility that depends on certain environmental conditions or triggers or another gene variation for expression.

The initial establishment of the broad categories of classical schizophrenia and affective, bipolar, or manic depressive, illness was largely based on descriptive symptoms. These categories have been further subdivided over time, but they still represent somewhat heterogenous subtypes that may, as in diabetes mellitus, represent more than one disease and etiology with different inheritance mechanisms. Previously, varying differences in nomenclature and in what was included in "schizophrenia" over the years has made genetic study and interpretation difficult. The major evidence for the role of genetic factors in schizophrenia and the mood disorders originally came from family studies, twin studies, adoption studies, and biochemical analyses. More recently, genetic modeling, linkage, whole-genome linkage and association studies, proteomic approaches, whole-network gene expression studies, and other molecular genetic techniques are being used to understand the genetic contribution. Most of the early studies and techniques suffered from methodological problems, but nearly all of them documented some type of genetic component. At this time, however, the exact nature of the genetic contribution to the major mental disorders remains unknown. Another way in which genetic contribution has been studied is by examining drug action and effects on psychiatric disorders and using that information to examine gene variations that might be relevant. Nurses practicing in the mental health area are integral to genetic-related issues in other ways. Counseling and therapy skills related to issues surrounding the diagnosis of a family member with a genetic disorder, whether it be a birth defect in an infant or another type of disorder in the adult, include feelings of shock, denial, stigma, guilt, depression, and anger. Genetic testing and treatment decisions, coping with the results, and deciding who and how to tell about the results are some of the psychological and interpersonal issues in which services may be needed.

SCHIZOPHRENIA

According to the American Psychiatric Association's *Diagnostic and Statistical Manual of Mental Disorders* (DSM IV-TR, 2000), schizophrenia is a psychotic disorder that "lasts for at least 6 months, and includes 1 month of active phase symptoms (i.e., two (or more) of the following: delusions, hallucinations, disorganized speech, grossly disorganized or catatonic behavior, negative symptoms)" (p. 273). Subtypes include paranoid, disorganized, catatonic, undifferentiated, and residual. In addition, schizoaffective disorder is a disturbance in which symptoms of schizophrenia and a mood disorder occur together. The worldwide prevalence is about 1%. Some estimate that schizophrenia has a

heritability at about 80%, but unequivocable single genes have not yet been identified.

Among the major issues in studies include whether pure schizophrenia has been analyzed or whether the clinical spectrum of schizophrenic disorders has been included. At least 40 family and twin studies have been conducted. The essence of these studies is the consistent finding that there is a higher prevalence of the respective illness among blood relatives. Those studies that have compared the concordance of monozygotic (MZ) twins for schizophrenia with that of dizygotic (DZ) twins have found in all cases that the concordance rate for MZ twins is higher than for DZ twins. Although the exact rates have varied from study to study, these findings provide support for a heritability component. Overall concordance rates have varied from 35% to 92% in MZ twins and from 7% to 26% for DZ twins, with an overall pooled rate of 45.6% for MZ and 13.7% for DZ. High concordance rates appear to be associated with severity of the illness. The age of the onset of illness shows greater association between twins than would be expected by chance. In both groups, twins who have lived apart generally show similar concordance rates to those who have been raised in the same environment.

General conclusions from adoption studies reveal that children born of schizophrenic parents developed schizophrenia at significantly higher rates than did adoptees born of normal parents. Biologic relatives of those adoptees who developed schizophrenia had higher rates of schizophrenia and suicide than did the adoptive relatives and the biologic and adoptive relatives of adoptees who did not become schizophrenic. Adoptees born of normal parents but raised by schizophrenic adoptive parents did not show an increase in schizophrenia. In order to rule out the intrauterine environment or early interaction with a schizophrenic mother, some researchers studied paternal half-siblings. These half-siblings had the same biologic schizophrenic father but a different biologic mother. The increased incidence of schizophrenia found was interpreted as ruling out early maternal influences.

More recent studies have looked at the candidate gene approach or linkage, often focusing on genes or markers having pharmacologic, immunological, and biochemical associations. Based on these, some of those explored have been the gene for catecholamine methyltransferase, which metabolizes the neurotransmitters dopamine, epinephrine, and norepinephrine, as well as both receptors and transmitters for these and for GABA (gamma-aminobutyric acid), serotonin, and monoamine oxidase. Other promising candidate genes for susceptibility include neuregulin (*NRG1*), dysbindin (*DTNBP1*), *G72*, *RGS4* (the regulator of G-protein signaling-4), proline dehydrogenase (*PRODH*) disrupted in schizophrenia 1 (*DISC1*), the gene encoding phosphodiesterase 48 (*PDE48*), and catechol-O-methyltransferease (*COMT*). Many of these are located in chromosomal areas that are linked to schizophrenia. Molecular and mapping techniques have been used. Newer strategies such as microarray technology to examine gene expression appear promising. At present, the most promising information appears to be an association or linkage for schizophrenia with the following chromosomal sites: 1q21-22, 6p22-24, 6q21-22, 8p21, 10p11-15, 13q32, and 22q11-13. A subtype of schizophrenia, periodic catatonia, was also found to be associated with chromosome 15q14. In the case of chromosome 22, chromosomal microdeletions in chromosome 22q11.21-q11.23 may increase susceptibility. A known genetic syndrome, velocardiofacial syndrome (an autosomal recessive disorder with cardiac anomalies, learning disabilities, and cleft palate, also known as DiGeorge syndrome, discussed in Chapter 9), which is associated with small deletions in chromosome 22q11, includes about 10% who develop psychiatric disorders such as chronic paranoid schizophrenia. A candidate for a susceptibility gene on 22q12-13 is the A2a adenosine receptor, one of the receptors mediating central nervous system effects of adenosine, which showed linkage to schizophrenia in some persons. There has also been the possibility for a vulnerability locus for schizophrenia located on chromosome 6p, which was first described in the Irish Study of High-Density Schizophrenia.

Another area of investigation for etiology is unstable tandem repeat expansion (Chapter 4). In at least some cases, anticipation (the appearance of more severe disease progressively earlier in successive generations) and a parent-of-origin effect has been noticed in schizophrenia, giving credence to the possible involvement of unstable tandem repeat nucleotide expansion in etiology. A theory that has had a resurgence of interest is that of events that disrupt neurodevelopment, and thus result in schiz-

ophrenia, such as Rh incompatibility and severe nutritional deficiencies. Advanced paternal age has also been associated with a higher risk for adult schizophrenia, perhaps due to de novo paternal mutations. Despite evidence for some yet unknown genetic basis for schizophrenia, environmental disturbances appear to be needed for ultimate expression. It is likely that there will be multiple susceptibility genes eventually identified that act in conjunction with other genetic configurations, epigenetic processes, and environmental factors to result in the phenotype of schizophrenia.

MOOD DISORDERS

The mood disorders (MD), formerly described as affective disorders, may consist of depressive disorders, bipolar disorders, and mood disorders secondary to a general medical condition or substance induced. They may affect at least 1% of the population. In many of the classic family, twin, and adoptive studies, results were reported in terms of unipolar illness (UP) or bipolar illness (BP). It has been proposed that there may be three distinct BP subgroups defined by age of onset with an early, middle, and late (over age 50 years) onset that might vary etiologically. In BP patients, first-degree relatives had a higher incidence of affective illness than those of UP patients, but both were higher than in the general population. If the index patient has BP disease, the risks to relatives are higher than if the index patient has UP disease state. Moreover, 80–90% of patients with BP disorders have a family history of an affective disorder, and 50% of UP patients have a family history of a UP disorder, with few having any BP disease. They believe that a family history of BP disorders is important in diagnosis of an individual with depression. There are more female relatives affected than male relatives. This may represent a sex-influenced gene or a sex-related liability threshold as seen in congenital hip disease. Twin studies over time reveal the potential of a hereditary component, and have been reported at about 70% for MZ twins and 20% for DZ twins. Concordance in MZ twins increases with the severity of the proband's illness.

Some adoption studies have been reported for the affective disorders. These basically found an excess of all psychopathology in the biologic parents of the MD adoptees as compared to their adoptive parents. This incidence has been reported as similar to that of the biologic parents of MD persons who were not adopted. The most important finding of the adoption studies is that the incidence of mental illness paralleled that of the biological relatives of the adoptee rather than the adoptive relatives.

Although biochemical and immunological studies have been investigated, linkage and molecular studies have been the most recent approaches. These have focused on susceptibility regions on chromosomes and on certain biochemical polymorphisms. The latter have included disturbances in dopaminergic and noradrenergic transmitter systems, serotonin 2A receptor (*HTR2A*) gene polymorphisms, GABA, and the glutaminergic pathways. Gene expression arrays offer new ways to look for associated differences in gene expression. Past reports of linkages in regard to chromosomes have been in conjunction with the X chromosome and chromosomes 11 and 21 but have been difficult to substantiate. X chromosome associations were suggested by an observed excess of females in mood disorders. Various studies have had contradictory findings, and a gene on the X chromosome may represent at least one susceptibility gene. The most significant linkage associations with chromosomal areas for bipolar disorder currently are as follows: 4p15-16, 9p22, 10q11, 12q23, 13q32, 14q, 18p11.2, 18q12, 18q22, 21q22, and 22q11-12. Recent approaches to depression consider it as a complex and multifactorial trait with newer ideas about the mechanisms behind it, which then suggest different candidate genes that could be investigated in a systematic way. The expansion of unstable tandem repeats has also been suggested as an etiology. In one family, Darier disease (an autosomal dominant skin disorder) has been shown to be associated with bipolar illness.

BEHAVIOR AND GENETICS

The field of behavioral genetics is complex and interesting. It is reasonable to suppose that there are genetic influences on parameters such as behavior as one considers the genetic influence on structural determination and patterning of anatomical configurations or of the regulation of neurotransmitters, for example. Many of the investigations have been carried out in animal models because of problems in studying human populations, which has been difficult because of the belief that finding a genetic component to a behavioral trait means that the trait is immutable. Rather, such traits can be molded and are indeed shaped by environmental influences. Often, understanding the genetics can lead to treatment advances. For example, persons with some types of dyslexia have responded to particular educational approaches that improve outcome. Distinct reading phenotypes may each be linked to different chromosomal regions. Mutation in the gene *FOXP2*, located on chromosome 7, which encodes a transcription factor, leads to a rare speech and language disorder. In addition, a duplication of a segment in the long arm of chromosome 7 (7q11.23) contains many genes but also corresponds to a deletion in the same region found in the Williams (also known as Williams Beuren) syndrome, which is a neurodevelopmental disorder with short stature and strong expressive language skills in addition to other features. More often, multiple genes are believed to be involved, with environmental influences as well. Genome-wide scans have identified regions on chromosomes 2, 13, 16, and 19 that may influence speech and language disorders. A recent finding in dyslexia is that about 17% had a deletion in a stretch of DNA in a gene known as *DCDC2*.

In one large family, a defect in the gene for monoamine oxidase A (MAOA) leading to deficiency resulted in an X-linked recessive mild mental retardation and a pattern of aggressive, impulsive, and violent behavior, including arson and exhibitionism. This disorder has been named Brunner syndrome. An animal model has also shown the association between deletion of the gene encoding MAOA and aggression in males. In animals, there are many examples of behavioral genetics. For example, ants can manipulate gene expression in developing juveniles so that some larvae that would have become docile workers are stimulated to become aggressive soldiers in response to a threat. A gene that controls social interactions has been found in mice. Dogs maintain specific behavioral traits within breeds. For example, a border collie will maintain eye contact with humans. If put at birth with a type of dog that does not, the border collie will continue this trait, and if another breed is put with border collies at birth, it will not develop the eye contact behavior. The eye contact behavior is an example of how a genetically determined trait may influence environment. People will respond differently to those who look directly at them as opposed to those who avoid eye contact, thus resulting in different interactions and experiences that shape development.

Persons with certain genotypes might create high-stress environments, thus increasing the probability of mental illness. A polymorphism in the dopamine D4 receptor gene that is related to novelty seeking has been reported. There has been considerable opposition to genetic study of some traits such as aggression, intelligence, criminality, personality, and sexual orientation. In one well-publicized incident, a conference on genes and criminality was postponed for a considerable time because of political issues. However, there has been a recent resurgence in the influence of genes in virtually every realm of behavior, including social attitudes, psychological interests, and even such traits as divorce (by virtue of biochemical and personality systems) and religiousness. A recent twin study found that the heritability of cognition in elderly twins was 62%. Other conditions such as alcoholism, panic disorder, and dyslexia appear to have substantial genetic components. Discussion of these is beyond this text, however. Although it seems likely that many traits have some type of genetic component, how heredity and environment build on each other in complex ways is not understood. Understanding of some of these aspects will make a real contribution to how we approach public policy issues.

Autism is a pervasive developmental disorder that usually has its onset before 3 years of age. It is characterized by impairments in reciprocal social interaction and communication and preferred repetitive, stereotyped behaviors. It may include developmental delay, dysmorphic features, and epilepsy. Autism is more frequent in males. Several closely related disorders such as Asperger syndrome and disintegrative disorder are said to comprise autism spectrum disorders. There are no biological markers for diagnosis. While observations suggest genetic effects, genome-wide linkage and candidate gene studies have shown some preliminary suggestions of the involvement of areas on chromosomes 2, 7, 13, and 15q11-13. Various gene variations have been implicated in autism, including the *RELN* gene, which codes for a protein that guides neuronal migration. As in other disorders, epigenetic and environmental factors appear to play a role, although these have not been identified.

ALCOHOLISM, SMOKING, AND ADDICTION

Not everyone who uses recreational drugs, including nicotine from smoking, meets criteria for substance abuse disorder. Thus, while variation in drug metabolism, neuronal physiology, and other biological factors is recognized as important, other factors in development and from the environment play a role. A complete discussion of these complex conditions is not possible here.

Alcoholism has been investigated in twin studies and in adoption studies, and these have provided evidence of a genetic component. Complex disorders are difficult to study, and in alcohol dependence, end points and definitions have varied. For example, items such as tolerance, acute intoxication, withdrawal symptoms, amount of alcohol consumed, and episodic versus steady consumption may be defined differently. Chief areas of interest have been variations in the gene for the mitochondrial aldehyde dehydrogenase (*ADLH2*), which converts an intermediate product of ethanol metabolism, acetaldehyde, to acetic acid. A mutation known as *ALDH2*2/*2*, and to a certain extent, the heterozygote, *ALDH2*1/*2*, results in elevated blood levels of acetaldehyde after ingesting alcohol, leading to a flushing reaction. Few with this genotype become alcohol dependent. In another example, the gene encoding the enzyme alcohol dehydrogenase (ADH) converts alcohol to acetaldehyde, and variations in its subunits also affect alcohol dependence risk in various ethnic groups. Another gene of interest has been the dopamine D2 receptor gene. A large long-term study, the Collaborative Study of the Genetics of Alcoholism, is being carried out.

Smoking behavior is thought to have both genetic and environmental components. Evidence for genetic components comes from twin studies and from variability in nicotine metabolism. Environmental and social influences are also known to be important, especially in the initiation of smoking. A group of enzymes (see Chapter 6) known as cytochrome P-450 (CYP) metabolizes nicotine to cotinine. Variations in the gene (*CYP2D6*) allow people to be poor, extensive, or ultrarapid metabolizers. People who metabolize nicotine more slowly appear less likely to become dependent, while those who are ultrarapid metabolizers may smoke more heavily to maintain their blood nicotine levels. Thus, while people may begin smoking for various reasons, becoming dependent may be related in part to metabolism. Polymorphisms of dopamine receptor genes as well as genes, encoding the opioid, cannabinoid, and glutamine receptors, may influence dependence on various drugs. Many of these genes interact with each other, influencing effects, as well as with the environment.

NURSES AND RISK REDUCTION

Nurses in this field may also be involved in assisting clients to decrease the psychological distress in individuals and families that may be associated with genetic testing, prenatal diagnosis, genetic screening, cancer risk assessment, genetic diagnoses, life adjustments, and genetic counseling. Nurses may do this in a number of ways depending on their preparation, including enhancing coping skills, stress and anxiety reduction, and providing actual counseling. For any client at risk, nurses may be able to intervene by maximizing positive environmental factors by providing or helping clients to find a supportive atmosphere and by providing access to ongoing counseling or development programs. Techniques for the reduction of stress and promotion of positive family interactions may also help to ameliorate effects due to genetic factors.

END NOTES

Behavioral genomics is an area of intense interest and renewed research now using molecular methodologies and complex data analysis made possible by technological advances such as the study of gene expression through microarrays. Currently it is believed that the contribution of single gene mutations to overall behavioral genetics is relatively rare, although such contributions illustrate that abnormal behaviors can result from these mutations. It is more widely believed that in the vast majority of cases, multiple genes contribute to behaviors and that these are influenced by both environmental factors and genes that may not appear to be directly connected with behaviors. However, when subgroups for psychiatric disorders such as bipolar disorder are examined by subcategories such as by early age of onset, there may be a greater contribution of single mutant genes such as is found in diabetes mellitus.

Genetic analysis of various behavioral phenotypes, including personality, learning disabilities, and psychiatric disorders, is still a sensitive research area because of ethical, social, and legal concerns. Various societal and ethical concerns include the introduction of behavioral genetics in the courts ("my genes made me do it") and the use in education and school settings as well as in respect to employment. For example, a gene variation may be associated with predisposition to a trait such as assertiveness. An employer might want to hire salespeople with predisposition for such a trait. In another theoretical situation, an employer might not want to hire employees with predisposition to a trait such as poor impulse control. It is expected that this area will grow in the future.

The occurrence of mental changes as side effects in drug therapy with agents such as the corticosteroids, reserpine, amphetamines, methyldopa, and others that occur in some patients receiving them may uncover further information about the etiology of mental disorders and also identify susceptible subgroups in the population.

THOUGHTS FOR DISCUSSION

- What would be the implications of genetic testing for behavioral and personality traits if such were available? Discuss in terms of both policy and health care issues.
- Should the results of genetic testing for behavioral and personality traits be made available to school principals, school nurses, and teachers if a child is found to be genetically predisposed to a trait such as shyness or hyperactivity?
- What are the implications of genetic enhancement of personality traits or intelligence?
- Would you support or oppose the use of such genetic enhancement? Why or why not?

12

Community and Public Health Nursing and Genomics

Major public health initiatives involving genomics have increased in recent years. Among the topics discussed in this chapter are screening programs, including newborn, carrier, and workplace screening; the concept of ecogenetics in relation to public health policies; the impact of environmental exposures on birth defects and genetic disorders; and exposures in the workplace.

GENETIC SCREENING

Genetic screening involves testing of populations or groups that is independent of a positive family history or symptom manifestations. Screening may include population-based programs that are commonly sponsored by hospitals, health centers, community groups, or governmental agencies and is usually conducted in individuals without symptoms to detect those who need further follow-up. Genetic testing is conducted in persons at elevated risk due to family history or to confirm diagnosis. (Genetic testing is discussed in Chapter 5.) The types of screening include:

- Heterozygote (carrier);
- Newborn screening;
- Prenatal screening aimed at all pregnant women for detection of fetal anomalies such as maternal serum screening for alpha-fetoprotein and other certain other markers discussed in Chapter 8;

- Predictive screening, which may be done in the workplace.

Although there can be differences in the use of the term *screening*, an acceptable definition is the "presumptive identification of an unrecognized disease or defect in an apparently healthy individual." Genetic screening was more specifically defined by the Committee for the Study of Inborn Errors of Metabolism (1975) of the National Academy of Sciences, and this is still the accepted definition. Essentially it is a search in a population for:

- Persons who possess genotypes that are associated with the development of genetic disease. The usual purpose is so that treatment can be instituted or the natural course of the disease altered. An example is screening newborns for phenylketonuria (PKU) in order to restrict phenylalanine in their diet to prevent intellectual disability.
- Persons with certain genotypes that are known to predispose the individual to illness. An example is the identification of individuals with G6PD deficiency who, after being identified, can avoid the precipitation of hemolytic anemia by avoiding certain foods and drugs, as discussed in Chapter 6.
- Persons who are the heterozygous carriers of recessively inherited genes that in autosomal recessive disorders (in double dose) can cause genetic disease in their descendants. An example is screening programs for the detection of Tay-Sachs carriers. This type of screening pro-

vides information to an individual so that he/she can make reproductive plans for the future. Genetic counseling, including the discussion of reproductive options and the availability of prenatal diagnosis, is an essential component of this type of screening.

- Persons with polymorphisms (variations) not now known to be associated with a disease state. This allows the gathering of information relative to the genetic makeup of the population. This may begin as research and later have therapeutic value. A common example is in the observed variation of the human blood groups.

Screening may be whole population based or may be more specifically directed, for example, to a particular ethnic group. Genetic testing is usually directed at specific persons at elevated risk.

As further technical advances in disease detection and diagnosis occur, the potential for the expansion of genetic testing and screening programs will grow. Therefore, nurses will be increasingly involved in such programs and in different practice settings. School nurses in some areas may be involved in screening programs or in the results of genetic tests for a specific child. Nurses may be responsible for or involved in planning for such a program, implementing it, and evaluating the outcomes. As genetic testing and screening become integral parts of primary care, health professionals themselves will need to understand the tests, the meaning of the results, the emotional and psychological impact of both positive and negative results, ethical and social issues engendered by testing or screening, the potential for impact on insurability and employment, and what options are available, and they must be able to provide education and interpretation of the results to clients and family members.

The major acceptable reasons for genetic screening include:

- Detection and ultimate diagnosis of a condition;
- Genetic counseling;
- Treatment;
- Supportive management;
- Successful adaptation;
- Education;

- Provision of reproductive option information;
- Offering of prenatal diagnosis and reproductive options;
- Implementation of preventive and prophylactic strategies, often to modify risk or disease severity or for early detection of disease;
- The description of the natural history of a genetic disease when no treatment is available;
- The gathering of information for research purposes such as enumeration.

The use of genetic screening for political or eugenic ends is never acceptable. Genetic screening and testing related to prenatal diagnosis, cancer, and Alzheimer disease are discussed in Chapters 5, 8, and 10.

INFORMATION BEFORE CHOOSING GENETIC TESTING OR SCREENING

Genetic testing and screening should take place within the context of adequate and appropriate education provided at the level of the client's understanding that takes into consideration and respects his/her ethnic and cultural values and beliefs. It should include access to genetic and other counseling, further diagnostic options if needed or appropriate, appropriate therapeutic interventions, and/or preventive or prophylactic strategies. The environment for informed consent and the decision to participate should be free of coercion, and understanding should be evaluated. Before undertaking testing or screening, information on health, medical, and life insurance coverage for both the testing and screening, for potential psychological consequences, and for follow-up care depending on the results should be ascertained.

PLANNING A GENETIC SCREENING PROGRAM

The stimulus to begin a specific screening program may originate in a variety of ways, and pressure for screening services often arises out of enthusiasm instead of reason. Programs may be initiated because a test for a condition has been developed, not by rational selection of a specific genetic disorder amenable to screening. Actual impetus may come from investigators or institutions interested in research or field testing, community groups at high risk for a specific disorder, legislators responding to constituent concerns, or general public pressure generated by mass media information or citizen groups interested in a specific condition. Different groups may wish to provide the screening services alone or in conjunction with a local or state health department, hospital, school, or community-based clinic, or these health care institutions may initiate screening. Important considerations in planning a genetic screening program are summarized in Table 12.1.

Because resources are not limitless and not every condition is amenable to screening, certain criteria should be considered when deciding if the disorder in question warrants the initiation of a new program or inclusion in a long-standing one. Genetic screening shares many principles and characteristics

with mass screening for nongenetic disorders, but some reflect the unique nature of genetic disorders. Genetic disorders are permanent, can be threatening to a person's self-esteem and identity, may have unintended consequences and implications for insurance and employment based on "preexisting" conditions, and have implications not only for the person being tested but also for his/her relatives and descendants because screening is not only for the actual disease state but also for the carrier condition. Several basic major questions (described next) should be addressed before making a decision on whether a mass screening program should be initiated for a particular genetic condition.

Importance of the Disorder

Is the disorder or condition for which screening is being considered an important problem? "Important" can be interpreted to mean either that it is prevalent in the population or that it is a serious

---

TABLE 12.1   Considerations in Planning a Genetic Screening Program

- Request for screening or recognition of the problem.
- Assess the need.
- Justify the need.
- Determine feasibility and appropriateness.
- Decide on the type of screening program.
- Designate the target population, its health status, and its use of the health system.
- Establish goals and objectives based on sound ethical principles.
- Consider the cultural, ethnic, and religious beliefs and practices of the population.
- Identify and seek the cooperation of both lay and professional community leaders.
- Plan the program in conjunction with these leaders (include a consumer representative).
- Rank and prioritize goals.
- Identify alternative courses of action.
- Determine the type and extent of program services to be provided.
- Identify program needs and resources—facilities, equipment personnel, and budget.
- Determine how program effectiveness will be measured and evaluated.
- Redefine objectives and goals in light of the above considerations.
- Establish policies and procedural guidelines.
- Assess the awareness and knowledge of lay and professional communities at large.
- Plan and implement the educational program using lay and professional workers.
- Recruit and train community volunteers.
- Plan publicity and media campaigns.
- Select a screening site, technique or test, and services to be offered.
- If possible, run a small trial program, evaluate it, and revise it based on the evaluation.
- Implement the screening program.
- Evaluate and revise constantly, including cost-benefit ratio and cost-effectiveness.

Note: The order of these considerations may vary. The available budget may determine the components of the program and the extent of the services or vice versa. Provision for education, counseling, follow-up of those with positive results, diagnostic referral, record keeping, privacy, and treatment provisions are essential.

problem. Individually, each genetic disease is relatively rare; however, as a group, the burden is significant. By preventing intellectual disabilities from occurring by neonatal screening for a disorder such as hypothyroidism, the cost to society of supportive or institutional care is eliminated, to say nothing of the elimination of financial and less tangible burdens to the family. Another way to evaluate the importance of a disorder is to examine its prevalence in a select high-risk population. An example would be considering the initiation of carrier testing for thalassemia in a community population of Greek ancestry in which the carrier rate would be substantially above that of the population as a whole. Such testing would consistently increase the cost-effectiveness and maximize the resources available. Another consideration includes, especially for newborn screening, questions of whether importance refers not only to high incidence but also to questions of seriousness and the potential for prevention or modification of complications, effects on short- and long-term morbidity, and potential impact and disability amelioration.

Availability of Screening Test

Is there a technique available that is suited for use in screening or detection as opposed to use in diagnosis? Such a test must meet certain criteria discussed later in this chapter. The test available may also determine the type of screening program to be offered. Testing should take place in an accredited, experienced laboratory to ensure the quality of the genetic tests. For some disorders, not every mutation known can be screened for due to logistical and cost considerations. There may also be variation in techniques used to screen for certain disorders—some may be more accurate than others.

Understanding and Potentially Altering the Natural History of the Disorder in Question

Can the disorder be favorably influenced by detection as opposed to later diagnosis? For example, would there be a point in screening all Jewish infants in a community for Tay-Sachs disease when there is no known treatment at present? Or would the maximum benefit be derived from carrier testing and prenatal diagnosis in a high-risk population subgroup? What is the appropriate population to screen for the condition in question? If a disease state itself is screened for, is there some presymptomatic or latent period that is detectable by a screening test? Another consideration that follows is whether there is an effective, acceptable, recognized treatment available that improves survival or function. If the carrier state is screened for, what are the implications of being a carrier? Is it acceptable to screen populations, identify individuals with a disorder, and then have nothing to offer them in regard to treatment? For genetic disorders, genetic counseling and the offering of reproductive options or prenatal diagnosis are usually considered legitimate screening goals. Some consider the opportunity for supportive and anticipatory management, successful adapatation, education, offering genetic counseling and prenatal diagnosis, allowing reproductive and life planning, and prevention strategies to modify risk and severity of illness as well as complications enough reason to screen. An example of the latter is the use of prophylactic treatment with penicillin and enrollment in comprehensive care to reduce the morbidity and mortality of children with sickle cell disease.

Appropriateness and Feasibility, Including Facilities for Diagnosis and Treatment

Assuming that the previous considerations are met, what facilities are needed? What are available? What other resources are needed? Are there available resources for diagnostic referral for patients with positive screening tests? What treatment facilities are available? Are laboratory facilities available and satisfactory? What else is needed? There needs to be a full program, including education, counseling, testing recalls and confirmatory testing, further diagnostic procedures, referrals to specialists, and comprehensive treatment, including a multidisciplinary approach. Is the agency considering screening the one that can best provide the service? Is the condition an appropriate one for the agency to expend resources on? Is the problem a major need for this population? Is there evidence of substantial benefit to the selected population? Is there evidence of acceptance on the part of the population? At a minimum, a screening program should:

- Have clear goals;
- Ensure appropriate education of the lay and professional segments of the target population;
- Have policies based on ethical principles;
- Provide informed consent;
- Provide privacy and confidentiality;
- Be voluntary, without coercion;
- Use a satisfactory, suitable screening technique;
- Have laboratory facilities available;
- Provide for diagnostic referral, follow-up, counseling, and record keeping;
- Have enough personnel to implement the program;
- Include a means for evaluation.

Questions have been raised whether screening programs, particularly for newborns, should be initiated for purposes of supportive and anticipatory management, life planning, and preventive strategies to modify risk and severity of illness as well as complications. Also in the case of newborns, the need for continued family-centered community coordinated treatment and care into adulthood is increasingly recognized.

Cost-Benefit and Cost-Effectiveness

A final consideration is that of program cost versus benefit. How can the cost of the screening program be justified when balanced against diagnosis after the disorder has manifested itself? For genetic disorders, the burden of disease is both tangible and intangible. A few recent cost-effectiveness studies have been undertaken. They demonstrate that the cost-benefit ratio is favorable in neonatal screening for congenital hypothyroidism. Others, like maple syrup urine disease (MSUD), may be cost-effective when it is included with other disorders in newborn screening programs but would be less cost-effective if a community at large was screened for carriers of MSUD given the low incidence and a relatively undefined population at risk. Also, using one specimen for multiple screening tests means that screening very early in life can miss some disorders such as PKU, whereas if it is done later, damage from others such as MSUD will already have occurred. Another issue is whether cost should include human suffering. Should, for example, newborn screening be done universally for all detectable metabolic conditions because no cost should be spared to detect even one affected newborn?

ELEMENTS IN ORGANIZATION OF THE PROGRAM

Once it has been determined that screening for a particular genetic disorder is appropriate, justified, and feasible, other planning should begin. These elements will vary depending on the type of program. Some of these are discussed next.

Types of Screening

The choice of a type of screening program evolves from the previously discussed definition of genetic screening. Of these, the two most frequent purposes of screening are for detection either of the disease state itself or the carrier state. The most common type of screening for genetic disease states is in newborns, usually to allow the earliest possible treatment and management to be instituted so that damage can be minimized. Programs for detection of carriers of deleterious autosomal or X-linked recessive disorders are most often conducted among young adults in specific population groups in outpatient or community settings in order to provide genetic counseling, give information on reproductive choices, and offer prenatal diagnostic services. Screening for the carrier state is not always as feasible as detecting the actual disease state, even if it is desirable. A test may not be able to distinguish between the normal state and the carrier state, only between normal and diseased. Specific aspects of carrier screening are discussed later. Knowledge of elements of the genetic disorder such as its frequency in different population subgroups, available test capability, and choice of screening program type help to determine the population that should be screened in a specific community, whether it be on the basis of age, race, ethnic origin, or some other parameter. Some are geared to young adults in specific ethnic groups, as in premarital screening, so reproductive options can be clarified.

Target Population

Delineation of a target group at whom the screening program is directed also helps to make decisions about other program elements, such as location, educational approach, time, format, types of counseling, facilities, equipment, and publicity. For example, if the screening is aimed at young adult couples, weekdays from 9:00 am to 5:00 pm will not yield the largest number of participants. If young children or mothers are part of the target group, child care facilities should be planned, perhaps in conjunction with volunteer groups in the community. Any particular social, cultural, or religious practices affecting the population to be screened should be identified. For example, a Tay-Sachs carrier screening program in an orthodox Jewish neighborhood held on a Saturday will show few, if any, attendees. These aspects are more important in screening populations other than newborns, as that setting (the hospital) usually is predetermined and the newborn is essentially a captive population, whereas for others, screening is voluntary. The geographic area covered by screening will also delineate the target group. For a young population of high school education or less, educational information may be presented in a multimedia format or use a "soap opera" or "true confession" approach.

Site, Facilities, and Resources

An appropriate screening site must be selected. It should be easily accessible to the target population. It should have the space to include all the resources that are deemed necessary for the program such as an area and facilities for activities in Box 12.1. Requirements may vary if the actual processing of the specimen takes place on-site or somewhere else and if diagnostic referral facilities, counseling and follow-up services, or other program components are located on-site or elsewhere. The screening site will also be influenced by whether plans are for an ongoing program, a short-term program, or a one-shot screening. Screening programs have been held in such diverse locations as shopping malls, churches, schools, neighborhood health centers, barber and beauty shops, laundromats, street corners, hospitals, clinics, physicians' offices, and work settings. Selection depends on the aims of the program, the needs of the targeted population, and accessibility for that population. Selected steps in a community screening program are shown in Figure 12.1.

While screening in a temporary site such as a neighborhood facility may help to increase participation in the screening program, disadvantages also are possible. One important consideration is establishing a permanent location or base for the data collected during screening, such as the person's personal information and test results. After an initial mass screening program, it may be most effective to incorporate screening in additional individuals into a permanent health-related institution. Records could then be maintained in one place, knowledgeable people could be available for later clarification about the disorder, and people needing further services could obtain them.

If personnel resources need supplementing, volunteers from the target population are sometimes used, but the clients' privacy and confidentiality should be maintained. These issues should be addressed before recruitment, not after.

Characteristics of a Suitable Screening Test

The qualities sought in selecting a test for use in a genetic screening program are listed in Box 12.2. Few tests fulfill all desired qualities equally well. Such qualities as absolute precision may be sacrificed for others such as low cost, as further confirmatory diagnostic workups need to be done anyway if positive results are found. The more quickly a test can be performed, the greater the benefit to both client and provider. Waiting time will be decreased, minimizing the number of clients who may decide not to participate. In addition, a greater volume of people can be served in a shorter time, adding to increased cost-effectiveness as fewer provider personnel may be needed.

The test procedure and specimen should be subject to as little clerical processing, handling, and

---

BOX 12.1

Facilities Needed for Screening Activities

- For intake and reception
- Where education before screening can be carried out
- Where needed personal data can be confidentially obtained
- For waiting before the actual screening test
- For child care facilities if needed
- Where the test procedure is done
- For administrative purposes
- For specimen collection and storage
- For maintenance of records
- For genetic counseling

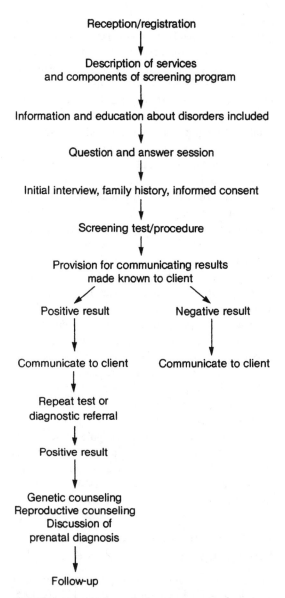

Reception/registration

↓

Description of services
and components of screening program

↓

Information and education about disorders included

↓

Question and answer session

↓

Initial interview, family history, informed consent

↓

Screening test/procedure

↓

Provision for communicating results
made known to client

↙   ↘

Positive result   Negative result

↓   ↓

Communicate to client   Communicate to client

↓

Repeat test or
diagnostic referral

↓

Positive result

↓

Genetic counseling
Reproductive counseling
Discussion of
prenatal diagnosis

↓

Follow-up

FIGURE 12.1   Selected steps in a community screening program at the site.

storage as possible in order to keep accuracy to a maximum. Simplicity in technique will also help to decrease error. Sensitivity and specificity are important in discussing screening tests, as are the related concepts of true positive, false positive, true negative, and false negative. Ideally, a screening test should be both highly sensitive and highly specific and have a low percentage of both false-positive and false-negative results. The sensitivity of a test measures the accuracy of the screening test in giving a

positive result in all subjects having the disease being screened for. For a test to be 100% sensitive, it must correctly identify all people having the disorder in question. The specificity of a test is its accuracy in giving a negative result in all those who do not have the disease being screened for. For a test to be 100% specific, it must correctly discriminate all those who do not have the disorder in question. A test that is not sufficiently sensitive does not recognize all those who do have the disease. A nonspecific test can falsely identify a healthy person as one who has the disease. In the apparently healthy population group being screened, there are actually two subgroups of people: those who have the disorder and those who do not. There are also two possible results of the screening test used to discriminate between these two groups of people: normal (negative) and abnormal (positive). The term *true positive* is used to denote those people who had a positive (abnormal) test result and also have the disorder. *False positive* is used for those who had a positive test result but do not have the disease. The term *true negative* is used to denote individuals who had a negative (normal) test result and are truly free of the disorder. *False negative* refers to individuals who have a negative test result but actually have the disorder in question. These relationships are illustrated in Table 12.2. Tests giving low rates of both false-positive and false-negatives are most desirable. A high level of false-positive results will result in

TABLE 12.2   Matrix Relating Health Status and Test Result

	Health Status	
Test result	Persons With Disease	Persons Without Disease
Positive (abnormal)	True Positives (A)	False Positives (B)
Negative (normal)	False Negatives (C)	True Negatives (D)

$$\frac{A}{A+C} \times 100 = \text{Sensitivity (in \%)} \qquad \frac{B}{B+D} \times 100 = \text{Specificity (in \%)}$$

overreferral for further diagnosis and a high cost, whereas a high number of false negatives will result in missing the individuals who are being sought, depriving them of treatments and thus decreasing the effectiveness of screening.

As an example, if one were setting up a blood pressure screening program for the detection of hypertension, a decision would have to be made as to what would constitute an abnormal blood pressure reading. If a reading of 130/80 mmHg were chosen, one would be relatively sure individuals with hypertension would be detected. However, one would also classify many individuals as hypertensive who were not (false positives). Thus, the detection program would be highly sensitive but nonspecific. If a reading of 160/100 mmHg were chosen, one would be relatively sure all those who did not have hypertension were not classified as positive, but many of those who were hypertensive would be missed (false negatives). Thus, there would be a high level of specificity but low sensitivity.

Another term also associated with the previous discussion is that of *predictive value. Positive predictive value* refers to the probability that the disorder screened for is present when the test is positive, while *negative predictive value* is the probability that disease is not present when the screening test is negative. The test or measure chosen for the screening program being established should be a valid indicator of the disease. It should be a true measure of the disorder in question. It should not be subject to a wide variety of interpretations. There should be agreement on what the results mean. Establishing ranges of normal and abnormal for the measure being used should be done before beginning a screening program. An accredited, reputable, experienced laboratory with established quality control standards should provide services. Despite all precautions, errors in results of tests can still occur. These are summarized in Table 12.3.

Several of these errors can be minimized by proper handling of the specimen. Others are dependent on the characteristics of the participant in screening such as diet and medication ingested. Information regarding these should accompany the specimen submitted. A not uncommon source of

TABLE 12.3   Factors Responsible for Inaccurate Screening Test Results

False Negatives
  Unusual variant present
  Too early for defect present to be manifested
  Disorder is detectable only under certain conditions (e.g., stress)
  Inadequate nutritional intake
  Loss of specimen material

False Positives
  Medications
  Special infant diets (e.g., soybean formulas)
  Hyperalimentation
  Transient metabolic aberration
  Production of a metabolite interfering with test
  Hypersensitivity of laboratory test used

Both
  Improper handling of specimen
  Improper storage of specimen
  Poor laboratory reliability
  Clerical error
  Delay in processing specimen
  Immature enzyme systems
  Improper laboratory procedures

error in newborn screening for metabolic errors occurs because the infant has not yet ingested enough formula or substrate to ascertain any abnormal processing. Another problem leading to false-positive findings results when a test is done early in life is that a particular infant has an immature enzyme system, which is not indicative of disease process but is only transient. An infant may need to be retested later if clinical evidence suggests the need, even if a screening test result was negative for the disorder in question. This is why further diagnostic investigation may be needed. Occasionally, missed detection results from failure to obtain a sample or failure to transport it to the lab. Regardless of the reason, nurses should anticipate that the parents will experience anxiety and apprehension when called for retesting. The qualities that most concern the client in a screening program are those of acceptability, convenience, comfort, and safety. Most clients participating in screening are volunteers who have been recruited. They usually feel well. Therefore, although they may be convinced to submit a urine specimen or allow venous blood to be drawn, it is less likely that they would allow a skin biopsy to be done or to submit to proctoscopy. For a screening program to attract large numbers of individuals from the group desired, specimens must be easily obtainable so there is a minimum of inconvenience and discomfort.

PLANNING PROGRAM COMPONENTS AND SERVICES

The aims, objectives, and policies of the specific program should be clearly delineated. The most effective way is to involve community representatives and leaders from the population group in which screening is contemplated, local health professional representatives, and representatives from local foundations for that disorder, if any exist.

These individuals should be able to assess the readiness of the population to be screened in terms of their knowledge of the condition in question. The kind of education needed prior to the screening can then be planned. Thus, education may be not only for the population being screened, but also for health professionals. For such professionals to participate by support, referral, and active involvement, they need to understand both the disorder and the aims, objectives, and components of the

screening program. Policy guidelines should be established. If a carrier screening program is aimed at young married couples, will a single person be allowed access? Will a couple in their 50s be allowed access? Equal access should be weighed against balancing harm and benefits, including test accuracy in different groups and cost-effectiveness. Such problems should be anticipated and discussed before program implementation.

The community advisory representatives will have knowledge of the sociocultural beliefs, practices, and language needs that may be unique or important to the population group and can seriously affect the success of the program. For example, who are the decision makers and authority figures in this ethnic group? What are the cultural beliefs about genetic disease? How is gender valued? Are individuals empowered in regard to decision making? How is the human body viewed and treated? Will interpreters be needed? Knowledge of these practices should be used in preparing materials and determining methods for publicity, education, counseling, follow-up, and referral. They also may affect the screening test format to be used and context in which it is explained.

Other decisions need to be made. What personal data will be collected from screening participants? What type and how long will records be kept? How will informed consent be obtained? How will results be communicated to participants? How will confidentiality be safeguarded? To whom will results be released? What will happen to the sample? Have appropriate arrangements been made for diagnostic testing for those with positive test results? What type and degree of counseling is needed? How many and what type of professionals are needed in the screening program? How will the program be evaluated? Will those with positive results be entered into a registry?

GENETIC TESTING AND SCREENING FOR HETEROZYGOTES (CARRIERS)

Each person is a carrier for 5 to 10 recessive harmful genes for rare disorders. These are so rare that usually one's chosen mate does not carry the same ones. When this does occur, genetic disease can occur in the offspring. Both carrier testing and carrier screening are available. Carrier testing is more usually done in a specialized setting and involves individuals already known to be of high risk because of family history, whereas screening usually involves those with no family history and takes place in other settings. Cystic fibrosis (CF) screening is possible, but at present there are more than 1,000 mutations of the *CFTR* gene that can result in CF, so widespread population testing is somewhat difficult, particularly in some ethnic groups, but mutation panels that identify a high percentage of carriers is possible. CF has been recommended for screening of the pregnant population and newborns. Within families, genetic testing can be much more accurate, basically directed at the most common mutation in that family, increasing the detection rate greatly, especially in non-White populations.

For carrier screening in which the person does not have the disease, the basic reasons for undertaking screening for detection of the heterozygous state are to provide genetic counseling, allow life and reproductive decision making, and prenatal diagnosis if desired later. The occurrence of genetic disease in the future children of someone who is a carrier for a specific recessively inherited disorder could be prevented in several ways. A future mate can be selected who is not a carrier for the same disorder. This can be known only if there is an accurate test for detection of the carrier state. If the person has selected or wishes to select a mate who is a carrier, prevention can be achieved through exercising various reproductive options. The couple can choose to have natural children or not. If they choose to have natural children, prenatal diagnosis can often be done to detect disease in the fetus. If the fetus is affected, they can then elect to terminate the pregnancy or continue it. If they choose not to have natural children, they could avoid conception, practice birth control, or select sterilization for either or both individuals. If they wanted children, they could either adopt them or elect reproductive options such as gamete (sperm or egg) donation, in vitro fertilization, or embryo implantation preceded by preimplantation diagnosis. These choices are illustrated in Figure 12.2 and can be discussed with the individuals involved in the genetic counseling that accompanies the carrier detection program.

Screening is not yet possible for many recessively inherited genetic disorders due to poor reliability of testing measures, lack of simple or acceptable techniques for screening, or expense resulting from lack of a defined population in which to screen. Carrier

screening for Tay-Sachs, CF, beta-thalassemia, and others have been carried out in high schools. There has been some concern regarding altered self-image, stigmatization, retention and understanding of information, understanding of impact, parental consent, the acting out of adolescents in relation to rebellion from parents, and need for self-identity as reasons for making a testing decision without regard to all the consequences, and others. On the other hand, adolescents may be sexually active, and proper genetic counseling following carrier screening may be important in some high-risk groups.

TAY-SACHS DISEASE: A PROTOTYPE

Tay-Sachs disease is considered to be the prototype for carrier screening. An infant born with this disease, in which GM_2 ganglioside accumulates in cells of the nervous system, appears normal until about 6 months of age. From then on, progressive mental and physical deterioration occurs, and death is inevitable, usually by 4 years of age. The basic defect is a lack of the enzyme hexosaminadase A (Hex A), which can result from a number of different mutations in the *HEXA* gene. The following characteristics made this disorder very amenable to heterozygote screening programs:

- There is a detectable reduction in Hex A activity in Tay-Sachs carriers, and DNA analysis is also possible.
- A simple, inexpensive test is available for detection of carriers that meets the criteria specified earlier for screening tests.
- Prenatal diagnosis is available.
- The mutant gene is concentrated in a specific population group: Jews of Eastern European (Ashkenazi) ancestry, particularly from one area of Poland and Lithuania.
- The carrier rate in Ashkenazi Jews is approximately 1 in 27–30 individuals, thus defining a high-risk population group.
- The natural course of the disease is progressive, inevitable, and fatal, thus making it a severe physical, emotional, and financial burden.
- The lack of any treatment has made the option of terminating an affected pregnancy a less controversial option than it might have been otherwise.

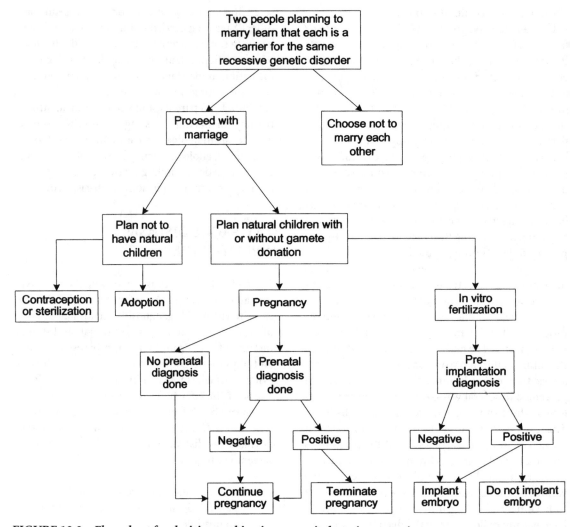

FIGURE 12.2   Flow chart for decision making in premarital carrier screening.

Jews who practice their religion according to the orthodox Jewish code do not generally subscribe to sterilization, abortion, or artificial insemination. Abortion can be permitted in specific cases with permission of rabbinical authorities. Conservative and reform Judaism take more liberal views. All three groups maintain interest in premarital Tay-Sachs disease screening. In some traditional Jewish communities, the results of Tay-Sachs screening are considered when marital matchmaking is undertaken by professional matchmakers. A special program begun in Israel, and offered in other places as well, the Chevra Dor Yeshorim Program, was designed to avoid Tay-Sachs disease in Hasidic Jews, who oppose abortion and contraception. In essence, in this program, when a woman or man turns 18 or 20 years of age, respectively, his/her blood is anonymously tested for Tay-Sachs and the number recorded in a registry. When a couple is about to arrange a match, the matchmaker or a couple can query the registry. If both are carriers, they are told that another match will be arranged.

All of these considerations led many years ago to the initiation of large-scale Tay-Sachs disease screening in Jewish communities in Baltimore and Washington, D.C. Since then, a large number of Jewish communities have participated in Tay-Sachs disease screening, and research has been conducted on various aspects of the program. This program has served as a model for others. Some of the points discovered in this program are of interest: word of mouth and media were the most effective ways of drawing participants; when new members joined a synagogue, the rabbi provided information about Tay-Sachs screening availability; the highest-ranking reasons for participation were desire to have children and perception of susceptibility.

SCREENING FOR SELECTED OTHER GENETIC DISEASES

A number of selected genetic diseases have been proposed for inclusion in population screening programs of various types, including those with recessive inheritance and those with pharmacogenomic implications. Some have been suggested for inclusion in newborn screening as discussed below, and others for later. These include factor V Leiden mutations, prothrombin 20210A mutation, methylenetetrahydrofolate reductase mutation C677T, polymorphism of the angiotensin I-converting enzyme, hereditary hemochromatosis as discussed in Chapter 10, and the A1555G mutation in the mitochondrial genome associated with aminoglycoside ototoxicity (see Chapter 6).

Factor V is part of the coagulation cascade eventually forming clots. The factor V Leiden mutation is present in about 2–15% of the general population, being most common in Caucasians, occurring in about 1.2% of African-Americans, and rare in Asian populations. It leads to a prevalent form of hereditary thrombophilia. It has a synergistic effect with certain environmental factors such as contraceptive drugs and other genes such as the prothrombin 21210A mutation. Factor V Leiden heterozygotes have a risk of about 10% for venous thrombosis, while it may be up to 80% for homozygotes. It is considered a risk factor for venous thromboembolism in pregnancy and needs to be assessed in the context of family history and past history of thrombosis. It can also result in pregnancy loss and placental abruption. It is still controversial as to whether to screen women for factor V Leiden mutations before prescribing oral contraceptives.

NEWBORN SCREENING

Newborn screening is one of the great genetic public health success stories. Once PKU was found to be associated with a type of intellectual disability that could be prevented if a low-phenylalanine diet was instituted soon after birth, a search began for a method to reliably detect PKU in newborns. Robert Guthrie developed such a test using blood taken from the neonate by heel stick with a few drops placed on filter paper and dried. Testing was based on a bacterial growth inhibition assay using the dried blood spot. This test became the prototype for screening virtually the entire newborn population. If an abnormal screening test was identified, a low phenylalanine (phe) diet could be instituted, further diagnostic confirmation could be initiated, and effective treatment put in place for those whose diagnosis was confirmed. In the early 1960s, newborn screening for PKU, after some initial opposition to the concept of government-mandated testing, rapidly became part of state maternal-child health programs. Newer technology, such as tandem mass spectrometry (MS/MS) and the expansion of molecular and DNA-based techniques, has identified additional mutations that fit accepted reasons for genetic screening and provided ways to detect them. Thus, the number of disorders that can be detected in the newborn has vastly increased to nearly 60, but states vary as to which disorders are included in their newborn screening panels.

The fact that some newborns will be screened for the full panel of available newborn screening tests, and some will not, depending on the state in which they are born, has been called a major public health inequity. Advocacy by parents has attracted popular press attention to this problem. Articles in the popular press and electronic media have highlighted cases of adverse consequences of potentially detectable metabolic disease in newborns that were not detected because the state in which the parents resided did not include those conditions in their state screening programs, as well as stories in which an infant was identified through newborn screening with a rare disorder and treated.

CASE EXAMPLE

One example that provoked activism by parents was that of a 6-month-old South Dakota infant who developed a rotavirus infection with diarrhea and vomiting. He took Pedialyte but had little else but was not dehydrated. He was found dead in his crib the next morning, and sudden infant death syndrome was thought to be the cause; however, autopsy revealed fatty accumulation in the liver. These changes plus the history of reduced caloric intake led to further testing, which revealed that he had medium chain acyl-CoA dehydrogenase (MCAD) deficiency, described below. One of the reasons for including this disorder in routine newborn screening programs is that affected children and families can receive necessary preventive education and therapy and in many cases avert untoward incidents.

The major reason for universal newborn screening is to identify at-risk infants who are apparently healthy, provide early treatment for certain disorders as soon as possible, and thereby prevent serious health consequences, especially severe intellectual disabilities. Infants with abnormal initial testing results usually have second screens and, depending on the results, further testing in order to confirm a diagnosis, but temporary treatment may be started in the interim if believed necessary. Many of the disorders detectable by newborn screening tests respond well to early treatment such as dietary restrictions.

Newborn screening must be concerned not only with screening and testing but with other components, such as:

- Education;
- Recalls and short-term follow up;
- Genetic counseling;
- Diagnosis;
- Referral to specialists;
- Management;
- Treatment;
- Nursing;
- Social and psychological services, in the short and long terms;
- Reproductive choices and life planning;
- Assistance in other areas such as schools, setting standards, quality assurance, and evaluation, ideally functioning as a coordinated system.

Newborn screening programs typically fall under a state's public health department. Typically states routinely screen newborns for a set of metabolic disorders and others as required by statute. States may also routinely screen newborns by blood specimen or other assessment for conditions of genetic or nongenetic causation such as congenital hearing loss, developmental hip dysplasia, human immunodeficiency virus (HIV) infection, and congenital toxoplasmosis. There have been a variety of standards and guidelines developed regarding criteria for inclusion of a disorder within screening programs, some specific to universal state newborn screening.

From time to time, states add disorders to mandated newborn screening programs, sometimes as a temporary pilot that may be:

- Universally applied;
- Applied for specific selected populations deemed to be at greatest risk;
- Included on a limited basis;
- Performed only by request.

For example, California recently added the option of additional screening for 25 more disorders but still does not implement biotinidase deficiency or congenital hearing loss as routine. The Save Babies Through Screening advocacy group (http://www.savebabies.org/release1-07.02.htm) recommends screening newborns for 55 diseases, which would require considerable cost and personnel, time as well as several procedures, and might engender parental anxiety. The following genetic disorders are mandated for newborn screening in most states:

- PKU
- Congenital hypothyroidism
- Hemoglobinopathies such as sickle cell disease
- Galactosemia
- Tyrosinemia
- Maple syrup urine disease
- Biotinidase deficiency
- Congenital adrenal hyperplasia
- Medium-chain acyl-CoA dehydrogenase (MCAD) deficiency
- Cystic fibrosis
- Homocystinuria

The District of Columbia screens for glucose-6-phosphate dehydrogenase (G6PD) deficiency (see Chapter 3). These are further discussed below. States also mandate screening for other conditions such as congenital hearing loss, which may be genetic or nongenetic, congenital toxoplasmosis (see

Chapter 8), and, in the case of New York, HIV infection. Other countries include conditions not currently mandated for inclusion in U.S. newborn screening programs and vice versa.

Changes and proposed adjustments are now being made in screening programs due to new genetic knowledge that:

- Has made detection of a given disorder possible;
- Allowed development of new technology for detection and analysis;
- Led to the availability of new or better treatment options, thus making a disorder fit the usual criteria for newborn screening.

These are reasons that assessment of which disorders to include or add must be an important component of the total program. The availability of MS/MS as an analytic technique allows about 30 different metabolic conditions to be screened for in the neonatal period using the same blood specimen. The technique does not, however, screen for every disorder included in screening programs such as galactosemia and biotinidase deficiency.

A mass spectrometer is a piece of equipment that separates and quantifies ions based on their mass/charge ratios that can use routinely obtained dried blood spot specimens. Data are transferred to a computer for analysis. Advantages include rapidity of analysis; greater accuracy than conventional methods, allowing screening for certain disorders to be more specific and sensitive; ability to detect disorders formerly difficult to detect; and the ability to screen for multiple diseases in a single run, including amino acid, fatty acid oxidation, and organic acid disorders. An issue is that some disorders can be detected at one or two days after birth by this means, but others are not detectable until the newborn is 5 days or older. This time is usually after hospital discharge, meaning that responsibility for additional specimen collection from a primary health provider or public health clinic is needed. Thus, primary care practitioners, including nurses, are responsible for ascertaining that newborns referred to their practices have been screened and results have been returned. Often nurses are instrumental in ensuring that these initial and follow-up specimens are collected.

The finding that in Virginia, undiagnosed metabolic diseases were identified in 1% of unexpected deaths during a 5-year study period and that 5% of all sudden infant deaths might be associated with metabolic diseases suggests that the use of tandem mass spectrometry routinely in newborn screening programs may have a positive impact. In some states, there is an option offered to parents to choose to test their newborn for additional disorders for an additional fee through the same channels that administer the mandated program or through other facilities such as private or university laboratories. Options for many of these tests are available directly to the consumer through Internet offerings as well, and regulation of this kind of test offering has been proposed. Eventually DNA-based technology will be used routinely for newborn screening, replacing or augmenting current technology.

State regulation of newborn screening is highly variable. There is no national policy that determines which disorders should be screened for or establishes uniform components of newborn screening programs such as procedures for the communication of test results, especially in cases where initial specimens yield a "panic" result requiring immediate notification and action. States may vary in which tests they use to detect a given condition and in what results or parameters constitute an abnormal test result. For example, states may define an abnormal screening test result for PKU as greater than 4, 10, 12, or 15 mg/dL or may state "as determined by metabolic specialists" (National Institutes of Health Consensus Development Panel, 2000). The end result is a great variety in newborn screening statutes, regulations, and requirements. Important elements of newborn screening programs are in Box 12.3. A detailed discussion is beyond the scope of this book. See Lashley (2005) for additional information.

In 2000, a report on newborn screening was issued by the Task Force on Newborn Screening of the American Academy of Pediatrics at the request of the Maternal and Child Health Bureau, Health Resources and Services Administration (HRSA), Department of Health and Human Services. This report did not specify which tests should be included nationally, although many expected that it would. The designation of tests was left to the states, although efforts to try to establish a minimum core set of tests for the nation are underway through the Maternal and Child Health Bureau. Some of the decision making of states has been based on the racial and ethnic population of those states and the most prevalent genetic disorders of those ethnic groups

---

BOX 12.3

Important Elements in Newborn Screening Programs

- Inclusion of all neonates before hospital discharge according to state laws and guidelines
- Provision to include neonates not tested before discharge and those born outside the hospital as soon as possible
- Education of parents about screening at appropriate educational levels considering cultural beliefs—reasons, what is involved, how the communication of results is handled, and others
- Informed parental consent within state laws
- Collection of appropriate specimens at proper times
- Reliable, accurate, standardized testing in a centralized laboratory
- Provision for rescreening if the infant is tested too early
- Communication of positive screening results to local physician or health care practitioner and parents quickly (by telephone with letter of confirmation), ideally with counseling and psychosocial support available to help with anxiety engendered
- Prompt follow-up of all newborns with positive screening tests
- Means of accurate diagnosis quickly available for all with confirmed positive screening tests
- Provision for genetic and other counseling that is culturally competent and educationally appropriate
- Provision for treatment and ongoing management of infant and family

---

since certain disorders are known to be prevalent in certain ethnic groups and rare in others, with cost-effectiveness as a driving force. Some have suggested that some disorders do not need to be universally tested for but can be targeted by ethnic group, a practice that in our ethnically mixed society may be genetically as well as ethically unsound, although some states are piloting targeted newborn screening for certain disorders. While the recommendations in this report are too numerous to cover in their entirety, following are some of the other major emphases in this report (American Academy of Pediatrics, 2000):

- Newborn screening is changing rapidly, and public health departments may not be keeping up with changes in technology, genetic discoveries, and increased advocacy efforts. There is a need for federal and state public health agencies in partnership with health professionals and consumers to better define responsibilities.
- Public health agencies need to involve families, health professionals, and the public in the development, operation, and oversight of newborn screening information.

- Effective newborn screening systems require an adequate public health infrastructure and must be integrated within the health care delivery system, with children being linked to a medical home to ensure appropriate care and treatment for medical, nonmedical, psychosocial, and educational needs of the child and family in the local community. This need for comprehensive long-term care was emphasized also by the Consensus Panel on Phenylketonuria (PKU): Screening and Management.
- Public health agencies need to ensure adequate financial mechanisms.
- Cost-effectiveness may be defined in various ways.
- The cost of screening has not included the needed infrastructure in most studies. Some studies have looked at cost only in regard to the screening test, but other elements, including cost of finding and informing families and reporting results, should be done.
- Model systems of care and support from infancy to adulthood for infants identified with disorders in newborn screening programs need to be designed and evaluated.

- National criteria need to be developed for adding disorders to state screening panels, but the report did not specify these or the disorders.
- Identified issues of state-to-state variance in uniformity about tests and educational information about the process are needed to be sure that prospective parents are aware of the process.
- Parents have the right to be informed about screening and the right to refuse it.
- Families have the right to confidentiality and privacy protections for newborn screening results.
- Parents need to be informed about benefits as well as potential risks of tests and treatments, use of specimens in the future, storage policies, and how they will receive test results.

In response to this report, the March of Dimes issued a statement in 2000 calling for nationally mandated newborn testing for the following diseases: PKU, hypothyroidism, galactosemia, sickle cell disease, congenital adrenal hyperplasia, biotinidase deficiency, maple syrup urine disease, and homocystinuria. Since that time, they have added MCAD and congenital hearing loss to this list.

The March of Dimes also called for:

- Abandoning currently available tests for new tests if the new test achieves a greater precision or a shorter turnaround time regardless of the cost differential;
- Putting safeguards in place for timely reporting of test results;
- Ensuring uniform quality of newborn screening tests nationwide, including an overarching authority to ensure this;
- Ensuring that every newborn have the same core of screening tests by mandate and that those be the best available even if the test is for a rare disease if that diagnosis can make a difference in the child's health (Howse & Katz, 2000).

The Maternal and Child Health Bureau commissioned the American College of Medical Genetics to address various issues in newborn screening including model policies and a recommended uniform core panel of genetic conditions that should be screened for nationally. They recommended 29 core conditions (Watson, Lloyd-Puryear, Mann, Rinaldo, & Howell, 2006) and online at www.mchb .hrsa.gov/screening (accessed August 17, 2006).

Some states have opted to allow parents to choose to have supplemental screening tests at outside labs at a moderate extra cost, such as $25. Some of the companies and universities offering this service advertise on the Internet with full instructions for parents. One of the problems identified is not the cost of the $25 for testing, but the money needed to fund the state infrastructure for recall and short-term follow-up, diagnosis, treatment, management, quality assurance, and program evaluation for many more conditions than originally planned.

Disorders Included in Newborn Screening

Because newborn screening is in an ever-changing state, additions may be made to the disorders in current detection programs. Disorders may also be discontinued if the detection rate is low in a particular state. Because nurses are likely to need information about disorders routinely screened for in newborns in order to assess the newborn intelligently, to communicate with and educate parents of newborns and infants, and to explain the need for further testing if an abnormal result is found, a brief synopsis of these are in Table 12.4. PKU is discussed in more detail below. The advent of mass newborn screening has shown that many of these disorders are more common than formerly believed. Infants dying from some inborn errors in the past were simply not diagnosed as having the disorder. Many were thought to have died of overwhelming sepsis, so the true disease incidence was not recognized. Some symptoms that should lead the nurse to consider recommending or referring the infant for screening test batteries for inherited biochemical disorders are discussed in Chapter 9. If the infant is diagnosed, siblings should be tested in case they have the disorder but have not manifested it, and they may benefit from treatment.

Another issue surrounding newborn screening is whether screening should be done for diseases that are not treatable or for those with no known clinical repercussions such as histidinemia, formerly included in some state newborn screening programs but now

TABLE 12.4 Disorders Commonly Included in Newborn Screening Programs

Disorder	Incidence	Number of States Requiring Inclusion[a]	Description
Biotinidase deficiency	1:60,000–1:137,000	40	AR disorder. Various degrees of severity. Typically symptoms begin at 3–5 months but can be as early as 1 week or even present at 10–12 years of age. Clinical picture includes myoclonic seizures, hypotonia, feeding difficulties, fungal infections, vomiting, diarrhea, ketoacidosis, coma, alopecia, skin rash, ataxia, developmental delay, lethargy, respiratory, vision and hearing problems. In severe cases can see acute metabolic decompensation. Treatment consists of daily free biotin supplementation.
Congenital adrenal hyperplasia	Depends on type, 1:10,000–1:18,000	45	AR inheritance for all types. 90% due to 21-hydroxylase deficiency; other types due to 11β-hydroxylate deficiency and 17α-hydroxylase deficiency. Several forms; some are mild, not appearing until adulthood. In the most common type, androgen hypersecretion results in masculinization of female fetuses and infants with ambiguous external genitalia, while in males premature pubic hair appears between 6 months and 2 years of age. Treatment is cortisol replacement therapy and correction of ambiguous genitalia.
Congenital hearing loss	1–3:1,000	28	Bilateral, profound congenital hearing loss can arise from a number of genetic causes with varying modes of transmission or infection such as cytomegalovirus. Connexin 26 gene mutations account for about 20% of childhood deafness. Early detection is important for optimal language development.
Congenital hypothyroidism	1:3,600–1:5,000	51	Congenital thyroid deficiency results from transient (prematurity and maternal antithyroid medications) and nontransient causes including congenital deficiency of thyroid tissue, deficiency of thyrotopin releasing hormone, thyroid stimulating hormone (TSH) deficiency, impaired response to TSH secretion, and more. States vary in test used. If needed, therapy should begin no later than 1 month of age to prevent intellectual disability. Confirmatory diagnosis must be done as quickly as possible and treatment started immediately. Can be from genetic or nongenetic causes. Inheritance depends on type.
Cystic fibrosis	Varies with population—for example, 1:2,500 in Whites; 1:323,000 in Japanese	33	See Chapter 8 for clinical description. Screening for CF has been somewhat controversial because there are more than 1,000 mutations of the CFTR gene and because there is a question of the advantages offered by early detection. Currently it is believed that benefits can include reproductive planning, implementation of therapy that can maximize health, and nutrition.
Galactosemia	1:40,000–1:60,000	51	Defect in metabolism of galactose has several variants. The classic deficiency is in galactose 1-phosphate uridyltransferase. AR inheritance. Infant appears normal until feeding begins, and galactose and other metabolites accumulate. Signs/symptoms include vomiting, diarrhea,

			jaundice, failure to thrive, cataract development, hepatomegaly, hypoglycemia, and eventually intellectual disability. Susceptible to *Escherichia coli* infections. Often mistaken for milk allergy. In the older child and adult, may see delayed speech and language, learning disabilities, ataxia, tremor, and behavioral disorders. In females, ovarian failure, premature menopause, amenorrhea, and hypogonadism may be seen. Early elimination of lactose from the diet is essential.
Hemoglobinopathies	51	Depends on type	Can include Hb SS, Hb SC, Hb S/β-thalassemia. See Chapters 3 and 9. No direct newborn treatment
Homocystinuria	41	1:150,000–1:200,000	AR inheritance. Deficiency or impairment of cystathionine beta-synthetase or methionine synthetase. Some are responsive to pyridoxine. More frequent in Ireland, England, and Australia; rare in Japan. Mild to moderate intellectual disability in about half. Clinical picture includes skeletal abnormalities such as kyphosis, scoliosis, pectus excavatum, tallness with excessively long limbs, osteoporosis, sparse and fragile hair; malar flush, spontaneous intravascular thromboses occur and in some cases lead to seizures. Dislocation of the lens occurs by 6 to 10 years of age. Often confused with Marfan disease. Treatment depends on cause but usually includes pyridoxine supplementation to responsive patients and dietary restrictions with betaine supplementation.
Maple syrup urine disease (MSUD)	42	1:100,000 but 1:176 among Old Order Mennonites	AR inheritance. Several forms. Most due to deficiency of decarboxylase leading to elevations of the branched chain amino acids leucine, isoleucine, and valine. One type is vitamin responsive. In classic type, at 3–7 days, infant shows poor sucking, poor feeding, vomiting, lethargy, hypotonia, and a high-pitched frequent cry with eventual hypoglycemia, acidosis, convulsions, alternating flaccidity and hypertonicity, and eventual intellectual disability if not treated early. A characteristic odor of maple syrup may be noticed in urine, sweat, and ear cerumen as early as fifth day. Permanent intellectual disability can occur by 1 week of age. Treatment is a newborn emergency. Consists of diet restricted in the branched chain amino acids, which is maintained to some degree throughout life.
Medium-chain acyl-CoA dehydrogenase (MCAD)	41	1: 6,500–1:20,000	AR inheritance. Disorder of mitochondrial fatty acid oxidation deficiency metabolism affecting cellular energy. Multiple allelic variants but *K3044E* accounts for the majority. Common in Northern European ancestry. Usually presents with crisis when infant/child has prolonged fasting, often due to illness, between 3 months and 6 years of age, and is often mistaken as SIDS or Reye syndrome. The picture can include any of the following: hypoglycemia, vomiting, lethargy, encephalopathy, respiratory arrest, hepatomegaly, seizures, apnea, comma, and long-term developmental and behavioral disabilities.
PKU	51	See text	See text.
Tyrosinemia	29	1:50,000–1:100,000 but 1:685 in one region in Quebec.	AR inheritance. Several types including a type that improves with ascorbic acid intake. Type I results from deficiency of fumarylacetoacetate hydrolase. Can begin in first month of life in acute type with failure to thrive, lethargy, irritability, vomiting, edema, ascites, hypophosphatemia, hepatomegaly, cirrhosis, and renal tubular abnormalities. Urine may have boiled cabbage odor. Presentation can also be with liver failure. Treatment includes diet low in tyrosine and phenylalanine but progresses, and liver transplantaion usually before 2 years of age is major treatment.

aSome states may not require but may offer universally or to select populations, or may require but not yet have implemented. Based on the 50 states and District of Columbia.

believed to be benign. Some believe that screening for those with no known clinical significance may allow long-term follow-up of such individuals and reveal hitherto unrecognized subtle consequences. This must be balanced against expense and anxiety engendered in the parents. Another issue is whether it is justifiable to screen for very rare disorders. Some believe that it yields a very low benefit-cost ratio, whereas others believe it is morally unjustifiable to do otherwise because of the potential to prevent adverse effects.

PKU

PKU was the first disorder to be included in mass newborn screening in the early 1960s. Years of experience with PKU screening revealed how little was known about hyperphenylalaninemia heterogeneity when screening was begun and points out the need for education of parents, informed consent for testing, and provision of genetic counseling services as

an integral part of treatment programs. Worldwide, more than 10 million newborns are now screened for PKU each year.

The amino acid phenylalanine (phe) is essential for protein synthesis in humans. A complex reaction is involved in the hepatic conversion of phenylalanine to tyrosine (see Figure 12.3), and blockage causes elevations collectively referred to as hyperphenylalaninemias. These include transient hyperphenylalaninemia, persistent non-PKU hyperphenylalaninemia, classic PKU, and deficient tetrabiopterin biosynthesis that may result from impaired recycling of tetrahydopterin due to dihydropeteridine reductase deficiency. Hyperphenylalaninemia refers to phe levels above 2 mg/dl (120 μM) and may result from various mutations interfering with the conversion of phe to tyrosine, including phenylalanine hydroxylase (PAH) deficiency resulting in classic PKU and a mild non-PKU hyperphenylalaninemia as well as several others.

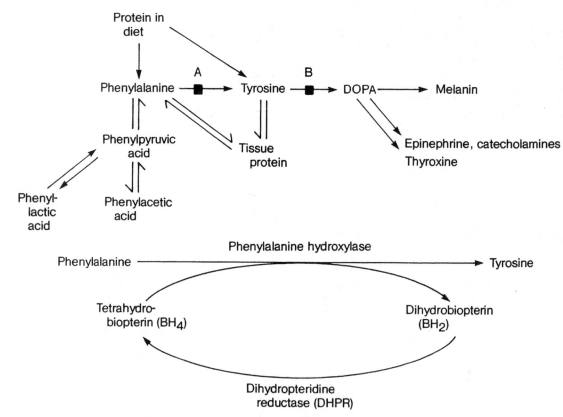

FIGURE 12.3   (*Top*) Abbreviated metabolism of phenylalanine and tyrosine. A = block in PKU (classical). B = block in albinism. (*Bottom*) Phenylalanine hydroxylating system (abbreviated). Some steps have been omitted for simplification.

Therefore, several defects in different steps in the metabolism of phenylalanine or its cofactor can result in elevated phe.

The most common of these forms is classic PKU characterized by less than 1% of PAH activity. Deficiencies of more than 1% PAH activity result in milder hyperphenylalaninemia noted as non-PKU hyperphenylalaninemia caused by PAH deficiency. Those with mild persistent hyperphenylalanemia (6 mg/dl or greater) may have a lower IQ if not treated, and so practitioners are being more aggressive in implementing diet therapy for these infants. More than 400 mutations of the PAH gene are known to result in classic PKU. Hyperphenylalanemia not resulting in classic PKU has different treatment approaches. It is important to rescreen infants who have positive early screening tests so that those with transient hyperphenylalaninemia are not placed on phenylalanine-restricted diets that could eventually be harmful to them.

It is now rare to see a child manifest the full spectrum of symptoms resulting from classic PKU because of screening programs and prompt treatment, but occasionally an affected infant is missed. Therefore, PKU should not be automatically ruled out in infants manifesting signs and symptoms associated with the disorder. Vomiting, eczema, and urine with a musty or mouselike odor are usually the only early symptoms. Delay in achieving developmental milestones may be noticed after 6 months of phenylalanine ingestion. Other symptoms that can occur are convulsions, increased muscle tone, agitated behavior, and delayed speech. A crossed-leg sitting position, tooth enamel hypoplasia, decalcification of the long bones, and a prominent maxilla are present. Pigment dilution occurs because of inhibition of tyrosinase by phenylalanine accumulation in the metabolic pathway leading to melanin synthesis (see Figure 12.3). Thus, affected untreated patients commonly have fair hair and blue eyes; in darkly pigmented families, the affected patient will be less pigmented than other family members.

It is very important to institute a phe-restricted diet as soon as possible and before 1 month. Continuous treatment throughout childhood, adolescence, and probably lifelong is now considered essential; diet restriction should be sufficient to keep plasma phe levels to normal ranges. Areas of controversy about the length of time to restrict phenylalanine in the infant's diet, the rigidity of restriction, and how to approach maternal PKU exist.

It is estimated that only 5% of infants who have presumptive positive tests are eventually proven to have PKU. False-negative results also occur because of early screening, especially if the infant is feeding poorly. Nurses can note those infants in whom this is true, so that extra emphasis can be placed on another test being done at about 3 weeks of age. The amount of formula ingested in the previous 24 hours, feeding difficulties, if any, and type of feeding (bottle or breast) should be noted on the form that is sent with the specimen for testing. Between 5% and 10% of infants eventually found to have PKU had negative results from screening tests. Any infant born into a family with a history of PKU needs more frequent than usual testing and monitoring. Another problem continuing to plague PKU screening has been the length of time taken to locate an infant with a positive screening test and conduct follow-up testing. This is problematic in instituting diet control to prevent retardation.

It has been suggested that all infants with persistent hyperphenylalaninemia and PKU be entered into a computerized registry for recontact in early adolescence in order to prevent the effects of maternal PKU on offspring. Questions of rights to privacy, confidentiality, and others must be balanced against the potential usefulness of such registry.

Infants found to have hyperphenylalaninemia on newborn screening may eventually be placed after diagnosis into one of several categories. The major ones are: classic PKU; transient hyperphenylalanemia without any further clinical significance; non-PKU hyperphenylalaninemia; and those with tetrabiopterin (BH_4) deficiency who need treatment for this.

The overall incidence of classic PKU in the general population in the United States is approximately 1 in 11,000 live births, whereas Irish and Scottish populations have an incidence as high as 1 in 5,000, and Black, Japanese, and Ashkenazi Jewish populations show an incidence as low as 1 in 100,000. Inheritance is by the autosomal recessive mode of transmission. Carrier detection and prenatal diagnosis of classic PKU are possible.

Other Disorders

With the advent of MS/MS technology, a large number of fatty acid oxidation defects, organic acidemias, aminoacidemias, and other disorders can be detected using a single sample. In several states, one or more of these are being included in pilot programs within state newborn screening. Most of these disorders are individually rare, but when looked at collectively are said to have an incidence of 1 in 4,000 to 1 in 5,000. A number of other genetic and nongenetic disorders have been suggested for potential inclusion in newborn screening programs. Examples include diabetes mellitus type 1, hyperlipidemia, familial hypercholesterolemia, neuroblastoma, fragile X and other chromosomal disorders, alpha-1-antitrypsin deficiency, Duchenne muscular dystrophy, hemochromatosis, *BRCA1* and other gene mutations predisposing to cancer, Tay-Sachs disease, tuberous sclerosis, and Huntington disease. Arguments against inclusion of some of these have to do with one or more of the following:

- The rarity of the disorder so that cost-effectiveness may be compromised
- The cost of the procedure, for example, in connection with chromosome analysis
- The lack of established ranges of normal
- Lack of agreement as to what the variation or disorder means relative to any disease process or harmful event
- Whether a disorder to which a genetic predisposition is identified will eventually become manifested (e.g., in *BRCA1* mutations, not all with the mutation eventually develop certain cancers)
- Disagreement on the need for early or even any therapeutic intervention
- Lack of treatment options available
- In the case of no available treatment options, the possibility of psychological harm, disruption of families, and discrimination
- For presymptomatic disorders such as Huntington disease, the possibility of psychological distress for a lifetime, as well as discrimination as to education, jobs, and insurance
- If screening for one type of chromosome disorder such as fragile X is done, and another finding is identified, whether to reveal the incidental finding
- Interference with the person's right not to know (in this case, the child might not want such information, but parents may already have obtained it)

- The inability to alter or affect the natural history of the disease

Not too long ago, some screening of newborns was done for chromosomal abnormalities. Questions of cost, ethics, and ambiguity of the meaning of results forced their discontinuation, but these have been suggested again. Hyperlipidemia and familial hypercholesterolemia had been suggested as appropriate for inclusion in newborn screening programs. Here again there is a lack of agreement on the meaning of the test result and what interventions (if any) would be appropriate to use. It is not clear whether a low-fat diet instituted early could retard the later development of coronary artery disease, especially for some underlying genetic causes. Part of the problem is the length of time involved in studying such cause and effect. In Britain and elsewhere, neonatal screening of male newborns is routine for Duchenne muscular dystrophy. Although no curative treatment is currently available, the family could receive genetic counseling, thereby possibly preventing repeat cases in a family, early planning could occur, and the family is spared anxiety during future diagnosis. However, they would have to live a longer time with the knowledge that their child is affected, and this could affect the entire family and familial relationships. Tuberous sclerosis is an autosomal dominant disorder characterized by white leaf-shaped macules visible under a Wood's light, epilepsy, intellectual disability, shagreen patches, and a typical rash on the nose and cheeks. It has been suggested for inclusion in newborn screening by using Wood's light for depigmented areas. Arguments against inclusion have included the argument that less than 100% show these "white nevi," and some would be missed, leading to false reassurance.

Conclusions

Newborn screening is not without problems. Changes in obstetric practice have shortened the hospital stay of both mother and infant. Thus, specimens are usually obtained just before the infant leaves the hospital, which can be as early as 24 hours after birth, and screening tests for some disorders may not be accurate this early. If they are not performed then, however, the compliance rate may be ubstantially lower. Infants transferred from one hospital to another might be missed. Many newborns will slip through the cracks in the health care system, not being detected until irreversible damage has occurred. An illustration of the need to still consider inherited metabolic diseases in an older person even in the era of newborn screening is illustrated by the case of a 17-year-old who presented with auditory and visual hallucinations and paranoia who was found to have the pyridoxine-responsive form of homocystinuria. His symptoms normalized within several weeks of pyridoxine therapy. Another criticism of mass newborn screening is the expense in screening low-risk infants for certain disorders. For example, it is relatively rare for a Black infant to have PKU. Should PKU testing thus be confined only to White infants in order to increase its cost-effectiveness? Is the expense justified if disease in any child can be prevented or treated? On the other hand, if one blood or urine specimen can be used for disease screening for many disorders, this reduces the expense, but such multiplex testing may compromise accuracy. In addition, screening for many disorders at a time when accuracy may not be optimal for all may later lead to their erroneously not being considered as diagnostic possibilities. However, after diagnosis is made and treatment begins, vigilant monitoring is necessary to ensure not only optimal treatment, but also the exclusion of unnecessary treatment or misdiagnosis, which also can be hazardous. There is a relatively high false positive rate for newborn screening tests in general.

Effective newborn screening requires a coordinated, comprehensive, multidisciplinary, integrated system for delivery of care so that complex systems function effectively. This includes specimen collection; transport; tracking; laboratory analysis; data collection and analysis; locating and contacting families of infants with abnormal results on initial and subsequent screening for further evaluation and testing; and provision of follow-up services, including diagnosis, treatment, and long-term management that encompasses education, psychological, nursing, and social services, genetic counseling, medical nutrition therapy, and medical foods. To date, parents have been minimally aware that their newborn has been screened for genetic disorders. As awareness of newborn screening opportunities and issues grows, public and professional voices will influence how newborn screening occurs in the United States in the future.

SOCIAL AND ETHICAL ISSUES ASSOCIATED WITH SCREENING

A variety of social, ethical, and legal issues arise from conducting screening. Potential risks and benefits associated with screening are summarized in Table 12.5. Various social and ethical issues are discussed more fully in Chapter 13. Of particular significance in screening are the right to refuse to participate, informed consent, right to privacy and confidentiality of information, ownership of samples and future use, disclosure of incidental or unexpected findings, access to information, and alteration of familial relationships. Individual feelings that may be seen with genetic testing, such as the possibility of stigmatization and reduced self-worth, are also a potential consequence. Some of these will be discussed below.

Although some newborn screening is compulsory, many states provide for exemption from screening of the newborn for genetic disorders if this is a violation of the parents' religious beliefs. This raises two interesting issues. The first is that parents are often not specifically asked to give informed consent for this type of screening, so they never have the opportunity to refuse their child's participation. They may either never find out that testing has been done or find out at the time of hospital discharge. The second point is whether the parents should have the right to deny the child the privilege of discovering whether he/she may have disorders such as PKU and hypothyroidism, which are amenable to early treatment, thus preventing retardation. How does the principle of causing no harm apply? Whose rights are most important in this instance? Should parental refusal be honored, or is it unjustifiable?

In other types of screening programs in which participation is purely voluntary, exercising the right to refuse to participate in screening should not result in the denial of any other services. Subtle coercion should also be avoided. This can inadvertently occur if screening is sponsored by a dominant social or religious institution in that culture or other perceived powerful group.

It is wise for health professionals to thoroughly discuss and have a policy on what is to be done with

TABLE 12.5   Potential Risks and Benefits Associated with Screening

	Type of Screening		
	Carrier	Newborn	Predictive
Potential risks			
Uncovering misattributed parenthood	X	X	X
Stigmatization	X		X
Impaired self-concept	X		X
Increased insurance rates or loss of benefits	X		X
Loss of chosen marital partner	X		X
Social and cultural consequences	X	X	X
Interference with parent-child bonding		X	
Imposition of sick role	X	X	X
Anxiety associated with false-positive results	X	X	X
False feeling of security associated with false-negative results	X	X	X
Loss of the right not to know	X		X
Overprotection of child		X	X
Guilt feelings	X	X (parent)	X
Potential benefits			
Improved self-image if not a carrier or affected	X		X
Recover potential productive member of society		X	
Data collection for health planning	X	X	X
Allows reproductive planning options	X	X	X
Institute plan for early detection of disease development			X
Initiation of early treatment		X	X
Alter disease process		X	X
Provide genetic counseling	X	X	X
Avoid costs associated with disease development		X	
Extend services to other relatives	X	X	X
If negative, avoidance of later unpleasant, expensive tests			X

unexpected findings before beginning testing or screening. Often a statement is included as part of informed consent as to what information will and will not be revealed. Incidental findings could also have an impact on stigmatization, insurance, and genetic discrimination issues.

One of the risks of screening is the discovery of misattributed parenthood, usually paternity. For example, if a screening program for sickle cell is undertaken in school screening and a child is discovered to have sickle cell trait, but neither putative parent has it, the chances are that one or both parents are not the natural parents of this child, barring a laboratory error. How is this situation to be handled? Does disclosure hold that such results must be shared? Can they be withheld? Can only the mother be informed of the result? The admonition to "do no harm" may be a guiding principle in making a decision. Again, incorporating a statement about

policy into a pretesting or screening consent can be valuable.

Several types of problems can arise in this area. The first is to whom the results of testing or screening can be released. Ideally, only the person undergoing the screening should be given these results. In practice, testing or screening records may be kept and handled by a wide variety of nonprofessional personnel and volunteers. They may have access to other persons' identity for billing, insurance, and follow-up purposes. In small communities or neighborhoods, anonymity is not possible, and unintended stigmatization may result. In some screening programs, such as those for sickle cell, the actual sponsorship may be under the auspices of lay community groups. Patients can consent to disclosure of the findings of screening. This may be specified. For example, the person may wish to have results sent to his/her physician or to certain relatives, which raises another issue. All records should be kept in such a way that the individual is not immediately identifiable. Therefore, a code number instead of names should be used. Special care must be taken when entering data in a central computer or data bank. Often these are accessible to individuals by means of telephone computer access.

Another type of a breach of confidentiality that can occur is by revealing statistical data that accidentally allow a person who has been tested to be identified. It is imperative that no individual can be identified in this way, even if it makes the research data presentation less detailed. Disclosure of information to unrelated third parties, such as insurance companies or employers, may have other consequences. These may include higher insurance rates, cancellation of insurance policies, or loss of job opportunities. Employers have long used various attributes in their selection process, and some now include genetic information.

Identification of a child with a genetic variant that has not been shown to have any definite correlation with clinical disease, the carrier state, or an actual genetic disorder itself can change the relationship between the child and his/her parents. In the newborn, disruption of parent-infant bonding can occur. Overprotectiveness can occur at any age, leading to impaired psychological development. Parents can experience guilt at having given this disorder to the child, whether or not there is any basis in fact for these feelings. A sick role may be imposed on the child. These issues may be particularly prominent in population testing or screening for disorders for which there is no present treatment such as Duchenne muscular dystrophy. The finding among siblings that one is a carrier and others are not can change their relationships with each other.

In the excitement of inducing participation in mass carrier screening or testing, it is easy to forget the risks that may occur. Impairment of self-image or self-worth is one such risk. Adolescents are particularly vulnerable because they are still searching for and developing their self-identity. Views of their peers are extremely important in this development. Thus, for example, the effect of identifying all Jewish students in a high school population to volunteer for Tay-Sachs carrier testing can be extreme. First, they are identified as "different." Second, many of those who are then identified as carriers have been shown to have an impaired self-concept.

Some researchers have attempted to justify this result by stating that many of the noncarriers had improved self-concepts. Because little long-term research has been done in this area, the long-term effects are not known. Nurses, with their understanding of growth and development, can assist in identifying these issues before screening begins. In a study of carrier testing for both Tay-Sachs disease and cystic fibrosis among Jewish high school students in Australia, another question that arises is whether the identification of carrier status is important to this age group. What are the anticipated uses to which it will be put? These young people can, however, begin to identify themselves in new and less favorable terms such as, "I am a Tay-Sachs carrier." In any school setting, it is difficult to prevent school officials from learning the results of the testing or screening. This should be considered in the planning phases of the program. Is it really the needs of the participants who are being met in the screening? Or is it the needs of the researchers? Once a person is identified as a carrier, regardless of age, there is no way to return to the pretesting or screening state of ignorance.

In a rural Greek population, an intensive educational effort and screening program were instituted for carriers of thalassemia in an effort to reduce the incidence. Carriers were identified, and the screeners left the village. When they returned several years later, they discovered that those individuals who were identified as carriers were virtually untouchable. Marriages could not be arranged for them as was the custom. The social status of their families was impaired, so that, in effect, all members were affected. It has been believed that education of an ethnic population as to the disorder will minimize stigmatization, but this might be a reflection of the culture of the health care provider, not the population being tested. It also emphasizes the importance of understanding the culture of the group in which screening is to be done before attempting to initiate a program. The participation of knowledgeable community individuals helps to minimize some of the negative aspects and alert the providers to potential cultural problems. Although the rationale for singling out ethnic groups for high-risk genetic screening centers on economic feasibility, the issue of discrimination can apply. Screening should be kept voluntary, and equal access for all to the screening should be allowed. Definition of groups on ethnic and racial lines may accrue both benefits and burdens for them. It was not long ago that arguments directed at improving the race through eugenics was popular in this country. The result of this thinking was the imposition of immigration restrictions, prohibitive marriage laws, sterilization acts, and the distraction from the real roots of labor and social problems. Between 1911 and 1930, about 30 states passed sterilization laws for a variety of conditions ranging from insanity to alcoholism to criminality. Thus, many fears are founded in history.

The misunderstanding of the health status of carriers, particularly in the case of sickle cell has also led to unintended consequences. Loss of employment; loss of access to certain jobs, educational opportunities, and professions; discrimination for entry to the Air Force Academy; and increased insurance rates have been but a few. In addition, some who are identified as carriers may not themselves understand the meaning of that status.

THE FUTURE

The potential for various types of genetic screening is expanding. These will include population and targeted genetic screening for actual diseases, carrier state, predictive screening, and newborn screening, as well as prenatal applications. Advances in scientific understanding and in the technology to translate the findings into practice will continue to grow. Many social, ethical, legal, and cultural factors impinge on genetic screening. They must be carefully considered before enthusiasm and good intentions lead unwittingly to harmful effects on individuals and groups. In regard to newborn screening, as there will be an increased ability to identify and treat an expanding list of disorders, there will be increased consumer advocacy to make broader universal detection available in a timely and responsible manner. As awareness of these issues grows, public policy decisions will increasingly influence genetic screening in the future. Nurses, among other health professionals, will need to be aware of the trends and issues surrounding screening, be informed so they can educate and interpret information correctly for their clients in a culturally sensitive and educationally appropriate manner, understand the emotional and psychological impact of results and the potential impact on such issues as

insurability and future life planning, and understand the need for a coordinated, comprehensive screening plan with appropriate follow-up of services.

GENETIC EFFECTS FROM ENVIRONMENTAL AGENTS

Potentially hazardous chemicals are present in our environment both deliberately, such as in food additives, agricultural chemicals, industrial compounds, and fuel, and inadvertently through contamination, pollution, and accidents. The effect of environmental agents on genetic material is an increasing source of public concern as well as a public health problem. Hazardous chemicals may cause:

- Damage to the developing fetus directly (teratogenesis; see Chapter 8);
- Somatic damage such as cancer;
- Mutation by direct damage of genetic material in the germ cells, resulting in hazards to future generations.

Numerous different chemicals are in worldwide use, with new ones added each year. They are distributed widely and are present in natural and synthetic forms, alone and in combination. Once in the environment, they may enter the food chain and attain greater concentration. A minimum safe dose or level or safe time exposure has not been established for most of these. Relatively few have been investigated with respect to their mutagenic, carcinogenic, or teratogenic effects. Most carcinogens (80–90%) are also mutagens, but mutagens are not necessarily carcinogens.

The term *toxicogenomics* has been defined as the study of genes and their products important in adaptive responses to toxic exposures. Exposures to certain environmental agents can result in genetic consequences to:

- The exposed individuals themselves;
- Their immediate offspring;
- Future generations.

This is because of structural or functional disruption of the genetic material or apparatus in germ or somatic cells. It is difficult to connect cause and efect between a specific agent and most birth defects, genetic disorders, and neoplasms. Agents with delayed, indirect, or subtle effects are hardest to identify.

Damage to genetic material may have different outcomes depending on the agent, exposure, and the person's genetic constitution. Each person has his/her own constellation of metabolizing enzymes and receptors. Therefore, each handles chemicals in a unique manner. Damage to the germ cells may result in a dominant or recessive single gene mutation; a chromosomal mutation involving gain, loss, or rearrangement of parts of chromosomes; or genomic mutation affecting chromosome number (gain or loss) but not structure. Agents can also cause changes in DNA functioning such as imprinting (see Chapter 4). A dominant gene mutation may result in visible anomalies in the offspring or infertility in the individual if the damage is so great that normal offspring cannot be produced. Production of abnormal germ cells may also result in repetitive spontaneous abortions or fetal death when reproduction is attempted. If the mutation is recessive, it may remain hidden for generations, being added to the genetic load of unfavorable genes for the population. Mutation in somatic cells may result in (1) carcinogenesis in individuals exposed, or by transplacental mechanisms in their offspring (e.g., vaginal cancer in daughters of women who took diethylstilbestrol (DES) during pregnancy) or (2) in structural or functional damage to the developing embryo or fetus, which may not be immediately evident. Somatic mutations may also contribute to aging and heart disease. Various databases exist for tracking environmental damage, including the Developmental and Reproductive Toxicology/Environmental Teratology Information Center (DART/ETIC), available from the National Library of Medicine's Toxicology Data Network (TOXNET).

Some issues that society must consider are how agents with the potential for harmful genetic, carcinogenic, or teratogenic effects can be identified before release into the environment; whether such agents should be used; assessment of the risks and evaluation of the benefits to be gained from their use; and the extent of evidence necessary in order to effect a public health decision on regulation and control. Society must ultimately balance the risks of adverse effects, such as environmental contamina-

tion and genetic damage, against utility, economic benefits, and comfort. For example, DDT is restricted in this country but is considered necessary in other parts of the world to control malaria, a major health problem. Persons also look at the utility of such agents differently; the farmer and the wildlife conservationist view the use of pesticides from different perspectives for example. What price will be considered reasonable for the use of genotoxic agents?

ECOGENETICS AND PUBLIC HEALTH GENOMICS

Ecogenetics may be defined as individual variation in response to agents in the environment causing genotoxic and other effects. Its importance lies in implications for policies that affect the public health. Because most individuals have some genetic differences from others, they may react in varying ways to their environment, which in a broad sense includes all chemical exposures, food and drug intake, exposure to infectious agents, and the like. (Aspects of individual susceptibility and response are discussed in Chapters 3 and 6.) In many instances, the person who has an unexpected response to a particular food (e.g., persons with G6PD deficiency to fava bean ingestion) can easily avoid it. A person who is susceptible to a certain drug, such as barbiturates in the genetic disorder of acute intermittent porphyria, can avoid the drug.

In the case of food additives, the picture is more complex. Food additives such as dyes and preservatives may act to modify the metabolism of chemicals. Well-known examples of individual responses include to monosodium glutamate (Chinese restaurant syndrome) and to foods containing nitrates and tyramine. Tartrazine (FD&C yellow no. 5), a color additive to food, drink, and pharmaceuticals, may cause the response of asthma, urticaria, rhinitis, or angioedema in susceptible persons. The Food and Drug Administration (FDA) estimates that 50,000 to 100,000 persons in the United States are intolerant to tartrazine. About 15% of those who are intolerant to aspirin are also affected by tartrazine. Recent labeling requirements have made products containing tartrazine easier to identify. However, the public health issue is whether additives that may benefit one group should be added to a wide range of food when they may not be tolerated by some individuals. Truly "one man's meat can be another's poison."

Such concerns are not limited to foods. As an example, a child who used an insect repellant containing N,N-diethyltoluamide (DEET) developed a Reye-like syndrome and died. She was heterozygous for ornithine carbamoyltransferase deficiency (a urea cycle enzyme disorder), which caused her to have a lower level of this enzyme. These decreased levels apparently did not allow her to metabolically process the chemicals in the repellant properly. Yet most people use the product without apparent effect, and it is particularly effective in repelling mosquitoes, some of which may carry diseases such as the West Nile virus.

PROBLEMS IN ASSOCIATING EFFECTS WITH ENVIRONMENTAL AGENTS

There are many difficulties in associating a particular agent with an adverse outcome, as shown in Box 12.4. Other difficulties that relate to teratogenic agents are discussed in Chapter 8.

HAZARDOUS EXPOSURES IN THE ENVIRONMENT AND WORKPLACE

Hazardous exposures to genotoxic agents may occur through the release of substances into the environment or exposure in the workplace. In fact, much of the information about the effects of such substances in humans has been obtained through unintentional exposure. Exposure is usually of two types: that of a low dosage over a long-term period or a short-term intense exposure such as occurs more often in accidents. There may be overlap in exposures between the workplace and environment, since those exposed to a toxic agent at work may also live near the workplace. Families of those working in certain industries are exposed to certain agents through contact with clothes and other articles of the worker. Sometimes hazardous workplaces, such as university chemistry laboratories, are hard to recognize.

Deleterious genetic effects can be manifested by adverse changes in the reproductive capacity or process in both males and females. This may be evidenced by impaired fertility (as seen in menstrual irregularities and abnormal sperm, for example), infertility, spontaneous abortion, fetal or perinatal death, stillbirth, intrauterine growth restriction, birth defects, or altered sex ratios in offspring. These may be used as end points in monitoring exposure effects. Some agents believed to cause such effects are listed in Table 12.6, but there is a lack of agreement as to most of these in the literature. Selected agents are discussed below.

Evidence of environmental contamination by toxic chemicals often comes to light because of the observation of what appears to be a high frequency or clustering of birth defects, spontaneous abortions, or miscarriages, and may be observed by citizens or professionals. One of the first widespread examples was discovered in 1956 in the Minamata Bay area of Japan. Industrial waste from a fertilizer company containing methylmercury was discharged into the bay that was used for fishing. In all these cases, some persons were more susceptible to the mercury, as not all those who ate contaminated products evidenced toxicity. (This is discussed in Chapter 8.)

High levels of mercury (above 1 ppm) are present in certain fish such as swordfish, shark, tilefish, whale, and mackerel in the United States. Pregnant women, nursing mothers, and young children should minimize the amount of these fish that they eat. Another source of mercury is thimerosal, used as a preservative in vaccines. This use has engendered concerns that have been somewhat controversial. While some have believed that the use of thimerosal in vaccines was associated with the development of autism spectrum disorders, the published research findings do not resolve the issue. In the United States, this use has virtually been eliminated. Use continues in other countries since the World Health Organization has indicated that thimerosal use in vaccines is safe. Dental amalgam fillings are a source of inorganic mercury exposure, often through inhalation during preparation or removal. Cultural practices such as in religious ceremonies in some sects such as voodoo and Santaria may also expose segments of the population, as may the use of cosmetic creams that contain calomel.

BOX 12.4

Some Difficulties in Associating Environmental Agents With Adverse Outcomes

- A particular agent may induce a specific genetic change that may be manifested in different phenotypic ways.
- Individual genetic differences can alter susceptibility and resistance.
- Effects may be removed from the obvious impact of the agent. For example, a chemical can change a person's ability to metabolize other substances.
- Chemicals in the environment are rarely present alone; rather, they are in mixture and can then interact with other substances.
- Past failure to appreciate that exposure of both males and females can result in germ cell mutations leading to adverse reproductive outcome as well as risk to future generations.
- Concentrations of a chemical may not reflect its biologic activity.
- There may be difficulty in detecting an increase in a birth defect that is rare or within a small population.
- There may be failure to account for synergistic and additive effects.
- There may be lack of knowledge of a person's past status (e.g., were chromosomes normal before exposure?).
- It is hard to pinpoint an exposure period to a specific agent retrospectively.
- Persons may not know that they were exposed to a particular agent.
- If they know they were exposed to a toxic agent, they may not know what it was.
- Influence of personal habits such as smoking on outcome is not always known or accounted for.
- There may be no available confirmatory records of either the exposure or the genotoxic outcome available.
- It is difficult to make an association between common exposures to an agent. For example, if several workers are exposed to one chemical and all of them developed a certain type of cancer but were seen by practitioners in towns many miles apart, the connection might not be made.
- There is a dependence on memory recall or incomplete or vague data.
- The duration, dosage, and concentration of the agent to which they were exposed may be unknown.
- The person may be embarrassed, may selectively omit vital information, may fear job loss, may feel an outcome is detrimental to his/her self-image, may have poor recall, or may not be aware of an adverse outcome in his/her spouse, and therefore may not reveal vital information.
- Political and economic pressure is brought to bear by private industry, health departments, the military, and the government because of fear of litigation, expediency, or perceived necessity for the use of a substance.
- Testing systems are insensitive.
- Long-term testing is not done because of high costs and time.
- It is difficult to extrapolate test results from animal studies to humans.
- An outcome that occurs years after exposure may not be associated with it, or if thought to be, may not be able to be proved.
- Information related to compliance with the use of protective measures may not be available.
- Companies may be reluctant to inform workers and others of all substances used in processing because of "trade secrets."

TABLE 12.6   Selected Environmental Agents With Reported Genotoxic and Reproductive Effects in Humans

Agents	Reported Effects[a]
Benzene	↑Chromosome aberrations including breaks; leukemia
Carbon disulfide	Sperm abnormalities, impotency, decreased libido (M); menstrual disorders (F); ↑spontaneous abortions; ↑prematurity
Chlordecone (Kepone)	↓Spermatogenesis; ↓libido (M)
Chlorinated hydrocarbon pesticides	↑Blood dyscrasias; ↑childhood neuroblastomas
Chloroprene	↑Spontaneous abortions in wives of male workers; ↑chromosome aberrations, disturbances in spermatogenesis
Dibromochloropropane (DBCP)	Low or absent sperm; infertility (M)
Formaldehyde	↑Spontaneous abortions; ↓birth weight in offspring
Hexachlorophene	↑Birth defects
(PCBs)	↓Birth weight in offspring; specific congenital anomalies such as brown pigmentation, gum hyperplasia, skull anomalies; developmental delay
Nonionizing radiation	↑Perinatal death; ↑congenital malformations; ↓birth weight; ↑congenital anomalies
Smelter emissions (mixed substances including arsenic, sulfur dioxide, cadmium, lead, mercury)	↑Spontaneous abortions; infertility (M); ↓birth weight; ↑congenital anomalies; ↑frequency of Wilms tumor in offspring
Vinyl chloride	↑Chromosome aberrations; ↑spontaneous abortions in wives of workers; carcinoginesis, ↑birth defects
High temperature exposure	↓spermatogenesis; ↑birth defects (?)

[a]For most of these agents, research reports vary: some report these effects and others report negative findings.
↑ = increased. ↓ = decreased. M = male. F = female.

Perhaps the most controversial and widely publicized episode of environmental exposure to hazardous wastes was that of the Love Canal neighborhood of Niagara Falls, New York. In the 1940s, chemical companies filled an abandoned canal with toxic wastes, including chlorinated hydrocarbons, amounting to more than 21,000 tons of more than 200 different chemicals. In 1953, Hooker Chemical and Plastics Company sold the property to the Niagara Falls Board of Education for one dollar. Hooker maintains that the board was told the site was not suitable for a school, and the deed apparently contains a clause indicating the presence of the waste with provisions that no claims could be filed. In the late 1950s, about 100 homes were built along the banks of the dirt-covered canal, with a school built in the center. Residents noticed chemicals migrating through the topsoil, children falling in the soil received chemical burns, and there were odors and seepage in basements. Eventually the anger and fears of the residents became largely directed at the state health department because the chemical companies were major employers in the area and the state was not perceived as taking adequate action. Differences also existed within the scientific community as to the handling, analysis, and interpretation of data. For example, data on spontaneous abortions and birth defects could be analyzed by simple proximity to the canal center or by those homes designated as "wet" (those that were on former streambeds from the canal) versus "dry" homes. A study that was about 15 years old was chosen as the control group for comparing the frequency of spontaneous abortions. This study had a preselected population and bias because it was done on a group of women with previous problem pregnancies. Debate also centered on the methods and results of chromosome studies, including the lack of a contemporary control group. Also controversial was the method of interpretation of data related to cancer development in the Love Canal area. Love Canal has now been deemed safe for occupancy by some, and new homes have been sold in that area.

Toxic exposure to lead has occurred by means of environmental pollution through air and contaminated water and agricultural soil, from substances such as lead-based paint in older homes, and also through the workplace, as people in many occupations are exposed to lead. Exposures from hobbies may also occur. This is discussed in Chapter 8 in regard to maternal-child health.

Prevention of lead exposure is critical, and if children live in areas of exposure, this exposure should be interrupted. This is not always easy to accomplish in a short period of time. In areas where the drinking water is high in lead, nurses can advise women planning pregnancy to have their water checked and use an alternate source, such as bottled water, for drinking, if necessary. Additionally, household substances such as paint, dust in contaminated areas, or contamination through employment such as construction work can pose a risk to the worker and the family. It is important to advocate safe environmental lead levels and provide the necessary education and resources such as public health departments to make homes and communities safe from lead contamination. Good preconceptional counseling and prenatal care can help the mother reduce lead exposure during and after pregnancy.

The largest radiation accident occurred at the Chernobyl nuclear power plant in the Ukraine on April 26, 1986. The most contaminated areas were the Ukraine, Belarus, and the Russian Federation, but other areas of Europe were also exposed. At least 5 million people were exposed to ionizing radiation as a result. One of the major outcomes was the increase in childhood thyroid cancer when compared with pre-Chernobyl figures. In addition, children exposed during early pregnancy in Greece were 2.6 times more likely to develop leukemia than those who were unexposed. Some children exposed in utero were said to exhibit mental retardation and behavioral effects. Excesses in unstable chromosome-type aberrations were seen but not chromatid-type aberrations.

There are more than 100,000 waste sites in the United States. Therefore, nurses should be prepared to deal with the types of issues identified by the Love Canal incident. These include inadequate communication among professionals and between professionals and residents, misconceptions about what the research studies could actually show, inadequate attention to the needs and fears of the residents, poor preparation and planning for the research needed to examine the impact of the wastes on the health problems present, and the political issues and legal liabilities that impinged on the entire investigation. Other exposures may occur in communities due to wastewater disposal or even the chlorination disinfection of drinking water, which suggests that by-products such as trihalomethanes and trichloroethylene may be associated with certain birth defects and adverse pregnancy outcomes.

The nurse who is involved with potential or actual hazardous exposures in the community or workplace may feel role conflict between responsibility to the employer and to the client. There are some ways in which he/she can participate in the prevention of such hazards and the protection of the client as both a citizen and a professional. Some ways involve consideration of the following questions:

- Which agents are of major concern in causing genetic damage or carcinogenesis?
- How can they be accurately identified before exposure occurs?
- What actions should be taken when a potential genotoxic agent is discovered?
- What are minimum safe levels of exposure?
- How can exposure be minimized?
- Are there protective devices and measures that can be taken?
- What are they?
- Are they likely to result in nonadherence?
- Can individuals who are susceptible to damage by a specific agent because of their genetic constitution be identified? If so, how should this information be used? What weight should it have?

- Does it affect males and females the same way? If not, what special precautions must be taken?
- What information should be given to workers? Should all workers know their genetic profile in relation to toxic chemicals? How should this information be presented?
- How can their risks be explained to them in a noncoercive, realistic manner?

Some of these issues are addressed in the next section. It is important for the nurse to have the deserved confidence of the client so that effective protection can take place.

TESTING, SURVEILLANCE, AND GENETIC MONITORING

There are several approaches that can be taken for the minimization of genetic hazards from agents used in the workplace and encountered in the environment—for example:

- Identifying agents with potential mutagenic, teratogenic, and carcinogenic effects before widespread human exposure occurs by the use of various types of assays and through the use of large toxicogenomic databases;
- Devising appropriate regulations, controls, standardization, and guidelines for the use of such agents;
- Monitoring the emission of toxic substances and the concentration and levels of toxic agents emitted into the atmosphere, water, food, and so on of the environment and workplace;
- Using protective practices and devices within the workplace;
- Using preemployment screening and testing;
- Using ongoing periodic genetic monitoring of those believed to be exposed to toxic agents.

New methods of monitoring and standardization are being developed using DNA and RNA microarray and profiling technology for detecting genetic variations and gene expression variations leading to risk assessment and monitoring.

WORKPLACE SCREENING AND TESTING

The use of genetic testing or screening before or during employment has been controversial. On the one hand, they could be used to minimize the deleterious genetic effects of agents used in the workplace by, in some cases, identifying the genetically predisposed or hypersusceptible individual before employment in the particular industry or before assignment to a new location where different potentially hazardous substances will be encountered. Only a small number of individuals who have genetically determined differences in susceptibility to environmental agents found in the workplace can be identified, but the potential is growing. In addition, the use of such testing to determine possession of genes for susceptibility to diseases such as colon or breast cancer or for the development of a late-onset disorder such as Huntington disease presents dilemmas. What is the potential for discrimination not only in terms of initial employment but also for promotion opportunities? Can a company refuse to hire a qualified individual because testing shows that person will eventually develop Huntington disease? Can such discrimination extend to family genetic testing?

The workplace may also be a site for population screening for genetic disorders or carrier conditions. For example, such screening has been conducted for hemochromatosis. However, while the usual standards for genetic screening must be met in such programs, maintaining privacy and confidentiality and protecting workers from any adverse effects on employment are extremely important. There may be some justification in determining susceptibility to agents used at the employment site. On one side is the argument that such identification diminishes health hazards, can prevent severe reactions or disease, and allows early diagnosis and ongoing monitoring for the identified individual. On the other side is concern about an approach that may "blame the victim" and decrease the responsibility of the industry to control hazardous environmental conditions. At one point, the Occupational Safety and Health Administration (OSHA) medical surveillance requirements and National Institute for Occupational Safety and Health (NIOSH) bulletin

ecommendations for preplacement for occupational exposure to certain chemicals required "genetic
factors" to be included in the personal, family, and
occupational history. Some U.S. companies use or
plan to use routine genetic screening and monitoring along with tests for genetic susceptibility.

Some of the known genetically determined differences in susceptibility that manifest problems after certain exposures that have been applied include
the following:

- Persons with G6PD deficiency (discussed in
  Chapter 6) may experience hemolysis on exposure to certain chemicals such as aniline,
  acetanilid, benzene, carbon tetrachloride, chlo-
  roprene, lead, nitrites, and toluidine.
- Exposure to respiratory irritants and cigarette
  smoke aggravates respiratory disease in persons with alpha-l-antitrypsin deficiency (discussed in Chapter 10).
- Hypersensitivity on immunologic skin tests
  can detect sensitivity to organic isocyanates
  and indicate which individuals are most likely
  to exhibit an asthma-like syndrome or a delayed hypersensitivity response when exposed.
- Persons who are slow acetylators of N-acetyltransferase (see Chapter 6), which inactivates
  chemical arylamines such as naphthylamine,
  benzidine, and others, may have higher risks
  of bladder cancer when exposed to these agents.
- Persons with the low-activity form of the
  enzyme paraoxinase, which inactivates the
  pesticide parathion, may be predisposed to developing poisoning at low levels of exposure,
  either as spray pilots, mixers, field hands, or
  from general environmental exposure. An interesting example followed the release of sarin,
  a nerve gas, in Tokyo in 1995. It is believed
  that those who died were more vulnerable
  than others because their paraoxinase activity
  was such that they did not convert the sarin to
  a less toxic chemical rapidly enough.
- Those with reduced capacity to metabolize
  carbon disulfide may develop sensitivities such
  as polyneuritis.

Regardless of the type of screening used, the
meaning of the test and what it shows must be understood. An example of recent widespread misun-

derstanding was the restriction of persons with sickle cell trait from becoming pilots in the U.S. Air
Force because of the inaccurate belief that high altitudes could not be tolerated. Genetic testing or
screening should not be used to discriminate. However, only relatively few states have laws prohibiting
employer discrimination on the basis of genetic
testing. A suit filed in California alleged that Black
employees had been tested for the sickle cell gene
mutation without their consent. The suit was dismissed on grounds that this did not constitute
employee privacy intrusion. While the Equal Employment Opportunity Commission (EEOC) states
that under the Americans with Disabilities Act
(ADA) compliance manual employers cannot discriminate on genetic information, how extensive
this is and whether full protection is offered is debated. National legislation is needed for protection.

In a case of genetic testing of employees in the
workplace, a legal challenge filed in 2001 stated that
the Burlington Northern Railway Company was requiring those who claimed work-related carpal tunnel syndrome to undergo DNA testing for a genetic
predisposition to this disorder, specifically deletion
of the peripheral myelin protein-22 gene. This deletion can result in hereditary neuropathy with a liability to pressure palsies that can result in carpal
tunnel syndrome. Brandt-Rauf and Brandt-Rauf
(2004) related that at least one person was not told
that blood samples requested were for genetic testing, and that one person who refused was threatened with firing if he did not comply. The company
agreed to stop such testing. On the other hand, employers might be expected to protect their employees from hazards in the workplace by use of genetic
testing. For example, the Dow Chemical Company
was sued by the widow of a worker who had died
from leukemia. She claimed that cytogenetic testing
might have detected early indications of leukemia
development secondary to the worker's exposure to
benzene in the workplace. It is expected that the use
of genetic testing in the workplace will grow and
that the issues engendered by such use must be sufficiently addressed before growth occurs.

Protective Devices and Practices

Concern about the effect of certain chemical and
physical agents on fertile women has also been a

source of some controversy. Regulations have been devised in regard to substances to which the pregnant worker cannot be exposed. In some cases, concern has also been directed to the employment of fertile women in certain industries or for work with certain agents. This is because in some cases, the agent in question is not universally recognized as having mutagenic or teratogenic effects and exposure may thus not be regulated; women may choose to work in such areas because of pay advantages and therefore assume risk, or they may even choose sterilization because they perceive the risk of job loss if they become pregnant. Some companies have offered comparable pay at other jobs for fertile or pregnant women when the substance is known to be fetotoxic. Others have instead immorally, and in some circumstances illegally, withheld raises or promotion unless women chose to be sterilized in order to stay at certain jobs with risky exposures. This issue is fraught with complexities about sex and job discrimination and legal compensation. Substances can be mutagenic or affect the fetus through the male directly or indirectly, such as secondary exposure of the wives of such employees through contaminated clothing and other items. Physical protective measures such as respirators and protective clothing may be used to minimize exposure to employees who handle some known toxic substances. In these instances, compliance may be an important factor because of the severe discomfort associated with such protection or because of failure to associate danger with substances that are odorless, colorless, and tasteless with no immediately apparent effect. Some employers consider employees responsible for their own protection in their adherence to safety regulations and in relation to personal habits such as cigarette smoking or alcohol consumption, which may increase their risk of carcinogenesis.

SURVEILLANCE

Surveillance for genetic effects of chemical agents may be done in the workplace or in the general environment. For example, monitoring the rates of spontaneous abortions, general or specific birth defects, and an increased incidence of specific cancers can be used to try to detect a change that may be attributed to a specific agent that has been previously undetected. This may be done among specifi workers and their spouses or in specific geographi areas. There can be difficulties in this effort, however

- There can be many different etiologies fo these outcomes.
- The exposed populations are too small to readily establish statistical significance.
- The effects seen are apparent only years o decades after the event. As one can imagine how easy would it be to connect a case of neu roblastoma in a child with his father's employ ment working with chlorinated hydrocarbor pesticides 4 years previously?

Various studies have looked at the parental occupations of children born with birth defects. A review of the studies and of limitations associated with them may be found in Shi and Chia (2001) Hewitt's (1992) secondary analysis of nurses working with antineoplastic drugs found a higher relative risk for the development of leukemia and othe cancers than in the controls. Nurses' risks with these drugs have also been found by many others. Nurses, like workers in any other industry where toxic agents are used, should be aware of specific hazard: and take advantage of protective measures. Some states are now acquiring detailed occupational data on birth certificates, but some view this as an invasion of privacy. When taking an occupational or recreational history, the nurse should be sensitive to potential exposures commonly found among certain occupations. Some of these are listed in Table 12.7. Questions pertinent to the histories are discussed in Chapter 7.

Chemical and physical agents in our environment constantly bombard us at home, at work, at school, and at leisure. Various genes are involved in the metabolism of such chemicals and in mechanisms of repair in response to them. Understanding has increased as to the role that genes play in the manifestation of effects from both short-term and long-term exposures, but there is still not a uniform consensus on the best ways to assess damage or interpret results. In addition to the projects of the Environmental Genome Project of the National Institute of Environmental Health Sciences, NIH, there is a proposed National Children's study protocol to examine childhood environmental exposures from prenatal through 21 years of age.

TABLE 12.7   Selected Occupations and Potential Exposures to Toxic Agents

Occupation	Possible Exposures
Barber, hairdresser, beautician	Aerosol propellants, hair dye, acetone, ethyl alcohol, benzyl alcohol, halogenated hydrocarbons, hair spray resins
Dentist, dental technicians	Mercury, nitrogen dioxide, anesthetics, X-rays, vibration
Farmer	Mercury, arsenic, lead, nitrogen dioxide, silica, pesticides, fertilizers
Dry cleaner	Benzene, contaminated clothing, trichloroethylene naphtha
Nurse	Anesthetic gases, alcohol, ethylene oxide, carcinogenic agents, radiation, infectious agents, nitrogen dioxide
Photographer	Mercury, bromides, iodides, silver nitrate, caustic agents, iron salts, lead
Printer	Inks, antimony, lead, noise, vibration, benzene, methylene chloride
Textile industry	Cotton dust, synthetic fiber dust, formaldehyde, benzene, toluene, chloroprene, styrene, carbon disulfide, heat

Nonetheless, education and prevention remain important components for addressing environmental hazards to health and reproduction.

KEY POINTS/ISSUES AND QUESTIONS TO CONSIDER

- What are the differences between genetic testing and genetic screening?
- Do most chemicals carry some risk to a few individuals?
- Should such products be removed from the market?
- Should warning labels be used?
- How many other products cause severe effects in a few susceptible individuals?
- Are current public policies to address these adequate?
- Should newborns be screened for every possible genetic disorder in an era of cost concern?
- What should the relative responsibilities of parents and the state be in the provision of medical and diet foods for children affected by genetic disease?
- For newborn screening, in disease conditions for which few data are available for long-term outlook and impact, should this influence decisions about screening? In other words, should a disorder be included in the routine newborn screening programs if there is no clear evidence that early detection and/or treatment have significant impact on the long-term outlook?
- What are the pros and cons of conducting screening for genetic conditions in the workplace?
- A couple has decided against having any newborn screening for their child in a state in which the parent may make that decision. What would you discuss with them supporting screening for their child and why?

13

Trends, Social Policies, and Ethical Issues in Genomics

Human genetics, perhaps more than any other science, has influenced and been influenced or manipulated by social, economic, political, and religious forces. The practical application of developments in genetics as seen in genetic testing, screening, counseling, prenatal diagnosis, advanced therapeutic management and the exercise of such reproductive options as gamete donation, in vitro fertilization, preimplantation diagnosis, selective embryo transfer and implantation, contraception, sterilization, gender selection, selective embryo reduction, abortion, and adoption affect both individuals and society, raising important questions of rights and responsibilities that bear on both present and future generations. Is the "brave new world" now? James Watson once said that our fate used to be thought of as being in the stars; now it is in our genes.

The results of the research under the auspices of the Human Genome Project have emphasized the influence of genetics. Moral, social, and ethical problems posed by human genetics have been discussed throughout this book, most specifically in Chapters 3, 5, 8, 10, and 12. The work of the Human Genome Project as discussed in Chapter 1 has brought to the forefront many of these issues. Early in the project, its significant impact on society was recognized, and therefore ethical, legal, and social implications were made an integral part of the project.

This chapter concentrates on the topics of cloning, transgenic plants, assisted reproductive technologies, eugenics, the effects of genetic practices on the gene pool (the collection of genes in a population) in this and future generations, th rights of the individual versus society, genetic dis crimination (defined by Natowicz, Alper, and Alper, 1992, as "discrimination against an individ ual or against members of that individual's famil solely because of real or perceived differences from the 'normal' genome in the genetic constitution o that individual," p. 466), and the implications of th "new genetics." While issues of gene patents and ownership have become important in this area, the are beyond the scope of this chapter.

CLONING

In February 1997, the cloning of a lamb (Dolly from an adult sheep cell caused considerable stir. A one university, human embryos were cloned from embryonic cells and grown to the 32-cell stage, a which point they could have been implanted in a woman's uterus, although they were not. Much discussion and speculation arose from the story, however, and the question is, "Will Mary follow Dolly? Since that time, other animals such as cows and mule have been cloned. There was even a report of the birth of a cloned infant in 2002 made by the religious cult the Raëlians, but it was not substantiated Cloned human cells are being used, however, for the production of embryonic stem cells, which are used for bone marrow transplantation and for the use of therapies for damaged cells and tissues. The embryo is sacrificed during harvesting of these cells.

Probably a clone would not be identical to its origin as an adult due to the environmental impact and shaping that occurs with every person. For example, if Beethoven had been raised in the Amazon basin, would his same talent have emerged and been recognized? Cloning, however, raises many issues and questions. Some have been tackled in books, movies, and other media such as *The Boys from Brazil* by Ira Levin in which multiple boys were cloned from Hitler. Other implications have to do with the possibility of raising cloned humans for spare body parts, for replacing a person with extraordinary talent or characteristics either "good" or "evil," or for many other reasons. Could a person be cloned without his or her knowledge or permission? What decisions should be made, if any? Who will make them? Who will enforce them and how?

GENETICALLY ALTERED AND TRANSGENIC PLANTS

Genetic alteration of plants has been a source of controversy, although humans have improved crops and domesticated animals by selective breeding for many years. Some of the ways to improve farm crops include making plants resistant to disease and predators, making plants resistant to weed killers, improving crop production, increasing the nutritional value, and altering features such as color, taste, and resistance to spoilage and freezing. While the National Research Council stated it was not aware of unsafe conditions brought on by genetically altered plants, the ecological impact and the impact of gene modification on the environment, the possibility of horizontal gene transfer, and other aspects are being examined. For example, soybeans modified with a Brazil nut gene, in one instance, caused allergic reactions in people who were allergic to the nut; thus, such modification could expose consumers to hidden allergies. There are also political and economic ramifications.

INFORMED CONSENT

Informed consent is an ethical issue that is applicable to genetic screening, testing, prenatal diagnosis, and more. The major hazards are in the social, economic, and psychological domains, and these should be discussed. Individuals should be informed of potential risks. The needed information should be described in terms understandable to the individual. The guidelines used nationally for the protection of human subjects are applicable to testing and screening even though they were developed for experimental research consents, as it can be legitimately argued that many potential short- and long-term risks of some genetic testing and screening are still not known. Thus, the nature and purposes of the genetic testing or screening should be clearly spelled out. What clients should know before consenting is discussed under the individual topics.

ISSUES OF PRIVACY, CONFIDENTIALITY, AND DISCLOSURE

These issues are inherent in genetic screening, genetic testing, prenatal diagnosis, and genetic counseling. Before availing themselves of such services, individuals should know who can gain access to the information and what confidentiality is in place. In regard to genetic counseling, most genetic counselors consider themselves responsible to the counselee. However, during the genetic testing or genetic counseling process, the counselor or provider may encounter information that is important to relatives of the counselee. By knowledge of the disorder and its pattern of transmission and by examining the pedigree of the family, other relatives at risk may be identified. Sometimes the counselee will not wish for such relatives to be contacted for several reasons: fear of stigmatization, a desire not to be in contact with certain relatives, a belief that the relative will not want the information obtained, and others. This is a delicate situation that deals with sensitive information. The President's Commission for the Study of Ethical Problems in Medicine and Biomedical and Behavioral Research (1983) recommended that under certain circumstances, the professional genetic counselor's primary obligation to a client may be subsumed. Their report stated:

> A professional's ethical duty of confidentiality to an immediate patient or client can be overridden only if several conditions are satisfied: 1) reasonable efforts to elicit voluntary consent to disclosure have failed; 2) there is a high probability both that harm will occur if the information is withheld and that the disclosed information will actually be used

to avert harm; 3) the harm that identifiable individuals would suffer would be serious; and 4) appropriate precautions are taken to ensure that only the genetic information needed for diagnosis and/or treatment of the disease in question is disclosed.

Because of the complexity of breaching professional confidentiality, even in the context of the "duty to warn," it has been suggested that the person contemplating such action seek review by "an appropriate third party." The Committee on Assessing Genetic Risks of the Institute of Medicine (Andrews, et al. 1994) has also commented. It believes that patients should be encouraged to share genetic status information with their spouse. This, however, can have later consequences. For example, in a case in South Carolina, the husband of a woman known to be at risk for Huntington disease sought to terminate her parental rights, and she was ordered by the court to undergo genetic testing. The committee also stated that while patients should share genetic information that would avert risk with relatives, that "confidentiality be breached and relatives informed about genetic risks only when attempts to elicit voluntary disclosure fail, there is a high probability of irreversible or fatal harm to the relative, the disclosure of the information will prevent harm, the disclosure is limited to the information necessary for diagnosis or treatment of the relative, and there is no other reasonable way to avert the harm" (p. 278). For example, a relative at risk for malignant hyperthermia (see Chapter 6) could have his or her life endangered by exposure to certain anesthetic agents if he/she possessed the mutant gene. In another situation, a pregnant woman whose male partner has a 50% chance for having Huntington disease wants to have prenatal diagnosis, but her male partner does not want to know his status, which could be revealed (but might not be) if the status of the fetus became known. They pose the question of whether the right of the pregnant mother to know the status of her fetus outweighs the right of the father at risk not to know his genetic status. In another case, one adult sibling could be diagnosed with Gaucher disease and not wish to inform the other siblings, who are patients of the same physician. The choices are to inform the siblings with appropriate education and counseling

and refer them for testing, perform such testing when other blood tests are being done without informing them of the reason, and not informing them. Does the health care provider have an overriding duty to warn them, and are such situations dependent on treatment options available? There are many such examples of ethical issues that advances in genetics engender.

Another statement on disclosure is by the American Society of Human Genetics (1998). The discussion includes the point that genetic information is both personal and familial, and the association provides a discussion of legal and ethical considerations, as well as international perspectives. Confidentiality is generally applied to genetic information like other medical information. It states, however, that "confidentiality is not absolute, and, in exceptional cases, ethical, legal, and statutory obligations may permit health-care professionals to disclose otherwise confidential information" (p. 474). It outlines exceptional circumstances that permit disclosure: "Disclosure should be permissible where attempts to encourage disclosure on the part of the patient have failed; where the harm is likely to occur and is serious and foreseeable; where the at-risk relative(s) is identifiable; and where either the disease is preventable/treatable or medically accepted standards indicate that early monitoring will reduce the genetic risk" and "The harm that may result from failure to disclose should outweigh the harm that may result from disclosure" (p. 474). Finally health care professionals are said to have a duty to inform counselees that information obtained may have familial implications. They further state that patients should be informed about the implications of their genetic test results and about potential risks to their family members. It is suggested that this be done both before genetic testing and when results are communicated. The American Society of Clinical Oncology (2003) states that the "health care provider's obligations (if any) to at-risk relatives are best fulfilled by communication of familial risk to the person undergoing testing, emphasizing the importance of sharing this information with family members so they may also benefit" (p. 2403). It also stated that there are differences in obligations when the at-risk relatives are also patients of the health care provider. Although case law is not clear, there have been lawuits because of physician failure to warn family members about their possible risk of genetic disease.

OWNERSHIP AND FUTURE USE OF SAMPLES TAKEN FOR TESTING/SCREENING

When blood or urine samples are used for testing or screening, these are often stored to use for additional testing. What happens to such samples? Such a use and its implications may be unknown to the person from whom it has been taken. Thus consent is not usual or may be buried in a complicated consent form. Could such samples be used for forensic or other legal identification reasons, and what does this mean in terms of the individual's right to privacy? Although these samples are generally considered to be a good source of material for research, certain questions are raised. What responsibilities are there if these samples are tested later and found to be positive for a different disorder or if a future test or treatment became available? Is the researcher then responsible for locating that individual and communicating results? Who actually owns these samples? The question of asking for the individual's consent for use in later testing could be obtained along with instructions for whether the individual wants to be informed of the results. This approach is being increasingly adopted. Individuals may also change their mind about the use of stored samples, and they should know the procedure for making their wishes known and acted on. If identifying information is erased from the sample, potential risks and benefits would be decreased, but again many issues are raised. One weighs the value of respecting individuality with the potential to discover potentially useful information. A controversy in the news media involved obtaining DNA samples from persons in armed services that were to be stored for 75 years. The reason given was for identification of combat casualties (see Chapter 3). In 1995, two members of the U.S. Marine Corps asserted that this violated their rights, but the military prevailed in a hearing. Statements on the storage and use of DNA samples have been formulated by various groups, but satisfactory legislation has not occurred.

EUGENICS, GENETIC DISCRIMINATION, AND GENETIC ENHANCEMENT

Eugenics refers to the improvement of a species through genetic manipulation. Positive eugenics seeks to accomplish this by increasing the frequency of traits considered desirable through encouraging selective mating and reproduction of those possessing such traits (the "fit"). Negative eugenics seeks to reduce the frequency of traits considered undesirable by preventing the reproduction of those persons possessing such traits (the "unfit"). Although plant and animal breeders have long practiced eugenics to improve crops and livestock, active advocation of formal programs in humans began in the latter part of the 19th century.

In America the Eugenics Record Office was established in Cold Spring Harbor, New York, in 1910. One of its major goals was the preservation of the "racial welfare" of the United States through the application of positive and negative eugenics by encouraging the propagation of those whom they considered to be fit and by preventing the propagation of those they considered unfit. Those whom they considered fit were individuals who were healthy, intelligent, of high moral character, of Anglo-Saxon or Nordic extraction, affluent, Protestant, and of the upper or upper-middle class. In fact, these characteristics were generally synonymous with those possessed by the eugenicists themselves. Although many proponents of eugenics were sincere in their intent to strengthen the human race and alleviate suffering, the movement was also a refuge for bigots, racists, and male supremists who came to dominate it. Genetics was used in an attempt to biologically justify the perceived inferiority of Blacks, Jews, and Southern and Eastern Europeans, including the Irish because they were Catholics. The activities and influence of the eugenicists ranged from sponsoring blue ribbon baby contests at county and state fairs to issues with a far more serious impact, such as eugenics sterilization laws and the Immigration Restriction Act of 1924 (the Johnson Act). The latter restricted immigration to 2% of the number of each nationality listed in the 1890 Census, a year that was well before the mass immigration of persons from Southern and Eastern Europe. This situation existed until passage of the Cellar Act of 1965.

Compulsory sterilization was seen as a way to prevent the propagation of the "unfit," a term that in its various interpretations included the mentally retarded (now called "persons with intellectual disabilities"), the insane, alcoholics, orphans, paupers, derelicts, epileptics, diseased and degenerate persons, and even chicken thieves. Campaigns for eugenics sterilization laws were launched, although some enthusiasts were already performing sterilizations in state institutions. The first state to institute involuntary sterilization laws was Indiana, in 1907. The wording and provisions of the laws varied greatly from state to state, and by 1935, more than 30 states had passed such laws. California was most active in their implementation and by 1935 had sterilized about 10,000 persons, whereas in the entire United States about 20,000 sterilizations were performed. Although these laws remain on the books in many states, they are rarely invoked. In Oregon, Governor Kitzhaber apologized for past abuses of sterilization occurring from 1923 to 1981. In addition to the institutionalized mentally retarded, involuntary sterilization abuses extended to those who were Black or poor. In the People's Republic of China, those persons with "a genetic disease of a serious nature" and those who are married and of childbearing age who are "considered to be inappropriate for childbearing" are asked to be sterilized or use long-term contraceptive methods (Beardsley, 1997; "Brave new now", 1997). The Minister of Public Health (Chen Mingzhang) in 1994 was quoted as saying that "births of inferior quality are serious among the old revolutionary base, ethnic minorities, the frontier and economically poor areas." Some have said that prenatal diagnosis with selective pregnancy termination already constitutes eugenics. Others believe these techniques constitute disease prevention instead. The question of preimplantation genetic diagnosis following in vitro fertilization to allow the selection and implantation of an unaffected embryo is generally considered more ethically acceptable than prenatal diagnosis followed by abortion. In the former case, spare embryos are not allowed to further develop, which many see as a more acceptable choice.

The misuse and misunderstanding of genetic knowledge coupled with an emerging doctrine of racial superiority led to disenchantment and de-

nouncement of the movement by many geneticists and citizens. By the 1930s, the visible abuse of genetics and eugenics for totalitarian aims and the flagrant disregard for human rights were so evident in Nazi Germany that not only did the movement die in the United States, but the discipline of human genetics itself was left with a tinge of suspicion that permeates many programs even today. Fears of genetic discrimination remain. For example, when it was discovered that a specific gene mutation for colon cancer was most common among Ashkenazi Jews, there were fears raised about discrimination that led to statements issued such as this one by Dr. Francis Collins: "I think it is very unlikely that the total number of genetic aberrations carried around by Jewish individuals is any greater than that of any other group" and "There is no perfect genetic specimen. We are all flawed" (Wade, 1997). However, as gene studies in Ashkenazi Jews continue, many leaders are refusing to participate, fearing vulnerability to discrimination. This is reminiscent of the feelings of many Black leaders in the early 1970s when screening programs for sickle cell anemia began.

As genetic applications to health care increase there are further concerns about genetic discrimination in relation to insurance issues and employment. Various pieces of legislation have been attempted since the mid-1990s when the Ethical, Legal and Social Implications (ELSI) Working Group of the Human Genome Project published on this concern, advocating that people be eligible for health insurance regardless of what is known about their past, present, or future health status. There are fears that health insurance coverage could be denied or excessive premiums charged for persons with genetic conditions that are actual or involve susceptibility. An example of the latter is a woman who carries a *BRCA1* mutation in which (as discussed in Chapter 10) susceptibility to cancers such as breast and ovarian is increased but not certain to develop. Potentially an individual or family member could be required to undergo genetic testing. While the Health Insurance Portability and Accountability Act (HIPAA) provided some protection against genetic discrimination in health insurance, it did not prohibit charging higher rates to persons based on genetic makeup, protect against disclosure of genetic information to insurers, or allow insurance applicants to be required to have genetic testing. The

Genetic Information Nondiscrimination Act of 2005 passed the Senate but was "held at the desk" at the House of Representatives. At this writing, important issues have not been addressed, and adequate and widespread protections have not been put in place.

As genetic manipulation and selective choice progress, the question of genetic enhancement has been raised. For example, certain characteristics are known to be associated with success in certain sports. In some instances, physicians have been asked to administer growth hormone not because the given individual is particularly short but in order to produce a taller individual so that he/she could play basketball, for example. The concept of "gene doping" is defined by the World Anti-Doping Agency as "the non-therapeutic use of genes, genetic elements, and or cells that have the capacity to enhance athletic performance" (Unal & Unal, 2004, p. 358). Examples include the potential for using gene therapy that encodes erythropoetin to increase oxygen transport in the tissues to increase aerobic capacity or the insulin-like growth factor-1 gene to stimulate muscle hypertrophy in specific muscles to enhance performance.

Athletes using such methods would be subjecting themselves to known and unknown health risks. Various agencies are developing warnings and standards. Another aspect is genotyping of athletes. It has been noted that certain gene variations might convey certain performance enhancements. For example, the R577X polymorphism in the gene that encodes for α-actinin-3, which is responsible for generating muscle force at high velocity, appears to produce advantages in performance. Conceivably using genotyping to select athletes early based on possession of identified favorable genetic polymorphisms and discouraging others has serious ethical and societal implications. It could even result in the planning of children who would carry a certain configuration of these polymorphisms to create a potential class of superathletes. As the future ability to perform genetic manipulations, gene therapy, and other direct and indirect genetic technologies is on the horizon, will we be asked to enhance human abilities and traits? Will embryo manipulation for enhancement and therapy become increasingly common? Will such options only be for those with the financial means to afford them? What kinds of discrimination could result?

INDIVIDUAL RIGHTS VERSUS THOSE OF OTHERS

The rights of individuals to make reproductive and other decisions are increasingly complicated by outside forces. For example, if a fetus is found to be affected with Down syndrome, the parents may decide to give birth to this child. If insurance companies or society said that if they knowingly gave birth to this child, no medical or health insurance coverage would apply for the birth or future care, how would that influence their decision? There are many issues regarding life insurance, disability income insurance, long-term-care insurance, critical illness coverage, and medical expense insurance in regard to genetics. In another instance, a Los Angeles TV anchorwoman, Bree Walker Lampley, was criticized on a talk show and elsewhere for deciding to have a child despite the fact that she has ectrodactyly, a hand deformity in which some digits are fused, known as "lobster claw," for which there is a 50% risk of transmission.

In order to provoke thought, some of the questions and problems relating to individual versus societal good and rights are exemplified by the following: Should society allow affected individuals to marry or mate if no prenatal diagnosis is available for the specific condition in question? Should they be prohibited from procreation? What should society do if a couple chooses not to abort an affected fetus? Should such measures be compulsory? Should there be more subtle pressures such as the refusal of society to contribute financially to the care and education of such children? How do these questions apply to women who are eligible for prenatal diagnosis because of advanced maternal age or because of other indications? Should prenatal diagnosis be mandatory for everyone? Should newborn screening be more inclusive, such as for adult-onset diseases and presymptomatic disorders? When one member of a couple is at high risk for inheriting the gene for a disorder such as Huntington disease, should that couple be "allowed" by society to have natural children without having molecular testing for the Huntington disease gene? And if the gene is present, does that person have the right to reproduce if he/she so chooses? Does he/she have a duty not to reproduce? Should society enforce sterilization of the person at risk? Does the right of the person to reproduce always supersede the possible burden to society? Does a person have the right to reproduce no matter what the effects are on his/her direct descendants? Should the right of the individual prevail?

Further advances in treatment will continue to reduce the burden of certain disorders. For example, the inborn inability to synthesize a certain vitamin may be compensated for relatively simply by taking a pill once a day. Would this disorder be considered a burden? What about other types of selection? For example, in one survey, a substantial percentage of respondents said they would want to choose a more intelligent or attractive fetus. How large a burden is the correction of a disorder such as pyloric stenosis by surgery? Would it be important enough to limit the reproduction of persons who have had this disorder? Who would make such decisions? On what basis? Should genetic counseling be firmly directive? Should it consider the interests of society or the interests of the individuals seeking counseling? Should the number of children a heterozygous couple is allowed to have be limited by law to reduce the frequency of the gene? What about all of the genotypes not detectable by current screening or diagnostic methods? What about possession of traits apart from the mainstream (including variations) whose meaning is unclear?

Other meanings are legal ones. Would criminals be able to mount a defense on the basis of their genetic constitution, for example, if they possessed genes with susceptibility to violence or aggression? In a California murder case, a woman was found not guilty because her violence was attributed to her having Huntington disease.

Other defenses have been mounted on the basis of genetic constitution. Should couples who decide to give birth to children with serious genetic conditions be criminally guilty of child abuse, as some have suggested? In a California case, the court stated that a child with a genetic condition could sue the parents for not having prenatal diagnosis and terminating the pregnancy.

New techniques are constantly raising new ethical questions. For example, should fetal oocytes be taken from the ovaries of aborted fetuses and used in assistive reproduction? What about posthumous reproduction? What should be done with embryos that have been cryopreserved? What do the terms *mother* and *father* mean?

FUTURE GENERATIONS

Suppose that it was decided that society could now think about instituting a type of eugenics program for the good of future generations. In addition to the problem of the inherent rights of the individual, some of the problems that could be identified at present are as follows:

- Knowledge about the inheritance of many traits is inadequate.
- It is not known what genotypes may be needed for humans coping with different environments in the future.
- It is not known what traits would be most desirable. For example, tallness might be a liability because of crowded conditions, whereas shortness might become highly valued.
- The consequences of the total elimination of a particular genotype cannot be foreseen.
- New mutations would probably continue to add new deleterious genes and traits to the population.
- Not all traits or genes are currently detectable or diagnosable.
- What traits should be included? Would late-onset diseases be detected presymptomatically? If so, perhaps no one would be free of such genetic susceptibility.
- The development of new treatments for disorders cannot be accurately predicted.
- Would the political and social ramifications of restricted reproduction compensate for perceived benefits?
- What would happen if harmful genes that were eliminated were tightly linked to essential ones?
- Who would make decisions about such programs?
- How could we reconcile such programs with the value we place on individual freedom in a democratic society?
- Have we already set foot down a eugenics path by offering testing, screening, prenatal diagnosis with the option of pregnancy termination, and assisted reproductive techniques?

These questions and problems are significant. Some have advocated the creation of a eugenics board to decide on traits amenable to and conditions for either a voluntary or compulsory eugenics program. Instead, it seems as if efforts should be concentrated on the support of society for a couple and family in making knowledgeable, voluntary decisions in their own best interests and in the elucidation and elimination of genetic disorders and birth defects.

END NOTES

This chapter has posed many questions and issues for discussion that are integrated throughout the text. Advances in genetics have profound impacts on contemporary society as well as future genera-

tions. Such advances include predictive susceptibility and other genetic testing and reproductive planning, prenatal diagnosis, assisted reproductive technologies, the potential for genetic manipulation and technology for both therapy and enhancement, the use of cloning, stem cell research and therapy, pharmacogenomic selection for therapy, cloning, use of population data bases such as in Iceland to search for variations, and use of genetic engineering in agriculture. What happens today affects both individuals and the larger society. It is important that we ensure that ethical standards and policies safeguard the rights of individuals as well as enable responsible scientific progress and research.

References

American Academy of Pediatrics. Committee on Genetics. Section on Hematology/Oncology. (2002). Health supervision for children with sickle cell disease. *Pediatrics, 109*, 526–535.

American Academy of Pediatrics. Committee on Genetics. (2001). Health supervision for children with Down syndrome. *Pediatrics, 107*, 442–449.

American Academy of Pediatrics. Newborn Screening Task Force. (2000). Serving the family from birth to the medical home. Newborn screening: A blueprint for the future. A call for a national agenda on state newborn screening programs. *Pediatrics, 106*, 389–427.

American Academy of Pediatrics. Committee on Genetics. (1995). Health supervision for children with neurofibromatosis. *Pediatrics, 96*, 368–372.

American Diabetes Association. (2006). Report of the Expert Committee on the diagnosis and classifications of diabetes mellitus. *Diabetes Care, 27*, S43–S48.

American Psychiatric Association. (2000). *Diagnostic and statistical manual of mental disorders: DSM-IV-TR 2000.* 4th ed. Washington, DC: American Psychiatric Publishing.

American Society of Clinical Oncology. (2003). American Society of Clinical Oncology policy statement update: Genetic testing for cancer susceptibility. *Journal of Clinical Oncology, 21*, 2397–2406.

American Society of Human Genetics Board of Directors and the American College of Medical Genetics Board of Directors. (1995). Points to consider: Ethical, legal, and psychosocial implications of genetic testing in children and adolescents. *American Journal of Human Genetics, 57*, 1233–1241.

American Society of Human Genetics Social Issue Committee on Familial Disclosure. (1998). Professional disclosure of familial genetic information. *American Journal of Human Genetics, 62*, 474–483.

American Society for Reproductive Medicine. (2004). Guidelines for sperm donation. *Fertility and Sterility, 82* (Suppl 1), S9–S12.

American Thoracic Society/European Respiratory Society Statement. (2003). Standards for the diagnosis and management of individuals with alpha-1-antitrypsin deficiency. *American Journal of Respiratory and Critical Care Medicine, 168*, 818–900.

Andrews, L. B., Fullarton, J. E., Holtzman, N. A., & Motulsky, A. G. (Eds.). (1994). *Assessing genetic risks. Implications for health and social policy.* Washington, DC: National Academy Press.

Barlow-Stewart, K., Burnett, L., Proos, A., Howell, V., Huq, F., Lazarus, R., et al. (2003). A genetic screening programme for Tay-Sachs disease and cystic fibrosis for Australian Jewish high school students. *Journal of Medical Genetics, 40*, e45–e57.

Beardsley, T. (1997). China syndrome. *Scientific American, 276*, 33–34.

Brandt-Rauf, P. W., & Brandt-Rauf, S. I. (2004). Genetic testing in the workplace: Ethical, legal, and social implications. *Annual Review of Public Health, 25*, 139–153.

Braude, P. (2006). Preimplantation diagnosis for genetic susceptibility. *New England Journal of Medicine, 355*, 541–543.

Brave new now. (1997). *Nature Genetics, 15*, 1–2.

Committee for the Study of Inborn Errors of Metabolism. (1975). *Genetic screening.* Washington DC: National Academy of Sciences.

Conway, G. S. (2002). The impact and management of Turner's syndrome in adult life. *Best Practice Research Clinical Endocrinology & Metabolism, 16*, 243–261.

Denborough, M. A. & Lovell, R. R. H. (1960). Anaesthetic deaths in a family. *Lancet, 2*, 45.

Doll, R., & Wakeford, R. (1997). Risk of childhood cancer from fetal irradiation. *British Journal of Radiology, 70*, 130–139.

Frías, J. L., Davenport, M. L., the Committee on Genetics, and the Section on Endocrinology. (2003). Health supervision for children with Turner syndrome. *Pediatrics, 111*, 692–702.

Gebhardt, D. O. (2002). Sperm donor suffers years later from inherited disease. *Journal of Medical Ethics, 28*, 213–214.

Genetic counseling. (1975). *American Journal of Human Genetics, 27*, 240–244.

Gerard, S., Hayes, M., & Rothstein, R. A. (2002). On the edge of tomorrow: Fitting genomics into public health policy. *Journal of Law and Medical Ethics, 30* (3 Suppl), 173–176.

Hewitt, J. B. (1992). *Cancer risks of nurses to assess the carcinogenic potential of antineoplastic drugs.* Unpublished doctoral dissertation. University of Illinois.

Holtzman, N. A., & Watson, M. S. (Eds.). (1997, September). *Promoting safe and effective genetic testing in the United States. Final Report of the Task Force on Genetic Testing.* Bethesda, MD: National Human Genome Research Institute.

Howse, J. L., & Katz, M. (2000). The importance of newborn screening. *Pediatrics, 106*, 595.

Hoyme, H. E., May, P. A., Kalberg, W. O, Kodituwakku, P., Gossage, J. P., Trujillo, P. M., et al. (2005). A practical clinical approach to diagnosis of fetal alcohol spectrum disorders: Clarification of the 1996 Institute of Medicine criteria. *Pediatrics, 115*, 39–47.

Lashley, F. R. (2005). *Clinical genetics in nursing practice.* (3rd ed.). New York: Springer Publishing.

McLeod, R., Boyer, K., Karrison, T., Kasza, K., Swisher, C., Roizen, N., et al. (2006). Outcome of treatment for congenital toxoplasmosis, 1981–2004: The National Collaborative Chicago-based Congenital Toxoplasmosis Study. *Clinical Infectious Diseases, 42*, 1381–1394.

National Institutes of Health Consensus Development Panel. (2000). National Institutes of Health Consensus Development Conference Statement: Phenylketonuria (PKU): Screening and management, October 16–18, 2000. *Pediatrics 106*, 972–982.

Natowicz, N. R., Alper, J. R., & Alper, J. S. (1992). Genetic discrimination and the law. *American Journal of Human Genetics, 50*, 465–475.

Practice Committee of the Society for Assisted Reproductive Technology; Practice Committee of the American Society for Reproductive Medicine. (2006). America Society for Reproductive Medicine/Society for Assisted Reproductive Technology position statement on West Nile virus. *Fertility and Sterility, 83*, 527–528.

Presidents Commission for the Study of Ethical Problems in Medicine and Biomedical and Behavioral Research. (1983). *Screening and counseling for genetic conditions.* Washington, DC: Government Printing Office.

Saenger, P., Wikland, K. A., Conway, G. S., Davenport, M., Gravholt, C. H., Hintz, R., et al. (2001). Recommendations for the diagnosis and management of Turner syndrome. *Journal of Clinical Endocrinology and Metabolism, 86*, 3061–3069.

Scheuner, M. T. (2003). Genetic evaluation for coronary artery disease. *Genetics in Medicine, 5*, 269–285.

Schwarz, E. B., Maselli, J., Norton, M., & Gonzalez, R. (2005). Prescription of teratogenic medications in United States ambulatory practices. *American Journal of Medicine, 118*, 1240–1249.

Shaffer, L. G., & Tommerup, N. (Eds.). (1995). *ISCN 2005. An international system for human cytogenetic nomenclature (2005).* Basel, Switzerland: S. Karger.

Shek, C. C., Ng, P. C., Fung, G. P., Cheng, F. W., Chan, P. K., Peiris, M. J., et al. (2003). Infants born to mothers with severe acute respiratory syndrome. *Pediatrics, 112*, e254–e256.

Shi, L., & Chia, S-E. (2001). A review of studies on maternal occupational exposures and birth defects, and the limitations associated with these studies. *Occupational Medicine, 51*, 230–244.

Theos, A., & Korf, B. R. (2006). Pathophysiology of neurofibromatosis type 1. *Annals of Internal Medicine, 144*, 842–849.

Unal, M., & Unal, D. O. (2004). Gene doping in sports. *Sports Medicine, 34*, 357–362.

Wade, N. (1997 Sept. 14). Testing genes to save a life without costing you a job. *New York Times*, 5.

Wald, N. J., Cuckle, H., Brock, J. H., Peto, R., Polani, P. E., & Woodford, F. P. (1977). Maternal serum-alpha-fetoprotein measurement in antenatal screening for anencephaly and spina bifida in early pregnancy. Report of UK collaborative study on alpha-fetoprotein in relation to neural-tube defects. *Lancet, 1(8026)*, 1323–1332.

Watson, M. S., Lloyd-Puryear, M. A., Mann, M. Y., Rinaldo, P., & Howell, R. R. (2006). Main report. *Genetic Medicine, 8(5 Suppl)*, 12S–252S.

Welsh, M. J. & Smith, A. E. (1995). Cystic fibrosis. *Scientific American, 273*(6), 52–59.

Wolfberg, A. J. (2006). Genes on the web—direct-to-consumer marketing of genetic testing. *New England Journal of Medicine, 355*, 543–545.

Working Party of the Clinical Genetics Society. (1994). the genetic testing of children. *Journal of Medical Genetics, 31*, 785–797.

World Health Organization Working Group. (1989). Glucose-6-phosphate dehydrogenase deficiency. *Bulletin of the World Health Organization, 67*(6), 601–611.

Further Reading

Almond, B. (2005). Genetic profiling of newborns: Ethical and social issues. *Nature Reviews Genetics, 7,* 67–71.

Blennow, K., de Leon, M. J., & Zetterberg, H. (2006). Alzheimer's disease. *Lancet, 368,* 387–403.

Brown, D. T., Herbert, M., Lamb, V. K., Chinnery, P. F., Taylor, R. W., Lightowlers, R. N., et al. (2006). Transmission of mitochondrial DNA disorders: Possibilities for the future. *Lancet, 368,* 87–89.

Centers for Disease Control and Prevention. (2006). Assisted reproductive technology surveillance—United States, 2003. *Morbidity and Mortality Weekly Report, 55 (SS-4),* 1–22.

Centers for Disease Control and Prevention. (2006). Recommendations to improve preconception health and health care—United States. *Morbidity and Mortality Weekly Report, 55 (RR-6),* 1–23.

De Boeck, K., Wilschanski, M., Castellani, C., Taylor, C., Cuppens, H., Dodge, J., et al. (2006). Cystic fibrosis: Terminology and diagnostic algorithms. *Thorax, 61,* 627–635.

Ferretti, P., Tickle, C., Copp, A., & Moore, G. (eds.). (2006). *Embryos, genes and birth defects.* New York: John Wiley & Sons.

Hadfield, S. G., & Humphries, S. E. (2005). Implementation of cascade testing for the detection of familial hypercholesterolaemia. *Current Opinion in Lipidology, 16,* 428–433.

Haines, J. L., & Pericak-Vance, M. A. (2006). *Genetic analysis of complex disease.* New York: John Wiley & Sons.

Hart, E. S., Albright, M. B., Rebello, G. N., & Grottkau, B. E. (2006). Developmental dysplasia of the hip: Nursing implications and anticipatory guidance for parents. *Orthopedic Nursing, 25,* 100–109.

Hoyme, H. E., May, P. A., Kalberg, W. O., Kodituwakku, P., Gossage, J. P., Trujillo, P. M., et al. (2005). A practical clinical approach to diagnosis of fetal alcohol spectrum disorders: Clarification of the 1996 Institute of Medicine criteria. *Pediatrics, 115,* 39–47.

Janssens, A. C. J. W., Aulchenko, Y. S., Elefante, S., Borsboom, G. J. J. M., Steyerberg, E. W., & van Duijn, C. M. (2006). Predictive testing for complex diseases using multiple genes: Fact or fiction? *Genetics in Medicine, 8,* 395–400.

Jones, K. (2005). *Smith's recognizable patterns of human malformation.* New York: Elsevier Health Sciences.

Lashley, F. R. (2001). Genetics and nursing: The interface in education, research, and practice. *Biological Research in Nursing, 3,* 13–23.

Lashley, F. R. (2005). *Clinical genetics in nursing practice.* 3rd ed. New York: Springer Publishing.

Lea, D. H., & Monsen, R. B. (2003). Preparing nurses for a 21st century role in genomics-based health care. *Nursing Education Perspectives, 24(2),* 75–80.

Lewis, J. A., Calzone, K. M., & Jenkins, J. (2006). Essential nursing competencies and curricula guidelines for genetics and genomics. *MCN American Journal of Maternal Child Nursing, 31,* 146–153.

Lewis, R. (2005). *Human genetics.* 7th ed. New York: McGraw-Hill.

Ludman, M. D., & Wynbrandt, J. (2006). *Encyclopedia of genetic disorders and birth defects.* New York: Facts on File, Inc.

Morton, C. C., Nance, W. E. (2006). Newborn hearing screening—a silent revolution. *New England Journal of Medicine, 354,* 2151–2164.

Nussbaum, R. L., Thompson, M. W., McInnes, R. R., & Willard, H. F. (2004). *Thompson & Thompson genetics in medicine.* New York: Elsevier Science.

Ornoy, A., & Tenenbaum, A. (2006). Pregnancy outcome following infections by coxsackie, echo, measles, mumps, hepatitis, polio and encephalitis viruses. *Reproductive Toxicology, 21,* 446–457.

Prows, C. A., & Prows, D. R. (2004). Medication selection by genotype: How genetics is changing drug prescribing and efficacy. *American Journal of Nursing, 104 (5),* 60–70.

Raghuveer, T. S., Garg, U., & Graf, W. D. (2006). Inborn errors of metabolism in infancy and early childhood: An update. *American Family Physician, 73,* 1981–1990.

Rasko, J. E., Ankeny, R. A., & O'Sullivan, G. M. (eds.) (2006). *The ethics of inheritable genetic modification: A dividing line?* Cambridge: Cambridge University Press.

Rhodes, R. (2006). Why test children for adult-onset genetic diseases? *Mt. Sinai Journal of Medicine, 73,* 609–616.

Roche, P. A., & Annas, G. J. (2006). DNA testing, banking and genetic privacy. *New England Journal of Medicine, 355,* 545–540.

Rutter, M. J., & Rutter, D. R. (2006). *Genes and behaviour: Nature-nurture interplay explained.* Oxford: Blackwell Publishers.

Schapira, A. H. V. (2006). Mitochondrial disease. *Lancet, 368,* 70–82.

Shannon, T. A. (2005). *Genetics: Science, ethics, and public policy.* Rowman & Littlefield Publishers, Inc.

Smith, G. D., Ebrahim, S., Lewis, S., Hansell, A. L., Palmer, L. J., & Burton, P. R. (2005). Genetic epidemiology and public health: Hope, hype, and future prospects. *Lancet, 366,* 1484–1498.

Stevenson, R. E., & Hall, J. G. (eds.). (2005). *Human malformations and related anomalies.* Oxford: Oxford University Press.

Strachan, T., & Read, A. P. (2004). *Human molecular genetics 3.* London: Garland Science.

Summers, K. M., West, J. A., Peterson, M. M., Stark, D., McGill, J. J., & West, M. J. (2006). Challenges in the diagnosis of Marfan syndrome. *Medical Journal of Australia, 184,* 627–631.

Therrell, B. L., Lloyd-Puryear, M. A., & Mann, M. Y. (2005). Understanding newborn screening system issues with emphasis on cystic fibrosis screening. *Journal of Pediatrics, 147,* S6–S10.

Toriello, H. V. for the Professional Practice and Guidelines Committee. (2005). Folic acid and neural tube defects. *Genetics in Medicine, 7,* 283–284.

Twomey, J. G. (2006). Issues in genetic testing of children. *MCN American Journal of Maternal Child Nursing, 31,* 156–163.

Van Cleve, S. N., & Cohen, W. I. (2006). Part I: Clinical practice guidelines for children with Down syndrome from birth to 12 years. *Journal of Pediatric Health Care, 20,* 37–54.

Van Cleve, S. N., & Cohen, W. I. (2006). Part II: Clinical practice guidelines for children with Down syndrome from 12 to 21 years. *Journal of Pediatric Health Care, 20,* 198–205.

van Esch, H. The fragile X premutation: New insights and clinical consequences. *European Journal of Medical Genetics, 49,* 1–8.

Vichinsky, E. P., MacKlin, E. A., Waye, J. S., Lorey, F., & Olivieri, N. F. (2005). Changes in the epidemiology of thalassemia in North America: A new minority disease. *Pediatrics, 116,* e818–e825.

Walsh, T., Casadei, S., Coats, K. H., Swisher, E., Stray, S. M., Higgins, J., et al. (2006). Spectrum of mutations in *BRCA1, BRCA2, CHEK2,* and *TP53* in families at high risk of breast cancer. *Journal of the American Medical Association, 295,* 1379–1388.

Watson, M. S., Mann, M. Y., Lloyd-Puryear, M. A., Rinaldo, P., Howell, R. H., & American College of Medical Genetics Newborn Screening Expert Group. (2006). Newborn Screening: Toward a uniform screening panel and system—executive summary. *Pediatrics, 117,* S296-S307.

Wattendorf, D. J., & Hadley, D. W. (2005). Family history: The three-generation pedigree. *American Family Physician, 72,* 441–448.

Wenstrom, K. D. (2005). Evaluation of Down syndrome screening strategies. *Seminars in Perinatology, 29,* 219–224.

Williams, J. K., Skirton, H., & Masny, A. (2006). Ethics, policy, and educational issues in genetic testing. *Journal of Nursing Scholarship, 38,* 119–125.

Working Party of the Clinical Genetics Society. (1994). The genetic testing of children. *Journal of Medical Genetics, 31,* 785–797.

Wright, L. (2005). Understanding genetics: A primer for occupational health practice. *American Association of Occupational Health Nursing Journal, 53,* 534–542.

Appendix A

Useful Genetic Web Sites for Professional Information

American Board of Genetic Counseling
http://www.abgc.net

American Board of Medical Genetics
http://www.abmg.org

American College of Medical Genetics
http://www.acmg.net

American Society of Human Genetics
http://www.faseb.org/genetics/ashg/ashgmenu.htm

Association of Professors of Human and Medical Genetics
http://www.faseb.org/genetics/aphmg/aphmgl.htm

Centers for Disease Control and Prevention, Office of Genomics and Disease Prevention
http://www.cdc.gov/genomics/

Genetic Alliance
http://www.geneticalliance.org

Genetics Education Center at the University of Kansas Medical Center
http://www.kumc.edu/gec

Genetics Education Partnership
http://genetics-education-partnership.mbt.washington.edu

Genetic Science Learning Center
http://gslc.genetics.utah.edu

HumGen
http://www.humgen.umontreal.ca/en/

International Society of Nurses in Genetics
http://www.isong.org

National Coalition for Health Professional Education in Genetics
http://www.nchpeg.org

National Human Genome Research Institute, National Institutes of Health
http://www.nhgri.nih.gov/

National Organization of Rare Disorders (NORD)
http://www.rarediseases.org

National Society of Genetic Counselors
http://www.nsgc.org

Online Mendelian Inheritance in Man (OMIM), National Center for Biotechnology Information
http://www.ncbi.nim.nih.gov/omim

Appendix B

Organizations and Groups With Web Sites That Provide Information, Products, and Services for Genetic Conditions

GROUPS PROVIDING A LARGE AMOUNT OF GENETIC SUPPORT GROUP INFORMATION

Canadian Directory of Genetic Support Groups
http://www.Ihsc.on.ca/programs/niedgenet/

Canadian Organization for Rare Disorders
http://www.cord.ca

Center for Jewish Genetic Diseases,
   Mt. Sinai School of Medicine
http://www.mssm.edu/jewish_genetic

Directory of Online Genetic Support Groups
http://www.mostgene.org/support/index.html

Easter Seal Society National Headquarters
http://www.easter-seals.org

European Organization for Rare Diseases
http://www.eurordis.org

Family Village
http://www.familyvillage.wisc.edu/index.html

Genetic Alliance
http://www.geneticalliance.org

Genetics Education Center at the University of
   Kansas Medical Center
http://www.kumc.edu/gec

Heredity Disease Foundation
http://www.hdfoundation.org

March of Dimes Birth Defects Foundation
http://www.modimes.org

Maternal and Child Health Bureau,
   Health Resources and Services Administration
http://mchb.hrsa.gov

National Center on Birth Defects and
   Developmental Disabilities
   Centers for Disease Control and Prevention
http://www.cdc.gov/ncbddd

National Coalition of Health Professionals in
   Genetics
http://www.nchpeg.org

National Organization for Rare Disorders
http://www.rarediseases.org

Office of Rare Diseases National Institutes of
   Health
http://rarediseases.info.nih.gov/

GROUPS PROVIDING SUPPORT INFORMATION ON SPECIFIC GENETIC DISORDERS

Aarskog Syndrome
   Aarskog Syndrome Parent Support Group
   http://www.familyvillage.wisc.edu/lib_aars.htm

Achondroplasia—See Short Stature

Acid Maltase Deficiency—See Muscular Dystrophy; Glycogen Storage Diseases; Liver Diseases

Acoustic Neuroma—Also see Neurofibromatosis
Acoustic Neuroma Association
http://anausa.org

Adrenal Disorders—Also see Ambiguous Genitalia; Growth Problems
National Adrenal Diseases Foundation*
http://www.medhelp.org/www/nadf
*Includes Addison disease, congenital adrenal hyperplasia, Cushing syndrome, and adrenal hyperplasia

Adrenoleukodystrophy and Adrenomyeloneuropathy
United Leukodystrophy Foundation
http://www.ulf.org

Agammaglobulinemia—See Immune Disorders

Alagille Syndrome—Also see Liver Diseases
Alagille Syndrome Alliance
http://www.alagille.org

Albinism
National Organization for Albinism and Hypopigmentation
http://www.albinism.org/

Alcohol and Drug Abuse, Including Fetal Alcohol Syndrome
AI-Anon/Alateen
http://www.al-anon.alateen.org

Alcoholics Anonymous
http://www.aa.org

National Organization on Fetal Alcohol Syndrome
http://www. nofas.org

SAMHSA's National Clearinghouse for Alcohol and Drug Information
http://ncadi.samhsa.gov

Alpha- l-Antitrypsin Deficiency—Also see Liver Diseases
Alpha-1 Association
http://www.alpha1.org/

Alzheimer Disease
Administration on Aging, Department of Health and Human Services
http://www.aoa.gov

Alzheimer's Association
http://www.alz.org/

Alzheimer's Disease Education and Referral Center
http://www.alzheimers.org

National Institute on Aging, National Institutes of Health
http://www.nia.nih.gov

Ambiguous Genitalia
Ambiguous Genitalia Support Network
http://www.isna.org/node/531

Intersex Society of North America*
http://www.isna.org
*Includes ambiguous genitalia, hermaphroditism, congenital adrenal hyperplasia, Klinefelter syndrome, and hypospadias

Amputees—Also see Disabilities, General
Amputee Coalition of America
http://www.isna.org/node/531

Amputee Information Network
http://amp-info.net

National Amputee Foundation, Inc.
http:/www.nationalamputation.org

Amyotrophic Lateral Sclerosis—Also see Muscular Dystrophy
ALS Association
http://www.alsa.org

Les Turner Amyotrophic Lateral Sclerosis Foundation, Ltd.
http://wwwlesturnerals.org

Anderson Disease—See Glycogen Storage Disorders

Angelman Syndrome
Angelman Syndrome Foundation
http://www.angelman.org

Angioedema—See Hereditary Angioedema; Immune Disorders

Ankylosing Spondylitis—Also see Arthritis
Spondylitis Association of America*
http://www.spondylitis.org
*Includes ankylosing spondylitis, Reiter syndrome, psoriatic arthritis, and arthritis associated with inflammatory bowel disease

Anophthalmia
  International Children's Anophthalmia
    Network
  http://www.ioi.com/ican

Apert Syndrome—Also see Craniofacial
    Anomalies
  Aperts Syndrome Pen Pals
  http://www.widesmiles.org/support/a.html

Argininosuccinic Aciduria—See Organic
    Acidemias

Arnold-Chiari Syndrome—Also see
    Hydrocephalus
  American Syringomyelia Alliance Project*
  http://www.asap4sm.com
  *Includes syringomyelia and Chiari I and II

  World Arnold-Chiari Malformation Association
  http://www.pressenter.com/~wacma/

Arrhythmias—Also see Heart Defects/Disease
  Cardiac Arrhythmias Research and Education
    Foundation
  http://www.longqt.org

  Sudden Arrhythmia Death Syndromes
    Foundation
  http://www.sads.org

Arthritis
  American Juvenile Arthritis Organization
  http://www.arthritis.org/communities/juvenile_
    arthritis/about_ajao

  Arthritis Foundation
  http://www.arthritis.org

  Arthritis Society (Canada)
  http://www.arthritis.ca/

  National Institute of Arthritis and
    Musculoskeletal and Skin Diseases
  National Institutes of Health
  http://www.niams.nih.gov

Arthrogryposis Multiplex Congenita—Also see
    Muscular Dystrophy
  AVENUES, National Support Group for
    Arthrogryposis Multiplex Congenita
  http://www.avenuesforamc.com

Ataxia—Also see Friedreich Ataxia; Muscular
    Dystrophy
  National Ataxia Foundation*

  http://www.ataxia.org
  *Includes ataxia telangiectasia, Charcot-Marie-
    Tooth disease, hereditary tremor, hereditary
    spastic paraplegia

Ataxia Telangiectasia (Louis Bar Disease)—Also
    see Ataxia; Tay-Sachs Disease
  A-T Children's Project
  http://www.atcp.org

Autism
  Autism Network International
  http://ani.autistics.org

  Autism Society of America
  http://www.autism-society.org/

  Cure Autism Now (CAN)
  http://www.canfoundation.org/

Barth Syndrome
  Barth Syndrome Foundation
  http://www.barthsyndrome.org

Batten Disease (Batten Vogt Syndrome)—Also see
    Tay-Sachs Disease
  Batten's Disease Support and Research
    Association
  http://www.bdsra.org

Beta-Glucuronidase Deficiency—See
    Mucopolysaccharidoses; Tay-Sachs Disease

Biedl-Bardet Syndrome—See Laurence-Moon
    Syndrome

BilaryAtresia—See Liver Diseases

Biotinidase Deficiency—See Metabolic Disorders

Birth Defects, General—Also see Disabilities;
    Genetic Disorders, General
  Birth Defect Research for Children
  http://www.birthdefects.org

  Center for Jewish Genetic Diseases
  http://www.mssm.edu/jewish_genetics

  Easter Seals
  http://www.easter-seals.org

  March of Dimes Birth Defects Foundation
  http://www.modimes.org

  National Center for Birth Defects and
    Developmental Disabilities, Centers for
    Disease Control and Prevention

http://www.cdc.gov/ncbddd

Blindness—See Vision Impairment

Bloom Syndrome
Center for Jewish Genetic Diseases
http://www.mssm.edu/jewish_genetics

Bone Diseases—Also see Osteogenesis Imperfecta;
Paget Disease; Osteoporosis; Osteoporosis and
Related Bone Diseases
National Resource Center, National Institutes of
Health
http://www.osteo.org/

Breast Cancer—Also see Cancer
National Breast Cancer Coalition
http://www.natlbcc.org

Susan G. Komen Breast Cancer Foundation
http://www.komen.org

Breast-Feeding
La Leche League International
http://www.lalecheleague.org

Burke Syndrome—See Schwachman Syndrome

Byler Disease—See Liver Diseases

Canavan Disease—See Tay-Sachs Disease

Cancer—also see specific type
American Cancer Society
http://www.cancer.org

Candlelighters Childhood Cancer Foundation
http://www.candlelighters.org

Kidscope
http://www.kidscope.org

National Cancer Institute, National Institutes of
Health
http://www.nci.nih.gov

National Childhood Cancer Foundation
http://www.curesearch.org/

Starlight Children's Foundation
http://www.starlight.org

Cardiac Arrhythmias/Diseases—See Heart
Defects/Disease

Carnitine Deficiency—Also see Muscular
Dystrophy
FOD Communication Network
http://www.fodsupport.org

Cartilage Hair Hypoplasia-—See Short Stature

Celiac Disease—See Gluten Intolerance

Central Core Disease—See Muscular Dystrophy

Cerebral Palsy
Easter Seals
http://www.easter-seals.org

UCP United Cerebral Palsy
http://www.ucp.org/

Charcot-Marie-Tooth Disease—Also see Muscular
Dystrophy; Ataxia
Charcot-Marie-Tooth Association
http://www.charcot-marie-tooth.org

CHARGE Syndrome
CHARGE Family Support Group (UK)
http://www.widerworld.co.uk/charge/index.htm

CHARGE Syndrome Foundation
http://www.chargesyndrome.org

Chromosome Abnormalities—Also see specific
disorder (e.g., Down Klinefelter, Turner, Cri-
du-Chat); Genetic Disorders; Mental
Retardation; Disabilities, General
11q Net (UK)
http://web.ukonline.co.uk/c.jones/11q/contents.
htm

4p-Support Group
http://www.4p-supportgroup.org

CHARGE Family Support Group
http://www.widerworld.co.uk/charge/index.htm

Chromosome 22 Central
http://www.nt.net/~a815/chr22.htm

Chromosome Deletion Outreach*
http://www.chromodisorder.org
*Includes chromosome deletions, chromosome
duplications, translocations, and inversions

Chromosome 18 Registry and Research Society
http://www.chromosome18.org

Chromosome and Genetic Links
http://www.trisomyonline.org/chromlinks.htm

Cri-du-Chat Syndrome Support Group
http://www.personal.u-net.com/~cridchat

IDEAS: IsoDicentric 15 Exchange Advocacy and
Support*
http://www.idic15.org

*Includes inverted duplication of chromosome 15, supernumerary marker chromosomes, duplication of chromosome 15, and chromosomal anomalies

Parents and Researchers Interested in Smith-Magenis Syndrome*
http://www.prisms.org
*Also includes deletion 17p11.2

SOFT (UK)
http://www.soft.org.uk

Support Organization for Trisomy (SOFT) 18, 13 and Related Disorders
http://www.trisomy.org

Trisomy 9 International Parent Support
http://www.trisomy9.org/9tips.htm

Unique, Rare Chromosome Disorder Support Group
http://www.rarechromo.org

Wolf Hirschhorn Support Group UK
http://www.whs.webk.co.uk

Cleft Lip/Palate—Also see Craniofacial Anomalies

Children's Craniofacial Association
http://www.ccakids.com

Cleft Palate Foundation
http://www.cleftline.org

Prescription Parents
http://www.samizdat.com/ppl.html

Smiles
http://www.cleft.org

Wide Smiles
http://www.widesmiles.org/

Cockayne Syndrome
Share and Care Cockayne Syndrome Network
http://www.cockayne-syndrome.org

Coffin-Lowry Syndrome
Coffin-Lowry Syndrome Foundation
http://www.clsf.info

Colorectal Cancer—Also see Cancer
Familial Gastrointestinal Registry (Canada)
http://www.mtsinai.on.cafamilialgican

Communicative Disorders—Also see Hearing Impairment
National Center for Stuttering
http://www.stuttering,com

Sensory Access Foundation
http://www.sensoryaccess.com

Sertoma International
http://sertoma.org/

Trace Center (communication devices and research), University of Wisconsin
http://www.tracecenter.org/

Congenital Adrenal Hyperplasia—See Adrenal Disorders; Ambiguous Genitalia; Growth Problems

Congenital Heart Disease—See Heart Defects/Diseases

Conjoined Twins
Conjoined Twins International
http://www.conjoinedtwinsint.com

Cooley Anemia—See Thalassemia

Cornelia de Lange Syndrome
Cornelia de Lange Syndrome Foundation
http://www.cdlsusa.org

Craniofacial Anomalies—Also see Cleft Lip/Palate
About Face, U.S.A.*
http://www.aboutfaceusa.org
*Includes facial anomalies, cleft lip/palate, Crouzon syndrome, Apert syndrome, Treacher Collins syndrome, hemangioma, and cystic hygroma

Children's Craniofacial Association
http://www.ccakids.com

Craniofacial Foundation of America
http://www.craniofacialcenter.com

Let's Face It
http://www.faceit.org

National Craniofacial Association
http:/www.faces-cranio.org

National Foundation for Facial Reconstruction
http://www.nffr.org

Cri-du-Chat—Also see Chromosome Abnormalities
5p– Society (Cri-du-Chat Syndrome)
http://www.fivepminus.org

Crohn Disease—Also see Inflammatory Bowel
Disease
Crohn's and Colitis Foundation of America
http://www.ccfc.org

Crohn's and Colitis Foundation of Canada
http://www.ccfc.ca

National Institute of Diabetes, Digestive and
Kidney Diseases, National Institutes of Health
http://www.niddk.nih.gov

Cutis Laxa—See Ehlers-Danlos Syndrome

Cystic Fibrosis
Cystic Fibrosis Foundation
http://www.cff.org

Cystic Fibrosis Trust England, United Kingdom
http://www.cftrust.org.uk

National Institute of Diabetes and Digestive and
Kidney Diseases, National Institutes of Health
http://www.niddk.nih.gov

Dandy-Walker Syndrome
Dandy-Walker Syndrome Network
http://www.familyvillage.wisc.edu/lib_dandy.htm

Darier Disease—See Ichthyosis; Skin Disorders

de Lange syndrome—See Cornelia de Lange
Syndrome

Deaf—See Hearing Impairment

Deaf-Blind—Also see Hearing Impairment; Usher
Syndrome; Visual Impairment
American Association of the Deaf-Blind
http://www.aadb.org

National Information Clearinghouse on
Children Who Are Deaf-Blind (DB-LINK)
http://www.tr.wou.edu/dblink/

Death, Neonatal and Infant—Also see Sudden
Infant Death Syndrome
A.M.E.N.D. (Aiding a Mother and Father
Experiencing Neonatal Death)
http://www.amendinc.com

Born Angels Pregnancy Loss Support
http://www.bornangels.com

Center for Loss in Multiple Birth (CLIMB)
http://www.climb-support.org

Compassionate Friends (TCF)
http://www.compassionatefriends.org

A Heartbreaking Choice
http://www.aheartbreakingchoice.com

SHARE
Pregnancy and Infant Loss Support
http://www.nationalshareoffice.com

Stork Net
http://www.storknet.com/cubbies/pil/

Dental Care
National Foundation of Dentistry for the
Handicapped
http://www.nfdh.org

Depression
Depression and Related Affective Disorders
Association
http://www.drada.org

National Institute of Mental Health, National
Institutes of Health
http://www.nimh.nih.gov

Diabetes Mellitus
American Diabetes Association
http://www.diabetes.org

Canadian Diabetes Association
http://www.diabetes.ca/

Juvenile Diabetes Research Foundation
International
http://www.jdfcure.org

National Institute of Diabetes and Digestive and
Kidney Diseases, National Institutes of Health
http://www.niddk.nih.gov

Diethylstilbesterol (DES)
DES Action, USA
http://www.desaction.org

National Women's Health Network
http://www.womenshealthnetwork.org

National Women's Health Resource Center
http://www.4woman.gov

Di George Syndrome—Also see Immune
Disorders; Chromosome Abnormalities
VCFS Educational Foundation*
http://www.vcfsef.org
*Includes DiGeorge syndrome, Shprintzen
syndrome, velocardiofacial syndrome, and
22q11.2 deletions

Disabilities, General—Also see Mental Retardation
  ADA & IT Technical Assistance Centers
  http://www.adata.org

  Administration on Developmental Disabilities
  http://www.acf.dhhs.gov/programs/add

  Association of University Centers on Disabilities
  http://www.aucd.org

  Council for Exceptional Children
  http://www.cec.sped.org

  Disability Connections
  http://www.disabilityconnections.org

  DisabilityInfo.gov
  http://www.disabilityinfo.gov

  Disability Rights Center
  http://www.drcme.org

  Exceptional Parent Magazine
  http://www.eparent.com

  Family Resource Center on Disabilities
  http://www.frcd.org

  Friends Health Connection
  http://www.friendshealthconnection.org

  Information Center for Individuals with
  Disabilities
  http://www.disability.net

  Maternal and Child Health Bureau, Health
  Resources and Services Administration
  http://mchb.hrsa.gov

  Medic Alert Foundation International
  http://www.medicalert.org

  Mobility International USA
  http://www.miusa.org

  National Association of the Physically
  Handicapped
  http://www.naph.net

  National Center for Education in Maternal and
  Child Health
  http://www.ncemch.org

  National Dissemination Center for Children
  with Disabilities
  http://www.nichcy.org

  National Clearinghouse on Disability and
  Exchange
  http://www.miusa.org/ncde/

  National Council on Independent Living
  http://www.ncil.org

  National Easter Seal Society
  http://www.easter-seals.org

  National Organization on Disability
  http://www.nod.org

  Parents Helping Parents*
  http://www.php.com
  *General disabilities, children with special needs,
  and tuberous sclerosis

  Social Security Administration Office of
  Communications
  http://www.ssa.gov

Down Syndrome—Also see Chromosome
  Abnormalities
  Association for Children with Down Syndrome
  http://www.acds.org

  Canadian Down Syndrome Society
  http://www.cdss.ca

  Caring
  http://www.caringinc.org

  Down Syndrome Research Foundation
  (Canada)
  http://www.dsrf.org

  Down's Syndrome Association (UK)
  http://www.downs-syndrome.org.uk

  National Down Syndrome Congress
  http://www.ndsccenter.org

  National Down Syndrome Society
  http://www.ndss.org

Dubowitz Syndrome
  Dubowitz Syndrome Parent Support Network
  http://dubowitz.org

Dwarfism—See Short Stature

Dysautonomia (Riley-Day Syndrome)
  Center for Jewish Genetic Diseases
  http://www.mssm.edu/jewish_genetics/

  Dysautonomia Foundation
  http://www.familialdysautonomia.org

Dysautonomia Treatment and Evaluation
    Center
    http://www.med.nyu.edu

Dyslexia—See Learning Disabilities

Dystonia (Torsion Dystonia)
    Center for Jewish Genetic Diseases
    http://www.mssm.edu/jewish_genetics/

    Dystonia Medical Research Foundation
    http:/www.dystonia-foundation.org

Ectodermal Dysplasia
    Ectodermal Dysplasia Society
    http://www.ectodermaldysplasia.org

    National Foundation for Ectodermal Dysplasias
    http://www.ednf.org

Edwards Syndrome—See Trisomy 18/13;
    Chromosome Abnormalities

Ehlers-Danlos Syndrome
    Ehlers-Danlos National Foundation
    http://www.ednf.org

Environmental Mutagens
    Centers for Disease Control and Prevention
    http://www.cdc.gov

    Clinical Teratology Web, Teratogen
        Information System (TERIS)
    http://depts.washington.edu/~terisweb/

    Environmental Health Clearinghouse National
        Institute of Environmental Health Sciences
    http://infoventures.com/e-hlth

    National Library of Medicine
    http://www.nlm.nih.gov/

Epidermolysis Bullosa
    Dystrophic Epidermolysis Bullosa Research
        Association of America
    http://www.debra.org

Epilepsy
    Epilepsy Canada
    http://www.epilepsy.ca

    Epilepsy Foundation
    http://www.epilepsyfoundation.org

    Epilepsy Information Service
    http://www.wfubmc.edu/neuro/epilepsy/
        information.htm

Fabry Disease—See Tay-Sachs Disease

Fanconi Anemia
    Fanconi Anemia Research Fund
    http://www.fanconi.org

Farber Syndrome—See Tay-Sachs Disease

Fetal Alcohol Syndrome—See Alcohol and Drug
    Abuse

Fibrodysplasia
    International Fibrodysplasia Ossificans
        Progressiva
    www.ifopa.org

Fragile X Syndrome—Also see Chromosome
    Abnormalities

    FRAXA Research Foundation
    http://www.fraxa.org

    National Fragile X Foundation
    http://www.nfxf.org/

Freeman–Sheldon Syndrome
    Freeman–Sheldon Parent Support Group*
    http://www.fspsg.org
    *Includes whistling face syndrome and
        craniocarpotarsal dysplasia.

Friedreich Ataxia—See Ataxia; Muscular
    Dystrophy

Fucosidosis—See Tay-Sachs Disease

Galactosemia—Also see Liver Diseases
    Parents of Galactosemic Children
    http://www.galactosemia.org

Gaucher Disease—Also see Tay-Sachs Disease
    Center for Jewish Genetic Diseases
    http://www.mssm.edu/jewish_genetics/

    National Gaucher Foundation
    http://www.gaucherdisease.org

Genetic Disorders, General—Also see Disabilities,
    General; Birth Defects, General
    Canadian Organization for Rare Disorders
    http://www.raredisorders.ca

    Center for Jewish Genetic Diseases
    http://www.mssm.edu/jewish_genetics/

    Genetic Alliance
    http://www.geneticalliance.org

    Heredity Disease Foundation
    http://www.hdfoundation.org

Maternal and Child Health Bureau, Health
    Resources and Services Administration
http://mchb.hrsa.gov

Med Help International
http://www.medhelp.org

MUMS National Parent-to-Parent Network
http://www.netnet.net/mums/

National Health Information Center
    Department of Health and Human Services
http://www.health.gov/nhic

National Organization for Rare Disorders
http://www.rarediseases.org

Office of Rare Diseases, National Institutes of
    Health
http://rarediseases.info.nih.gov/

Gluten Intolerance
    Celiac Sprue Association USA (CSA/USA)
    http://www.csaceliacs.org

    Gluten Intolerance Group of North America
        (GIG)
    http://www.gluten.net

    National Digestive Diseases Information
        Clearinghouse
    http://digestive.niddk.nih.gov

Glycogen Storage Disorders—See Liver Diseases
    Association for Glycogen Storage Disease*
    http://www.agsdus.org
    *Glycogen storage disease, acid maltase deficiency,
    Anderson disease, and amlopectinosis

Goldenhar Syndrome
    Goldenhar Syndrome Support Network
    http://www.goldenharsyndrome.org

Granulomatous Disease—Also see Immune
    Disorders
    Chronic Granulomatous Disease Association
    http://home.socal.rr.com/cgda

Growth Problems—Also see Short Stature; Tall
    Stature; specific disorder
    Human Growth Foundation (HGF)
    http://www.hgfound.org

    MAGIC Foundation*
    http://www.magicfoundation.org
    *Includes growth disorders, growth hormone

deficiency, McCune-Albright syndrome,
congenital adrenal hyperplasia, precocious
puberty, growth retardation in Down syndrome

Handicapped—See Disabilities, General

Hearing Impairment
    Alexander Graham Bell Association for the Deaf
    http://www.agbell.org

    American Society for Deaf Children
    http://www.deafchildren.org

    Better Hearing Institute
    http://www.betterhearing.org

    Canadian Hearing Society
    http://www.chs.ca/

    Deafness Research Foundation
    http://www.drf.org

    International Hearing Society
    http://www.ihsinfo.org

    Laurent Clerc Deaf Education Center
    http://clerccenter.gallaudet.edu/InfoToGo

    National Association for the Deaf
    http://www.nad.org

    National Institute on Deafness and Other
        Communication Disorders Information,
        National Institutes of Health
    http://www.nidcd.nih.gov/health

    Self Help for Hard of Hearing People
    http://www.shhh.org

Heart Defects/Diseases
    American Heart Association
    http://www.americanheart.org/

    Cardiac Arrhythmias Research and Education
        Foundation
    http://www.longqt.org

    Congenital Heart Anomalies-Support,
        Education, and Resources (CHASER, Inc.)
    http://www.csun.edu/~hcmth011

    Congenital Heart Information Network
    http://www.tchin.org

    National Heart, Lung, and Blood Institute,
        National Institutes of Health
    http://www.nhlbi.nih.gov

QTsyndrome.ch Group
http://www.qtsyndrome.ch

Sudden Arrhythmia Death Syndrome
   Foundation
http://www.sads.org

Hemangiomas—See Vascular Birthmarks and
Malformations

Hemochromatosis—Also see Iron Overload
Diseases
   Canadian Hemochromatosis Society
   http://www.cdnhemochromatosis.ca

   Hemochromatosis Foundation
   http://www.hemochromatosis.org

   Iron Overload Diseases Association
   http://www.ironoverload.org

Hemophilia
   National Hemophilia Foundation*
   http://www.hemophilia.org/
   *Includes von Willebrand disease and other
   clotting disorders

   World Federation of Hemophilia
   http://www.wfh.org/

Hereditary Angioedema—Also see Immune
Disorders
   U.S. Hereditary Angioedema Association
   http://www.hereditaryangioedema.com

Hereditary Exostoses, Multiple
   Multiple Hereditary Exostoses Family Support
      Group
   http://www.radix.net/~hogue/mhe.htm

Hereditary Hemorrhagic Telangiectasia
   Hereditary Hemorrhagic Telangiectasia
      Foundation International*
   http://www.hht.org
   *Also includes Osler-Weber-Rendu syndrome

Hermansky-Pudlak Syndrome—See Albinism

Hirschsprung Disease
   International Foundation for Functional
      Gastrointestinal Disorders
   http://www.aboutkidsgi.org

   National Institute of Diabetes, Digestive and
      Kidney Diseases, National Institutes of Health
   http://www.niddk.nih.gov

Homocystinuria—See Metabolic Disorders

Hunter Disease—See Mucopolysaccharide
Disorders; Tay-Sachs Disease

Huntington Disease
   Heredity Disease Foundation
   http://www.hdfoundation.org

   Huntington Society of Canada
   http://www.hsc-ca.org

   Huntington's Disease Society of America
   http://www.hdsa.org

Hurler Disease—See Mucopolysaccharide
Disorders; Tay-Sachs Disease

Hydrocephalus—Also see Arnold-Chiari
Syndrome
   Association for Spina Bifida and Hydrocephalus
   http://www.asbah.org

   Hydrocephalus Association
   http://www.hydroassoc.org

   National Hydrocephalus Foundation
   http://www.nhfonline.org

Hypercholesterolemia—Also see Heart
Defects/Diseases
   Inherited High Cholesterol Foundation
   http://www.medped.org/

I-cell Disease—See Mucolipidoses

Ichthyosis—Also see Skin Disorders
   Foundation for Ichthyosis and Related Skin
      Types*
   http://www.scalyskin.org
   *Includes skin disorders, ichthyosis, Darier
   disease, Sjögren–Larsson syndrome,
   erythrokeratodermas, peeling skin syndrome,
   acquired ichthyosis, bullous ichthyosis
   (epidermolytic hyperkeratosis), Chanarin-
   Dorfman syndrome, CHILD syndrome
   (unilateral CIE), epiderma nevus syndrome,
   progressiva symmetrica, harlequin fetus,
   ichthyosis linearis circumflexa, ichthyosis
   vulgaris, keratitis-ichthyosis deafness
   syndrome, lammellar ichthyosis/congenital
   ichthyosiform erythroderma

   National Registry for Ichthyosis and Related
      Disorders
   http://depts.washington.edu/ichreg/ichthyosis
      .registry

Immune Disorders
Immune Deficiency Foundation
http://www.primaryimmune.org

National Jewish Center for Immunology and
Respiratory Medicine
http://www.njc.org

U.S. Hereditary Angioedema Association
http://www.hereditaryangioedema.com

Incest
Clearinghouse on Child Abuse and Neglect
Information
http://childwelfare.gov

Survivors of Incest Anonymous
http://www.siawso.org

Incontinentia Pigmenti
Incontinentia Pigmenti International
Foundation
http://imgen.bcm.tmc.edu/IPIF

Infertility
International Council on Infertility Information
Dissemination
http://www.inciid.org

Resolve, The National Infertility Association
http://www.resolve.org/

Inflammatory Bowel Disease—Also see Crohn's
Disease
National Digestive Diseases Education
Information Clearinghouse, National
Institutes of Health
http://www.niddk.nih.gov

Iron Overload Diseases—Also see
Hemochromatosis; Thalassemia
Iron Overload Diseases Association
http://www.ironoverload.org

Isovaleric Acidemia—See Organic Acidemias

Joseph Disease
International Joseph Diseases Foundation
http://69.10.163.110/bastiana

Joubert Syndrome
Joubert Syndrome Foundation
http://www.joubertfoundation.com

Kearn-Sayre—See Mitochondrial Diseases

Kidney Diseases
American Association of Kidney Patients
http://www.aakp.org/

National Institute of Diabetes and Digestive
and Kidney Diseases, National Institutes of
Health
http://www.niddk.nih.gov/

National Kidney Foundation
http://www.kidney.org/

Klinefelter Syndrome—Also see Chromosome
Abnormalities
Klinefelter Syndrome and Associates
http://www.genetic.org/ks

Klinefelter Syndrome Support Group
http://klinefeltersyndrome.org

Klippel-Trenaunay Syndrome
Klippel-Trenaunay Support Group
http://www.k-t.org

Krabbe Disease—See Tay-Sachs Disease

Kugelberg-Welander Disease—See Muscular
Dystrophy

Lactic Acidosis
Congenital Lactic Acidosis Support Group
http://www.Kumc.edu/gec/support/lactic_a.html

Laurence-Moon Syndrome—Also see Retinitis
Pigmentosa; Vision Impairment
Foundation Fighting Blindness
http://www.blindness.org/laurence-moon-
bardet-biedel-syndrome.asp

Laurence Moon Bardet Biedl Syndrome
Network
http://mlmorris.com/lmbbs

Learning Disabilities
Council for Learning Disabilities
http://www.cldinternational.org

Learning Disabilities Association of America
http://www.danatl.org

Learning Disabilities Association of Canada
http://www.ldac-taac.ca

National Attention Deficit Disorder Association
http://www.add.org

NLDline (nonverbal learning disorders)
http://www.nldline.com

Orton Dyslexia Society
http://www2.selu.edu/Academics/Education/TEC/
orton.htm

Recording for the Blind and Dyslexic
http://www.rfbd.org

Leigh Disease—Also see Mitochondrial Disorders
National Leigh's Disease Foundation
http://www.kumc.edu/gec/support/leigh_di.html

Leukemia—Also see Cancer
Leukemia and Lymphoma Society of America
http://www.leukemia.org/

National Children's Leukemia Foundation
http://www.leukemiafoundation.org

Leukodystrophy—See Adrenoleukodystrophy and
Adrenomyeloneuropathy

Lissencephaly
Lissencephaly Network
http://www.lissencephaly.org

Liver Diseases
American Liver Foundation
http://www.liverfoundation.org

Biliary Atresia and Liver Transplant Network*
http://www.transweb.org/people/recips/resources/
support/oldbilitree.html
*Also includes Alagille syndrome, alpha-1-anti-
trypsin deficiency, Byler disease, galactosemia,
glycogen storage diseases, tyrosinemia, Wilson
disease, and acid maltase deficiency

Long QT Syndrome
Cardiac Arrhythmias Research and Education
Foundation
http://www.longqt.org

QTsyndrome.ch Group
http://www.qtsyndrome.ch

Sudden Arrhythmia Death Syndromes
Foundation
http://www.sads.org

Lowe Syndrome (Oculocerebrorenal Disease)
Lowe Syndrome Association
http://www.lowesyndrome.org

Lupus Erythematosus—Also see Arthritis
Lupus Foundation of America
http://www.lupus.org

Lymphangioleiomyomatosis LAM Foundation
http://lam.uc.edu

Lymphedema
National Lymphedema Network
http://www.lymphnet.org

Lymphoma—Also see Cancer
Leukemia and Lymphoma Society of America
http://www.leukemia.org/

Machado-Joseph Disease—See Joseph Disease

Macular Diseases—Also see Vision Impairment
Association for Macular Diseases
http://www.macula.org

Macular Degeneration International
http://www.maculardegeneration.org

Maffucci Disease—See Oilier Disease

Malignant Hyperthermia—Also see Muscular
Dystrophy
Malignant Hyperthermia Association of the
United States
http://www.mhaus.org

Mannosidosis—See Tay-Sachs Disease

Maple Syrup Urine Disease—Also see Metabolic
Disorders
Maple Syrup Urine Disease Family Support
Group
http://www.msud-support.org

Marfan Syndrome—Also see Tall Stature
National Marfan Foundation
http://www.marfan.org

Canadian Marfan Association
http://www.marfan.ca

Marfan Association (United Kingdom)
http://www.marfan.org.uk

Maroteaux-Lamy Disease—See Tay-Sachs Disease;
Mucopolysaccharide Disorders

McArdle Disease—See Muscular Dystrophy

McCune-Albright Syndrome—See Growth
Problems

Medium Chain Acyl-CoEnzyme A Dehydrogenase
(MCAD) Deficiency—Also see Mitochondrial
Diseases
Fatty Oxidation Disorders (FOD) Family
Support Group
http://www.fodsupport.org

Save Babies Through Screening
http://www.savebabies.org/

MELAS—See Mitochondrial Diseases

Menke Disease
Corporation for Menke's Disease
http://www.familyvillage.wisc.edu/lib_menk.htm

National Institute of Neurological Disorders
and Stroke, National Institutes of Health
http://www.ninds.nih.gov

Mental Retardation—Also see Disabilities,
General; specific disorders
American Association on Mental Retardation
http://www.aamr.org/

Arc of the United States (formerly Association
for Retarded Citizens of the United States)
http://TheArc.org/

President's Committee for People with
Intellectual Disabilities
http://www.acf.hhs.gov/programs/pcpid

Mental Retardation/Mental Illness
National Organization of the Dually Diagnosed
http://www.thenadd.org

MERFF—See Mitochondrial Disorders

Metabolic Disorders—Also see specific disorder
Association for Neuro-Metabolic Diseases*
http://www.kumc.edu/gec/supportJmetaboli.html
*Includes biotinidase deficiency, methylenete-
trahydrofolatereductase deficiency, phenylketonuria, maple syrup urine disease, propionic
acidemia, galactosemia, and others

Children Living with Inherited Metabolic
Disease (United Kingdom)
http://www.climb.org.uk

Fatty Oxidation Disorders Family Support Group*
http://www.fodsupport.org
*Includes medium chain acyl-CoA dehydro-
genase deficiency, short chain acyl-CoA
dehydrogenase deficiency, long chain
3–hydroxyacyl-CoA dehydrogenase deficiency,
very long chain acyl-CoA dehydrogenase
deficiency, electron transfer flavoprotein
dehydrogenase deficiency, carnitine palmitoyl
transferase I & II deficiency

National Institute of Diabetes, Digestive &
Kidney Diseases, National Institutes of Health
http://www.niddk.nih.gov

National Urea Cycle Disorders Foundation
http://www.nucdf.org

Organic Acidemia Asssociation
http://www.oaanews.org

Oxalosis and Hyperoxaluria Foundation
http://www.ohf.org

Purine Research Society
http://purineresearchsociety.org

Save Babies Through Screening
http://www.savebabies.org/

Metachromatic Leukodystrophy—See Tay-Sachs
Disease

Methylenetetrahydrofolate Reductase
Deficiency—See Metabolic Disorders

Methylmalonic Acidemia—See Organic Acidemias

Microphthalmia—See Anophthalmia

Miller Syndrome
Foundation for Nager & Miller Syndromes
http://www.nagerormillersynd.com

Miscarriages—See Death, Neonatal and Infant

Mitochondrial Diseases
Children's Mitochondrial Disease Network*
http://www.emdn.mitonet.co.uk
*Includes Leigh disease; Kearns-Sayre syndrome;
Pearson marrow-pancreas syndrome; mitochondrial encephalomyopathy/lactic acidosis
and strokelike episodes; myoclonic epilepsy/
ragged red fibers; neurogenic weakness, ataxia,
retinitis pigmentosa.

United Mitochondrial Disease Foundation*
http://www.umdf.org
*Includes Alpers disease (progressive infantile
poliodystrophy)

Moebius Syndrome
Moebius Syndrome Foundation
http://www.ciaccess.com/moebius/

Morquio Disease—See Tay-Sachs Disease

Mucolipidoses—Also see Tay-Sachs Disease
ML4 Foundation
http://www.ml4.org

National MPS Society*
http://www.mpssociety.org
*Includes mucopolysaccharidosis, mucolipidosis,
Hunter syndrome, Hurler syndrome,
Maroteaux-Lamy syndrome, Sanfilippo
syndrome, and Scheie syndrome

Mucopolysaccharide Disorders—Also see Tay-
Sachs Disease
National MPS Society
http://www.mpssociety.org

Multiple Births
International Twins Association
http://www.intltwins.org

Mothers of Supertwins (MOST)
http://www.MOSTonline.org

Multiple Births Foundation (UK)
http://www.multiplebirths.org.uk

National Organization of Mothers of Twins
Clubs
http://www.nomotc.org

Twins Clubs (UK)
http://www.twinsclubs.co.uk

The Twins Foundation
http://www.twinsfoundation.com

Twins and Multiple Births Association
http://www.tamba.org.uk

Multiple Sclerosis
International MS Support Foundation
http://www.msnews.org

Multiple Sclerosis Society of Canada
http://www.mssociety.ca

National Multiple Sclerosis Society
http://www.nmss.org/

Muscular Dystrophy
FacioScapuloHumeral Muscular Dystrophy
Society*
http://www.fshsociety.org
*Includes muscular dystrophy, facioscapulohu-
meral muscular dystrophy, Landouzy-Dejerine
facioscapulohumeral muscular dystrophy

Families of Spinal Muscular Atrophy*
http://www.fsma.org
*Includes spinal muscular atrophy, Werdnig-

Hoffmann disease, Oppenheim disease,
Kugelberg-Welander disease, Aran-Duchenne
type

Muscular Dystrophy Association*
http://www.mdausa.org/
*Includes many muscle diseases such as Becker,
Duchenne, congenital, facioscapulohumeral,
limb-girdle muscular dystrophy, myotonic
dystrophy; amyotophic lateral sclerosis;
Werdnig-Hoffmann, Kugelberg-Welander,
Charcot-Marie-Tooth diseases; Friedreich
ataxia; myasthenia gravis; McArdle, Pompe,
Cori diseases; phosphofructokinase deficiency;
carnitine palmityltransferase deficiency;
malignant hyperthermia; arthrogryposis;
miscellaneous myopathies

Muscular Dystrophy Association of Canada
http://www.mdac.ca

Parent Project Muscular Dystrophy
http://www.parentprojectmd.org

Myasthenia Gravis—Also see Muscular Dystrophy
Myasthenia Gravis Foundation of America
http://www.myasthenia.org

Myelin Disorders
Organization for Myelin Disorders Research
and Support*
http://www.familyvillage.wisc.edu/lib.myel.htm
*Also includes hypomyelination, delayed
myelination, dysmyelination, periventricular
leukomylasia, macroencephaly, microencephaly

Myoclonus
Myoclonus Research Foundation
http://www.myoclonus.com

Worldwide Education for Movement Disorders
http://www.wemove.org/myo

Myotonia Congenita—See Muscular Dystrophy

Myotubular Myopathy
Centronuclear and Myotubular Myopathy (UK)
http://tonilouise.tripod.com

Myotubular Myopathy Resource Group*
http://www.mtmrg.org
*Includes centronuclear myopathy

Nager Syndrome
Foundation for Nager and Miller Syndromes
http://www.nagerormillersynd.com

Nail-Patella Syndrome
  Nail-Patella Syndrome Worldwide
  http://www.nailpatella.org

Narcolepsy
  Narcolepsy Network
  http://www.narcolepsynetwork.org

  Narcolepsy & Sleep Disorders: An International
      Newsletter
  http://www.narcolepsy.com

  National Institute of Neurological Disorders
      and Stroke, National Institutes of Health
  http://www.ninds.nih.gov

  National Sleep Foundation
  http://www.sleepfoundation.org

Neural Tube Defects—See Hydrocephalus; Spina
  Bifida

Neurofibromatosis
  National Neurofibromatosis Foundation
  http://www.nf.org/

  Neurofibromatosis, Inc.
  http://www.nfinc.org

Neurological Disorders—Also see specific disorder
  National Institute of Neurological Disorders
      and Stroke, National Institutes of Health
  http://www.ninds.nih.gov

Nevoid Basal Cell Carcinoma Syndrome—Also see
  Cancer
  BCCNS Life Support Network
  http://www.bccns.org

Niemann-Pick Disease—Also see Tay-Sachs
  Disease
  Center for Jewish Genetic Diseases
  http://www.mssm.edu/jewish_genetics/

  National Niemann-Pick Disease Foundation
  http://www.nnpdf.org

Noonan Syndrome
  Noonan Syndrome Support Group
  http://www.noonansyndrome.org

Oilier Disease
  American Association of Multiple
      Enchondroma Disease*
  http:/www.aamed.net
  *Also includes multiple cartilaginous enchondro-
    matosis, Oilier osteochondromatosis, Maffucci
    syndrome

Oppenheim Disease—See Muscular Dystrophy

OptizG/BBB, Opitz G and Related Syndromes
  Opitz G/BBB Family Network
  http://www.opitznet.org

Organic Acidemias—Also see Metabolic Disorders
  Organic Acidemia Association*
  http://www.oaanews.org
  *Includes organic aciduria, isovaleric acidemia,
    methylmalonic acidemia, proprionic acidemia,
    acidemia, and errors of amino and fatty acid
    metabolism

Osler Weber Rendu Syndrome—See Hereditary
  Hemorrhagic Telangiectasia

Osteogenesis Imperfecta—Also see Bone Diseases
  Osteogenesis Imperfecta Foundation
  http://www.oif.org

Osteoporosis
  National Osteoporosis Foundation
  http://www.nof.org/

  Osteoporosis and Related Bone Diseases,
      National Research Center, National Institutes
      of Health
  http://www.osteo.org/

Ovarian Cancer—Also see Cancer
  Gilda Radner Familial Ovarian Cancer Registry
  http://www.ovariancancer.com

Oxalosis—Also see Kidney Diseases
  Oxalosis and Hyperoxaluria Foundation*
  http://www.ohf.org
  *Also includes primary hyperoxaluria (PH),
    hyperoxaluria, oxaluria, calcium-oxalate kidney
    stones

Paget Disease (of the Bone)
  Paget Foundation
  http://www.paget.org

Pallister-Hall Syndrome
  Pallister Hall Foundation (Australia)
  http://www.pallisterhall.com

Pallister-Killian Syndrome
  Pallister-Killian Syndrome Support Group
  http://www.pk-syndrome.org

Parkinson Disease
  American Parkinson Disease Association
  http://www.apdaparkinson.org

National Parkinson Foundation
http://www.parkinson.org/

Parkinson's Action Network
http://www.parkinsonsaction.org

Parkinson's Disease Foundation
http://www.pdf.org

Parkinson's Disease Information
http://www.parkinsons.org

Patau Syndrome—See Trisomy 18/13;
Chromosome Abnormalities

Peutz-Jeghers Syndrome—See Polyposis

Phenylketonuria (PKU)—Also see Metabolic
Disorders
Children's PKU Network (CPN)
http://www.pkunetwork.org

National Coalition for PKU and Allied
Disorders
http://www.pku-allieddisorders.org

National PKU News
http://www.pkunews.org

Pierre Robin Syndrome—See Stickler Syndrome

Pigment Disorders—See specific disorder such as
Albinism; Vitiligo

Polycystic Kidney Disease—Also see Kidney
Diseases

National Institute of Diabetes, Digestive and
Kidney Diseases, National Institutes of Health
http://www.niddk.nih.gov

Polycystic Kidney Research Foundation
http://www.pkdcure.org

Polyposis
Familial Gastrointestinal Cancer Registry
(Canada)
http://www.mtsinai.on.ca/familialgicancer

Porphyria—Also see Iron Overload Diseases
American Porphyria Foundation
http://www.porphyriafoundation.com/

Prader-Willi Syndrome
Prader-Willi Syndrome Association (UK)
http://www.pwsa.co.uk/

Prader-Willi Syndrome Association (USA)
http://www.pwsausa.org

Progeria
Progeria Research Foundation*
http://www.progeriaresearch.org
*Includes progeria, Cockayne syndrome,
Werner syndrome

Propionic Acidemia—See Organic Acidemias;
Metabolic Disorders

Prune Belly Syndrome
Prune Belly Syndrome Network*
http://www.prunebelly.org
*Also includes Eagle Barrett syndrome

Pseudoxanthoma Elasticum
National Association for Pseudoxanthoma
Elasticum
http://www.pxenape.org

PXE International (PXE)
http://www.pxe.org

Rare Disorders—See Genetic Disorders, General

Recreation and Leisure
Canadian Wheelchair Basketball Association
http://www.cwha.ca

Cooperative Wilderness Handicapped Outdoor
Group (CWHOG)
Idaho State University
http://www.isu.edu/cwhog/

Disabled Sports, USA
http://www.dsusa.org

HSA International (Handicapped Scuba
Association)
http://www.hsascuba.com

National Disability Sports Alliance
http://www.ndsaonline.org

North American Riding for the Handicapped
Association
http://www.narha.org

Special Equestrian Riding Therapy
http://www.sert.org/main.html

Special Olympics International
http://www.specialolympics.org/

WheelchairSports USA
http://www.wsusa.org

Wilderness on Wheels
http://www.wildernessonwheels.org

Refsum Disease—See Tay-Sachs Disease

Rehabilitation
    National Clearinghouse of Rehabilitation
        Training Materials
    http://www.ncrtm.okstate.edu/

    National Rehabilitation Association
    http://www.nationalrehab.org

    National Rehabilitation Information Center
    http://www.naric.com/

    Rehabilitation International
    http://www.rehab-international.org

    Resources for Rehabilitation
    http://www.rfr.org

Reiter Syndrome—See Ankylosing Spondylitis;
    Arthritis

Renal Disorders—See Kidney Disorders; specific
    disease

Respite
    National Respite Network
    http://www.arctirespite.org

Retinitis Pigmentosa—Also see Visual Impairment
    Foundation Fighting Blindness
    http://www.blindness.org

    Laurence Moon Bardet Biedl Syndrome
        Network
    http://www.mlmorris.com/lmbbs/

    RP International
    http://www.rpinternational.org

Rett Syndrome
    International Rett Syndrome Association
    http://www.rettsyndrome.org

Rubinstein-Taybi Syndrome
    Rubinstein-Taybi Parent Group
    http://www.rubinstein-taybi.org

Russell-Silver Syndrome
    Magic Foundation*
    http://www.magicfoundation.org
    *Also includes Silver syndrome, Russell syndrome,
    Silver-Russell syndrome

Sandhoff Disease—See Tay-Sachs Disease

Sanfillippo Disease—See Tay-Sachs Disease;
    Mucopolysaccharide Disorders

Scheie Disease—See Mucopolysaccharide
    Disorders

Scleroderma
    Scleroderma Foundation
    http://www.scleroderma.org

Scoliosis
    National Scoliosis Foundation
    http://www.scoliosis.org

    Scoliosis Association
    http://www.scoliosis-assoc.org

    Scoliosis Research Society
    http://www.srs.org

    Scoliosis Treatment Advanced Recovery System
        (STARS)
    http://www.scoliosis.com/

Self-Help Clearinghouses
    American Self-Help Group Clearinghouse
    http://www.mentalhelp.net/selfhelp

    National Self-Help Clearinghouse
    http://www.selfhelpweb.org

Sexuality
    Sexuality Information and Education Council of
        the U.S.
    http://www.siecus.org

Short Stature—Also see Growth Problems
    Human Growth Foundation
    http://www.hgfound.org

    Little People of America
    http://www.lpaonline.org

    MAGIC Foundation for Children's Growth
    http://www.magicfoundation.org

    Short Persons Support
    http://www.shortsupport.org

Shprintzen Syndrome—See Chromosome
    Abnormalities

Shwachman Syndrome
    Shwachman-Diamond Syndrome International*
    http://www.shwachman-diamond.org
    *Also includes Shwachman-Diamond syndrome,
    Burke's syndrome, Shwachman-Vodian
    syndrome

Shy-Drager Syndrome
    Shy-Drager Syndrome Support Group
    http://www.shy-drager.org

Siblings
Siblings for Significant Change
http://www.med.umich.edu/1libr/yourchild/
specneed.htm

Sibling Support Project
http://www.thearc.org/siblingsupport

Sickle Cell Disease
American Sickle Cell Anemia Association
http://www.ascaa.org

National Heart, Lung, and Blood Institute
National Institutes of Health
http:/www.nhlbi.nih.gov

Sickle Cell Disease Association of America
http://www.sicklecelldisease.org

Silver-Russell Syndrome—See Russell-Silver
Syndrome

Sjögren Syndrome
National Sjögren's Syndrome Association
http://www.sjogrenssyndrome.org

Sjögren's Syndrome Foundation
http:/www.sjogrens.com

Skeletal Dysplasias
Greenberg Center for Skeletal Dysplasias
http://www.hopkinsmedicine.org/
greenbergcenter/Greenbrg.htm

Skin Disorders—Also see specific disorder
Foundation for Ichthyosis and Related Skin
Types
http://www.scalyskin.org

Smith-Magenis Syndrome—See also Chromosome
Abnormalities
Parents and Researchers Interested in Smith-
Magenis Syndrome*
http://www.prisms.org
*Also includes deletion 17p11.2

Sotos Syndrome
Sotos Syndrome Support Association
http://www.well.com/user/sssa

Sotos Syndrome Support Group of Canada
http://www.sssac.com

Spina Bifida
Association for Spina Bifida and Hydrocephalus
(UK)
http://www.asbah.org

Spina Bifida Association of America
http://www.sbaa.org

Spina Bifida and Hydrocephalus Association of
Canada
http://www.sbhac.ca

Hydrocephalus Support Group
http://www.hydrosupport.org

Spinal Muscular Atrophy
Families of Spinal Muscular Atrophy
http://www.fsma.org

Sprue—See Gluten Intolerance

Stickler Syndrome
Stickler Involved People*
http://www.sticklers.org
*Includes Stickler syndrome, hereditary progres-
sive arthro-ophthalmopathy, Pierre Robin
syndrome

Sturge-Weber Syndrome—Also see Vascular
Birthmarks and Malformations
Sturge-Weber Foundation
http://www.sturge-weber.com

Sudden Infant Death Syndrome—Also see Death,
Neonatal and Infant
First Candle/SIDS Alliance
http://www.sidsalliance.org

National SIDS/Infant Death Resource Center
http://www.sidscenter.org

Syringornyelia
American Syringomyelia Alliance Project
http://www.asap4sm.com

Tall Stature—Also see Growth Problems
Tall Clubs International
http:/www.tall.org

Tangier Disease—See Tay-Sachs Disease

Tay-Sachs Disease
Center for Jewish Genetic Diseases
http://www.mssm.edu/jewish_genetics/
National Tay-Sachs and Allied Diseases
Association*
http:/www.ntsad.org
*Includes the following disorders: Batten, Cana-
van, Fabry, Farber, fucosidosis, Gaucher, Krabbe,
Landing, mannosidosis, metachromatic
leukodystrophy, mucolipidoses I–IV (sialidosis,
1-cell disease, etc.), mucopolysaccharidoses

(Hunter, Hurler, Scheie, Maroteaux-Lamy, Morquio, Sanfillippo, Sly or beta-glucuronidase deficiency), Niemann-Pick, Pompe, Refsum, Tangier, Tay-Sachs, Wolman disease, and others

Thalassemia—Also see Iron Overload Diseases
AHEPA-American Hellenic Educational Progressive Association*
http://www.ahcpa.org
*Thalassemia minor, thalassemia major, thalassemia intermedia, beta-thalassemia, Cooley's anemia

Cooley's Anemia Foundation
http://www.thalassemia.org

Thrombocytopenia Absent Radius (TAR) Syndrome
Thrombocytopenia Absent Radius Syndrome Association
http://www.kumc.edu/gec/support/tarsynd.html

Thyroid Disorders
American Foundation of Thyroid Patients
http://www.thyroidfoundation.org

National Graves' Disease Foundation
http://www.ngdf.org

Thyroid Foundation of America
http://www.tsh.org

Torsion Dystonia—See Dystonia

Tourette Syndrome
Tourette Syndrome Association
http://www.tsa-usa.org

National Institute of Neurological Disorders and Stroke, National Institutes of Health
http://www.ninds.nih.gov

Travel
AccessAbility Travel
http://www.access-ability.org/travel.html

Handicapped Travel Club
http://www.handicappedtravelclub.com

Mobility International
http://www.miusa.org

Society for Accessible Travel and Hospitality
http://www.sath.org

Travel Outlet
http://www.traveloutlet.org

Travelin' Talk
http://www.travelintalk.net

Treacher Collins Syndrome
Treacher Collins Foundation
http://www.treachercollins.org

Tremor, Familial
Coping With Essential Tremor
http://www.essentialtremor.org

Triple X Syndrome—See also Chromosome Disorders
Triple-X Syndrome
http://www.triplo-x.org

Trisomy 9—See Chromosome Disorders

Trisomy 18/13—See also Chromosome Disorders
Chromosome 18 Registry and Research Society
http://www.chromosome18.org

Support Organization for Trisomy (SOFT) 18, 13, and Related Disorders
http://www.trisomy.org

Tuberous Sclerosis
Tuberous Sclerosis Alliance
http://www.tsalliance.org

Turner Syndrome—Also see Short Stature; Chromosome Disorders
Turner's Syndrome Society of Canada
http:/www.turnersyndrome.ca

Turner Syndrome Society of the United States
http://www.turner-syndrome-us.org/

Turner Syndrome Support Society
http://www.tss.org.uk

Twins—See Multiple Births

Tyrosinemia—See Liver Diseases; Metabolic Disorders

Tyrosinosis—See Liver Diseases

Ulcerative Colitis—See Inflammatory Bowel Disease

Urea Cycle Disorders—Also see Organic Acidemias; Metabolic Disorders
National Urea Cycle Disorders Foundation
http://www.nucdf.org

Usher Syndrome—See Deaf-Blind; Hearing Impairment; Retinitis Pigmentosa; Vision Impairment

Vascular Birthmarks and Malformations—Also see Sturge-Weber Syndrome; Von Hippel–Lindau Syndrome

Vascular Birthmarks Foundation*
http:/www.birthmark.org
*Includes vascular malformations, port wine
  stain, Klippel-Trenaunay syndrome, hereditary
  hemorrhagic telangiectasia, Sturge-Weber
  syndrome, arteriovenous malformations, Von
  Hippel–Lindau syndrome, lymphangiomas

VATER Syndrome and Association
  TEF VATER National Support Network
  http://www.tefvater.org

Velo-Cardio Facial Syndrome
  Velo-Cardio Facial Syndrome Educational
    Foundation
  http://www.vcfsef.org

Vision Impairment—Also see Disabilities
  American Council of the Blind
  http://www.acb.org/

American Foundation for the Blind
http://www.afb.org

Association for Education and Rehabilitation of
  the Blind and Visually Impaired
  http://www.aerbvi.org

Blind Children's Center
http://www.blindcntr.org

Braille Institute
http://www.brailleinstitute.org

Canadian National Institute for the Blind
http://www.cnib.ca

Carroll Center for the Blind
http://www.carroll.org

Center for the Partially Sighted
http://www.low-vision.org

Choice Magazine Listening
http://www.choicemagazinelistening.org

Foundation Fighting Blindness
http://www.blindness.org/

Guide Dog Foundation for the Blind
http://www.guidedog.org

Guide Dogs for the Blind
http://www.guidedogs.com

Guiding Eyes for the Blind
http://www.guiding-eyes.org

Jewish Guild for the Blind
http:/www.jgb.org

Leader Dogs for the Blind
http://www.leaderdog.org

Library of Congress-Persons with Disabilities
http://www.loc.gov/access

National Association for the Visually
  Handicapped
  http://www.navh.org

National Association for Parents of the Visually
  Impaired
  http://www.spedex.com/napvi

National Braille Association
http://www.nationalbraille.org

National Federation of the Blind
http://www.nfb.org

Recording for the Blind and Dyslexic
http://www.rfbd.org

The Seeing Eye
http://www.seeingeye.org

Vision Council of America
http://www.visionsite.org

Vitiligo
  National Vitiligo Foundation
  http://www.nvfi.org

Von Hippel-Lindau Syndrome—Also see Sturge-
  Weber Syndrome; Vascular Birthmarks and
  Malformations; Cancer
  VHL Family Alliance
  http://www.vhl.org

Von Willebrand Disease—See Hemophilia

Werdnig-Hoffman Disease—See Muscular
  Dystrophy

Werner Syndrome—See Progeria

Williams Syndrome
  Williams Syndrome Association
  http://www.williams-syndrome.org

Wilson Disease—Also see Liver Diseases
  Wilson's Disease Association
  http://www.wilsonsdisease.org

Wolf-Hirschhorn Disease—Also see Chromosome
Abnormalities
4p–Support Group
http://www.4p-supportgroup.org

Wolf Hirschhorn Support Group UK
http://www.whs.webk.co.uk

Wolman Disease—See Tay-Sachs Disease

Xeroderma Pigmentosum
Share and Care Cockayne Syndrome Network
http://www.cockayne-syndrome.org

Xeroderma Pigmentosum Society
http://www.xps.org

Glossary

All terms in this section refer to their application in humans and human genetics.

aberration—any abnormality of chromosome structure or number

acentric fragment—a chromosome piece without a centromere due to breakage

acrocentric chromosome—one in which the centromere is near the end of the chromosome

agenesis—imperfect development or absence of an organ or its failure to form

allele—any one of two or more alternate forms of a gene located at the same locus

allozymes—enzymes that differ in electrophoretic mobility because of different alleles at a gene locus

amelia—complete congenital absence of one or more limbs

amnion—the innermost membrane of the amniotic sac that surrounds the fetus

amplification—the production of extra copies of genes or a section of DNA

anencephaly—a neural tube defect with partial or complete absence of the cranial vault and a rudimentary brain

aneuploid—any chromosome number that is not an exact multiple of the haploid (N) set; thus, trisomy 18 with 47 chromosomes is an aneuploidy, but triploidy with 69 chromosomes is a polyploidy

anhidrosis—absence of sweating

aniridia—absence of the iris of the eye

anodontia—absence of teeth

anomaly—abnormal variation in form or structure

anotia—absence of pinna of the ear

anticipation—refers to the occurrence of a trait or disorder at an earlier age with each successive generation and/or the increased severity of a disorder with each successive generation

antimongoloid slant—downward slant of palpebral fissures of eye

aplasia—absence of or irregular structure of tissue or an organ

apoenzyme—the protein part of a complex (conjugated) holoenzyme

apoptosis—the normal cellular process of programmed cell death

arcus cornae—an opaque ring seen in the cornea that is caused by a deposit of cholesteryl esters

ascertainment—the process of finding individuals or families for inclusion in genetic studies

association—anomalies that occur together more often than would be expected by chance but have not yet been recognized as a syndrome

assortative mating—nonrandom mating practices based on choosing or rejecting mates with certain traits

atresia—absence or closure of a normal opening

autosome(al)—any chromosome that is not a sex chromosome (X or Y); in normal human somatic cells, there are 22 pairs (44) of autosomes and 2 sex chromosomes (XX or XY)

Barr body—sex chromatin found at the edge of the cell nucleus in normal females that represents the genetically inactive X chromosome

base pair—two nitrogenous bases bonded together; in DNA, adenine pairs with thymine and cytosine pairs with guanine

base sequence—the order of bases on a chromosome or DNA fragment

brachydactyly—abnormally shortened digits

Brushfield spots—speckled areas noted on the iris in a small percentage of normal individuals and a large percentage of persons with Down syndrome

camptodactyly—flexion contracture or curvature of finger(s), usually the fifth finger

candidate gene—one that may be the site of causation for a given disease

canthus—outer or inner corner of the eye where upper and lower lids meet

carrier—a person who is heterozygous, possessing two different alleles of a gene pair (e.g., Aa as opposed to aa or AA)

centromere—the primary constriction of a chromosome where the long and short arms meet

CHARGE association—the nonrandom association of coloboma, heart disease, atresia choanal, retarded growth, and/or nervous system anomalies, genital anomalies, and ear anomalies or deafness

chimera—an organism composed of two or more cell lines; the product of the fusion of embryos

chromatid—after replication of a chromosome, two subunits attached by the centromere can be seen; each is called a chromatid, and after separation each becomes a chromosome of a daughter cell

chromatin—the material of which chromosomes are composed; contains DNA, RNA, histones, and nonhistone proteins

chromosome—microscopic structures in the cell nucleus composed of chromatin that contain genetic information and are constant in number in a species; humans have 46 chromosomes, 22 autosome pairs, and 2 sex chromosomes

clinodactyly—crooked finger that is curved inward sideways—usually the fifth digit

clone—a genetically identical cell population derived from a common ancestor; to clone an organism is to make a genetically identical copy of it

cloning DNA—manipulation to produce multiple copies of a single gene or groups of genetically identical cells from the same ancestor

codominance—the expression of each of a pair of alleles when present in the heterozygous state

codon—triplet bases in nucleic acids specifying placement of a specific amino acid in a polypeptide chain

coenzyme—an organic molecule that acts as a cofactor (e.g., vitamin B_{12})

cofactor—the nonprotein component of a conjugated enzyme that is required for activity; it can be organic or inorganic; if organic, often called coenzyme

coloboma—defect in or absence of tissue, usually in the iris of the eye; usually seen as a gap

complementary DNA (cDNA)—DNA that is synthesized from an mRNA template; usually used as a probe in physical mapping

complementation—ability of cells with different gene mutations to cross-correct in cell culture

compound heterozygote—presence of two different mutations of a given gene, one on each allele on each chromosome

concordance—the presence of a certain trait in two individuals, usually twins

congenital—present at birth; a congenital trait may or may not be caused by genetic factors

consanguinous—related by descent from a common ancestor, usually in the preceding few generations; blood relatives

consultand—the person whose genotype is of primary importance to the genetic counseling problem at hand; in practice, often used synonymously with *counselee*

contiguous gene syndrome—name given to disorders arising from small chromosome deletions or duplications of adjacent but functionally unrelated genes

crossing over—the physical event or exchange that gives rise to recombinant chromatids

crossovers—chromatid with genetic material from each homologous chromosome

deformation—anomaly resulting from mechanical forces causing constraint on the fetus

deletion—loss of all or part of a chromosome

diploid—the number of chromosomes normally present in somatic cells; in humans, this is 46, and is sometimes symbolized as 2N

deoxyribonucleic acid—the primary genetic material in humans consisting of nitrogenous bases, a sugar group, and phosphate combined into a double helix

discordance—when two members of a twin pair do not exhibit the same trait

dizygotic—twins originating from two different fertilized eggs; fraternal twins

DNA—deoxyribonucleic acid

DNA fingerprint—a person's unique pattern in regard to a selected section or total DNA

DNA hybridization—the process of the joining of two complementary DNA strands to form a double-stranded molecule

DNA probe—a selected fragment of DNA that is labeled, often with a radioactive isotope, and, through molecular hybridization, is used to find very similar or complementary regions of DNA in a sample

dominant—a trait is considered dominant if it is expressed when one copy of the gene determining it is present

dyshistogenesis—result from aberrant development of a specific tissue type

dysplasia—developmental abnormality of a tissue, for example, a nevus

empiric risk—one based on observed data, not theoretical models

epigenetics—alterations in a gene that do not involve the DNA sequence.

epistasis—the prevention of the expression of one gene by another gene at a different locus

eugenics—improvement of a species by genetic manipulations

euploidy—having a complete correct chromosome set

exons—structural gene sequences retained in messenger RNA and eventually translated into amino acids

expressivity—variation in the degree to which a trait is manifested; clinical severity

familial—the occurrence of more than one case of an anomaly in a family; a trait that appears with a higher frequency in close relatives than in the general population; it is not synonymous with *hereditary*

fitness—ability of a person with a certain genotype to reproduce and pass his/her genes to the next generation

flanking region—DNA on either side of a particular locus

forme fruste—minimal manifestation or mild form of a disorder

gamete—mature reproductive cells containing the haploid number of chromosomes (sperm or ovum)

gastroschisis—a congenital abdominal wall defect characterized by antenatal evisceration of the intestine through a small opening

gene—the functional unit of heredity; a sequence of nucleotides along the DNA of a chromosome that codes for a functional product such as RNA or a polypeptide

gene mapping—assignment of genes to specific sites on specific chromosomes

gene pool—all of the genes in a specific breeding population at a certain time

genetic code—nucleotide base sequence in DNA or RNA coding for specific amino acids

genetic constitution—a person's genetic makeup; refers to either one gene pair or all

genetic load—the recessive deleterious genes concealed in the heterozygous state within a population

genocopy—the production of the same phenotypic appearance by different genes

genome—the total genetic complement of an individual genotype—a person's genetic constitution at one locus or in total

genomic imprinting—differences in gene expression depending on whether the gene in question is inherited from the individual's mother or father

genomics—the study of the genome including gene sequencing, mapping, and function

hallux—big toe

hamartoma—an overgrowth of tissue normally present but in abnormal proportion and distribution; it is not malignant

haploid—the number of chromosomes present in the gamete; in humans this is 23, and can be symbolized as N

haploinsufficiency—the condition wherein one copy of a specific gene is not enough for normal development or function if one copy of that gene has been inactivated or deleted

haplotype—the set of alloantigens produced by the closely linked HLA complex genes located on chromosome 6

hemizygous—the condition in which only one copy of a gene pair is normally present, and so its effect is expressed (e.g., the genes on the X chromosome of the male as there is no counterpart present)

heterogeneity—in genetic use, the production of the same phenotype by different genetic mutations; in clinical use, differences within the same disorder

heteromorphism—morphologic chromosome polymorphism or variant

heterozygous—state in which the two alleles of a gene pair are different (e.g., Aa as opposed to aa or M)

HLA complex—the major histocompatibility region on chromosome 6

holandric—a trait controlled by genes on the Y chromosome; Y-linked inheritance

holoenzyme—a conjugated or complex enzyme consisting of an apoenzyme and cofactor

homologous chromosomes—chromosomes that are members of the same pair and normally have the same number and arrangement of genes

homozygous—state in which both alleles of a given gene pair are identical (e.g., AA or aa as opposed to Aa)

hydrocephalus—abnormal accumulation of fluid in the cranium, usually in ventricles or subarachnoid space, leading to an enlarged head and pressure on the brain

hyperlipidemia—increased blood lipid levels

hyperlipoproteinemia—elevation of blood lipoproteins

hypertrichosis—excessive hair growth

inborn errors of metabolism—inherited biochemical disorders caused by single gene mutations affecting enzymes involved in metabolic pathways

introns—intervening gene sequences in messenger RNA that are "cut out" and are not translated into amino acids

inversion—a chromosome aberration in which a segment has become reversed due to breakage, 180 degrees rotation, and reunion

in vivo—in the living organism

in vitro—in the test tube or laboratory

ion channel—a protein tunnel that crosses the cell membrane and changes conformation as it opens and closes in response to various signals; ion channels exist for such ions as calcium, chloride, potassium, and sodium

isochromosome—chromosome composed of either two long or two short arms due to abnormal separation during division

karyotype—the arrangement of chromosome pairs by number according to centromere position and length

Kayser-Fleischer ring—pigmented brownish-gold ring resulting from copper deposition in the cornea and seen in Wilson disease

library—a collection of cloned DNA probes

linked genes—genes located on the same chromosome within 50 map units of each other; they do not assort independently, and the closer they are to each other, the more frequently they are transmitted together

locus—the place on a chromosome where a gene resides

Lyon hypothesis—in the normal female (46,XX), one of the two X chromosomes is randomly inactivated and appears in somatic cells as sex chromatin

macroglossia—an unusually large tongue

macrosomia—growth excess of prenatal onset associated with several genetic disorders and seen in infants of diabetic mothers

malformation—morphologic defect of an organ resulting from an intrinsically abnormal developmental process

meiosis—reduction division of diploid germ cells resulting in haploid gametes

meiotic drive—mechanism resulting in unequal, nonrandom, or preferential assortment of chromosomes into gametes during meiosis

meningocele—bulging of meninges without involvement of the spinal cord

metabolome—the complement of all metabolites in the genome

metacentric chromosome—one in which the centromere is in the center of the chromosome

methylation—attachment of a methyl group to cytosine in DNA

microcephaly—small head circumference, usually defined as below the third percentile for age, height, and weight; associated with intellectual disability in most cases

micrognathia—undersized jaws, especially the mandible

microstomia—unusually small mouth

microtia—unusually small external ear

minute—a very small chromosome fragment

missense mutation—one in which the nucleotide alteration results in the placement of a different amino acid in the polypeptide chain from the one originally specified

mitosis—somatic cell division that normally results in no change from the usual diploid number of chromosomes

monosomy—missing one of a chromosome pair in normally diploid cells ($2N - 1 = 45$); a person with Turner syndrome (45,X) has a chromosome number of 45 instead of 46 and is monosomic for the X chromosome

monozygotic—twins originating from one fertilized egg; identical twins

mosaic—presence in the same individual of two or more cell lines that differ in chromosome or gene number or structure but are derived from a single zygote

multifactorial—determined by the interaction of several genes with environmental factors

multiple alleles—the occurrence of more than two alternate forms of a gene that can occupy the same locus, although only one can be present on each chromosome at a time

multiplexing—using several pooled samples simultaneously in analysis

MURCS association—nonrandom association of Mullerian duct aplasia, renal aplasia, and cervicothoracic somite dysplasia

mutagen—any agent that causes mutation or increases the mutation rate above the usual background rate existing

mutation—a heritable alteration in the genetic material

myelomeningocele—spina bifida with cord and membranes protruding

nondisjunction—the failure of two homologous chromosomes or of sister chromatids to separate in meiosis appropriately during cell division, resulting in abnormal chromosome numbers in gametes or cells

nuchal translucency—a thickening of the fetal neck seen on ultrasound examinination in the first trimester; called *cystic hygroma* and *nuchal fold* when seen in the later trimesters

nucleotide—a nucleic acid building block comprising a nitrogenous base, a five-carbon sugar, and a phosphate group

oligonucleotide—a short segment of nucleotides

omphalocele—congenital abdominal wall defect, commonly known as umbilical hernia

p—in cytogenetics, refers to the short arms of a chromosome; in population genetics, stands for the gene frequency of the dominant allele

PCR—polymerase chain reaction

pedigree—a diagrammatic representation of the family history

penetrance—fraction of individuals known to carry the gene for a trait who manifest the condition; a trait with 90% penetrance will not be manifested by 10% of the persons possessing the gene

phenocopy—a phenotype that mimics one that is genetically determined but is actually due to nongenetic causes

philtrum—vertical groove between upper lip and nose

phocomelia—a type of limb defect in which proximal parts of extremities are missing so that a hand might be directly attached to the shoulder or attached by a single irregular bone

pleiotropy—the production of multiple phenotype effects by a single gene

polydactyly—presence of extra (supernumerary) digits

polygenic—a phenotypic trait whose expression is controlled by several genes at different loci, each having an additive effect.

polymerase chain reaction—a technique to amplify a sequence of DNA and/or detect a specific DNA sequence in a sample

polymorphism—a genetic variation with two or more alleles that is maintained in a population so that the frequency of the most common one is not more than 0.99 and the frequency of one of the uncommon ones is maintained at at least 0.01

polypeptide—chain of amino acids formed during protein synthesis; may be a complete protein molecule or combined with other polypeptides to form one

polyploidy—a cell or individual having more than two haploid sets in an exact multiple; examples are triploidy and tetraploidy

proband—the index patient; the person who brings the family to the attention of the geneticist

probe—*see* DNA probe

promotor—DNA site where the enzyme RNA polymerase binds to initiate transcription

propositus—essentially the same as *proband*

proteome—the complete set of all proteins in the genome

q—in cytogenetics, refers to the long arms of a chromosome; in population genetics, stands for the gene frequency of the recessive allele

recessive—when the effect of a gene is expressed phenotypically only when two copies are present, as in the homozygous recessive state (aa)

recombinant DNA—hybrid produced by combining DNA pieces from different sources

recombination—reassortment of genes to form new nonparental types

restriction enzymes—enzymes that recognize a specific base sequence in DNA and cut the DNA everywhere that the sequence occurs

restriction fragment length polymorphism—variation in a restriction enzyme recognition site in the fragments of DNA that have been cut by a restriction enzyme

RFLP—restriction fragment length polymorphism

RNA—ribonucleic acid

sentinel phenotype—disorders followed to monitor populations for genetic damage as an early warning system; usually refers to sporadic disorders that follow an autosomal dominant mode of inheritance

sequence—a pattern of multiple anomalies derived from a single prior anomaly; order of nucleotide bases in DNA or RNA

sequencing—a method to determine the order of bases in DNA or RNA

sex chromatin—the inactive X chromosome

sex chromosome—the X or the Y chromosome

sex influenced—an autosomally inherited trait whose degree of phenotypic expression is controlled by the sex of the individual

sex limited—an autosomally inherited trait that is manifested only in one sex

shagreen patch—raised, thickened skin plaque commonly seen in tuberous sclerosis

short tandem repeats—*see* STRs

siblings—brothers and sisters from the same natural parents

sister chromatids—identical chromatids of the same duplicated chromosome before cell division

spina bifida—neural tube defect of the spinal column through which the cord or the membranes can protrude

sporadic—an isolated occurrence of a trait in a family

STRs—short tandem repeats; the STRs usually comprise pairs such as CG of two bases (although three to five pairs have been noted) that are repeated a few to many times.

structural gene—one that determines the amino acid sequence of the polypeptide chain

submetacentric chromosome—one in which the centromere is between the metacentric and acrocentric position

syndactyly—webbing or fusion of adjacent fingers or toes

syndrome—recognizable pattern of multiple anomalies, presumed to have the same etiology

syntenic—genes on the same chromosome that are more than 50 map units apart

tandem repeats—multiple copies of the same base sequence in a segment of DNA

teratogen—an agent acting on the embryo or fetus prenatally, altering morphology or subsequent function; causes teratogenesis

teratogenesis—exogenous induction of structural, functional, or developmental abnormalities caused by agents acting during embryonic or fetal development

tetraploid-cell or person with four copies of each chromosome, having a chromosome number of 4N = 96.

TORCH—abbreviation for the following organisms: toxoplasmosis, rubella, cytomegalovirus, and herpes simplex

transcription—the process by which complementary mRNA is synthesized from a DNA template

transcriptome—the complete set of RNA in the genome

translation—the process whereby the amino acids in a given polypeptide are synthesized from the mRNA template

translocation—transfer of all or part of a chromosome to another chromosome

transposable element—segment of DNA that can move from place to place in the genome; a jumping gene

triploid—cell or person with three copies of each chromosome, having a chromosome number of 3N = 69

trisomy—the presence of one extra chromosome in an otherwise diploid chromosome complement (2N + I = 47); the most common autosomal trisomy is trisomy 21, or Down syndrome

uniparental disomy—both chromosomal homologues are inherited from the same parent instead of inheriting one copy of each chromosome pair from the mother and the father

VACTERL association—the nonrandom finding of vertebral, anal, cardiac, tracheoesophageal, renal, and limb anomalies

variable number of tandem repeats—*see* VNTRs

VATER association—a nonrandom association of vertebral defects, anal atresia, tracheoesophageal fistula, and radial or renal anomalies

VNTRs—variable number of tandem repeats; short sequences of base pairs in DNA (such as CAG) that are repeated in order a varying number of times

wild type—the form of a gene or characteristic usually found in nature and thus usually considered the "normal" one; usually the most common as well

X-linked—located on the X chromosome

Y-linked—located on the Y chromosome

zygote—the diploid (2N) cell formed by fusion of a haploid egg and a haploid sperm during fertilization that develops into the embryo

Index